Evidence-Based Hyperbaric Medicine

António Gandra D'Almeida • Jorge Hidalgo
Editors

Evidence-Based Hyperbaric Medicine

Concepts and Clinical Application

Springer

Editors
António Gandra D'Almeida
Portuguese Army
Porto, Portugal

Jorge Hidalgo
Department of Critical Care
Karl Heusner Memorial Hospital
Belize City, Belize

ISBN 978-3-032-06345-8 ISBN 978-3-032-06346-5 (eBook)
https://doi.org/10.1007/978-3-032-06346-5

This Springer imprint is published by the registered company Springer Nature Switzerland AG
The registered company address is: Gewerbestrasse 11, 6330 Cham, Switzerland

To my family,
whose unwavering love and encouragement have been the steady light guiding me through every moment of this journey. Your belief in me has been my greatest strength, and your laughter, wisdom, and kindness are woven into every page.

To my friends,
who have inspired me with their stories, supported me with their patience, and reminded me that even on the hardest days, there is always joy to be found in shared moments and honest conversations.

To the teachers and mentors
who opened doors to new worlds with their passion for learning and their generosity of spirit. Your lessons echo far beyond the classroom, shaping the way I see, feel, and write.

To the readers—both known and unknown—who pick up this book with curiosity and hope. May you find something within these words that resonates, comforts, or challenges you, and may you always feel empowered to chase your own dreams.

—António Gandra D'Almeida

To my family
Your love has been my compass and your strength, my anchor.

To Antonio
Your passion, resilience, and generosity have been the driving force behind this work. This book carries your spirit—curious, kind, and committed to making a difference.

—Jorge Hidalgo

Contents

About the Editors

António Gandra D'Almeida is a doctor in the Portuguese Armed Forces, with areas of interest in general surgery, critical care patients, and catastrophe. He has a European Masters in Catastrophe, is a Fellow of the Society of Critical Care Medicine, a Fellow of the American College of Surgeons, a Trainer of several courses in his areas of interest, and an Editor of FCCS Surgical who has collaborated on several books.

Jorge Hidalgo is a Professor of Critical Care and Head of the Division of Critical Care at Belize Healthcare Partners. He currently serves as President of the World Federation of Societies of Intensive and Critical Care Medicine (WFSICCM).

In 2012, he was awarded the Master of the American College of Physicians (MACP), the highest recognition the College bestows upon its members. For over a decade, he has been the Director of the prestigious ACP Review Course hosted by the Paraguayan Society of Internal Medicine.

In recognition of his outstanding contributions to the Society of Critical Care Medicine (SCCM), he has received the Presidential Citation Award for ten consecutive years. He is also a two-time recipient (2016 and 2023) of the Global Safar Award, and in 2016 became the first Latin American intensivist to receive the title Master of the American College of Critical Care Medicine (MACCCM).

A Fellow of the American College of Chest Physicians (FCCP), he is an accomplished author and editor of numerous books and chapters on Critical Care Medicine. His recent publications with Springer include *Critical Care Administration* and *Highly Infectious Diseases in Critical Care*. He serves as Editor of *Fundamental Critical Care Support (FCCS) – Tropical* and actively contributes to the review and development of the MCCRC, FCCS, FCCS Obstetrics, and FCCS Surgical courses for the SCCM.

He is the SCCM Co-Chair of the Surviving Sepsis Campaign for Low-Resource Settings and is a regular international speaker, sharing his expertise and advancing critical care globally.

Chapter 1
History of Hyperbaric and Diving Medicine

Chamin Weerasekera

1.1 History of Diving Medicine

The earliest records of breath-holding dives for mother-of-pearl date back to 4500 BC, when divers would descend to the ocean floor to collect shells. These early divers soon discovered that staying underwater for extended periods of time posed serious risks, such as decompression sickness and lung injuries. As a result, ancient civilizations began experimenting with different techniques and equipment to mitigate these dangers. Historical artifacts and writings from ancient civilizations, such as the ancient Egyptians and Greeks, have been discovered that depict divers using specialized equipment and techniques for breath-holding dives. For instance, paintings on the walls of ancient Egyptian tombs show divers wearing primitive nose clips and using hollow reeds to breathe underwater. These artifacts and writings provide concrete evidence of the early experimentation and development of techniques and equipment for breath-holding dives.

The diving bell is one of the earliest types of equipment for underwater work and exploration. Its use dates back to ancient times, with references to the diving bell being made as early as the fourth century BC by Aristotle [1]. The first recorded use of a diving bell, however, was by Alexander the Great in 320 BC [2]. Since then, the design and functionality of diving bells have evolved significantly. From early iterations like those described by Guglielmo de Lorena in 1535, diving bells have been refined to allow for longer periods of underwater exploration and the ability to maintain an air supply within the bell [3]. This evolution has paved the way for advancements in underwater research and exploration. With the ability to descend to greater depths and stay underwater for longer periods of time, scientists and explorers have been able to make groundbreaking discoveries and gain a deeper

C. Weerasekera (✉)
Department of Anaesthesiology and Critical Care, Shrewsbury and Telford NHS Trust, Shrewsbury, UK

A. G. D'Almeida, J. Hidalgo (eds.), *Evidence-Based Hyperbaric Medicine*,
https://doi.org/10.1007/978-3-032-06346-5_1

understanding of the marine environment. For example, the use of diving bells has allowed researchers to study deep-sea organisms in their natural habitats, uncovering new species and documenting unique adaptations. Diving bells have also played a crucial role in underwater archaeological expeditions, enabling archaeologists to explore and document ancient shipwrecks and submerged structures. Without the advancements in diving bell technology, many of these important discoveries would not have been possible. Apart from underwater research and exploration, diving bells have been used for a wide range of purposes. One notable example is the use of diving bells during the construction of bridges and other underwater structures. By allowing workers to descend to the depths of the construction site, diving bells facilitated the construction process and made it possible to build structures that would otherwise be impractical. Another example is the use of diving bells in salvage operations, where they have been used to recover sunken ships and valuable cargo from the ocean floor.

The history of decompression research is closely associated with diving medicine. Sir Robert Boyle was the first person to give a description of the decompression phenomenon when he performed an experiment with a viper in a vacuum [4]. A bubble was observed in the eye of the viper, and it displayed extreme signs of discomfort.

It was not until the nineteenth century that the phenomenon of recompression was discovered. In 1841, Pol and Watelle of France observed that recompression relieved the symptoms of decompression sickness [4]. They pointed out that the danger did not lie in entering a shaft containing compressed air nor in remaining there, but rapid decompression alone was responsible for the sickness. They reported pain in the limbs, cerebral and respiratory symptoms, and the fact that some men died. They rightly recommended recompression as a therapeutic modality.

Paul Bert, a French professor of physiology and a student of Claude Bernard, is considered the father of pressure physiology. In 1878, while working closely with Dr. Alphonse Gal, the first doctor to actually dive in order to study how the body reacted underwater, Bert studied Gal's reports on divers who became symptomatic or died while surfacing. He conducted a series of dog experiments, exposing them to 7–9 atmospheres and subjecting them to rapid decompression. A majority of them died and exhibited grossly distended bodies with their right heart chambers filled with gas. When decompression was done slowly over 1–2 h after exposure to similar pressures, none of the dogs succumbed. Applying Dalton's and Henry's gas laws, Bert concluded that too rapid a decompression induced a pathophysiologic insult secondary to the supersaturation of body tissues with nitrogen, causing the formation of nitrogen bubbles. He also went on to suggest that divers stop halfway to the surface to allow for slow decompression after a deep dive—what is now known as deep stops [5].

The application of compressed oxygen in decompression sickness was initially investigated by Heinrich Drager. Following his methods, Behnke and Shaw employed hyperbaric oxygen treatment (HBOT) to treat decompression sickness in the late 1930s [6]. Through their efforts, compressed air was substituted for oxygen, and the first nitrogen–oxygen mixes were used. Additionally, hyperbaric treatment was adjusted based on the degree of the injury. HBOT was first used by the US Navy to treat decompression sickness in divers in 1939. Following World War II, the US military carried out a great deal of research on HBOT, which increased our understanding of surviving pressures and helped to popularize HBOT in the late 1950s and early 1960s. The military's research focused on investigating the physiological effects of different pressures and oxygen concentrations on divers, as well as developing protocols and equipment for safe and effective HBOT. This research not only improved the treatment of decompression sickness in divers but also had broader implications for the medical field, leading to advancements in the use of HBOT for various other conditions, such as carbon monoxide poisoning and non-healing wounds.

The establishment of the Undersea Medical Society in 1967 [7] was a significant milestone in the history of diving medicine. This society played a crucial role in advancing the field by promoting research, education, and collaboration among medical professionals specializing in undersea and hyperbaric medicine. The society provided a platform for sharing knowledge and best practices, leading to advancements in the understanding and treatment of diving-related illnesses and injuries. Additionally, society played a key role in advocating for the recognition of undersea medicine as a specialized field, leading to the establishment of certification programs and professional standards.

1.2 The Development of Hyperbaric Air Therapy

The development of hyperbaric therapy has a rich history that spans several centuries. Understanding the historical context of these developments is important to appreciate the significance of hyperbaric therapy today. For example, Henshaw's initial hyperbaric chamber in the seventeenth century laid the foundation for future experimentation and exploration of the potential benefits of altered air pressure. Despite the lack of empirical support, Henshaw's assertion that higher air pressure could treat acute illnesses demonstrates the early recognition of the potential therapeutic effects of hyperbaric therapy. He controlled the air pressure inside a sealed chamber called a domicilium by utilizing unidirectional valves on an organ bellows system. Henshaw asserted—without providing any empirical support—that while lower air pressure would be preferable for chronic problems, higher air pressure would treat acute illnesses [8]. Henshaw thought that the domicillium aided in digestion and protected the lungs from the majority of lung affections.

Henshaw's work did not gain much attention or contribute much to the advancement of the therapy. The main reason for this might have been the limited scientific understanding at that time, as it took over a century for oxygen to be discovered.

Henshaw's concept was not renewed until 1832, when Emile Tabarie in France submitted a project to the French Academy of Scientists. Taberie created an iron-based pneumatic chamber with two tubes: one for ventilation and the other for hydraulic pressure produced by a compressor. The doctor could enter and depart it through an antechamber without stopping the pressurization process. Tabarie claimed to have successfully treated 49 cases of mostly respiratory diseases [8].

A few more hyperbaric chambers have reportedly been developed after Tabarie.

There was a rebirth of interest in hyperbaric therapy in the treatment of respiratory diseases when Junod built a hyperbaric chamber. Junod named his technique "Le Bain d'Air Comprimé" (the compressed air bath), claiming that by boosting circulation to the brain and internal organs, it enhanced general health and feelings of well-being.

Lange ordered a cylindrical, wrought-iron room that could accommodate four people. The compressed air inside the chamber was cooled using one of two techniques. In the first instance, a stream of cold water was directed toward the force pump and the supply pipelines. The second method was to fill a cup-shaped hole at the top of the chamber with cold water, let it drip down the sides and soak the linen sheets, and then allow the water to evaporate, cooling the air. In order to keep the chamber at a comfortable temperature during the winter, heating was employed. The chamber also featured a device that regulated the airflow entering it so that it came in a steady stream as opposed to brief spurts.

Dianabad was the location of Leibig's pneumatic chamber in Reichenhall, Bavaria, Germany. Three people could fit in each of the three rooms in this pneumatic chamber. All three rooms were joined by a single antechamber, which made it possible for the doctor to come and go without changing the surrounding pressure. Additionally, the antechamber served as a sizable pressure regulator, shielding the patients from abrupt pressure spikes. Good ventilation was provided by a ventilation pipe that was inserted through a ceiling aperture.

Pravaz constructed the biggest chamber complex of this era in 1837, and it was located in the French city of Lyon. A total of 12 patients might be accommodated there. This treatment was dubbed "le bain d'air comprime" by Pravaz. According to him, these "compressed air baths" helped to expand the bronchi, which was beneficial in treating a variety of pulmonary and associated illnesses, such as tuberculosis.

J.L. Corning brought compressed air therapy to the United States for the first time in 1871 [8]. Corning's trips to the Hudson River Tunnel construction site sparked his interest in hyperbaric medicine. He saw many cases of paralytic decompression sickness, which made him believe that the illness was mostly a spinal cord ailment. Corning decided to employ compressed air therapy for a wider variety of nondecompression-related brain and spinal cord illnesses and diseases because he could clearly see potential in the ability of air recompression to resolve many of these instances. Kelly used a "compressed air bath apparatus" in 1876 to treat a patient. The apparatus had two locking plates that were controlled from the outside to seal pressures. French physician Fontaine created the first transportable hyperbaric operating room in 1877. It was stated that the high surrounding pressure would help patients with lung conditions and reduce hernias. Notably, 27 procedures were successfully completed in this mobile hyperbaric chamber over the course of the following 3 months. Inspired by the outcomes, Fontaine took the risk of building a massive hyperbaric surgical amphitheater large enough to receive 300 patients at a time. This was never implemented, as Fontaine became the first person to die in an accident at the Pneumatic Institute.

The British Medical Journal published C. Theodore Williams' 1885 paper, "Lectures on the Compressed Air Bath and its Uses in the Treatment of Disease," which promoted the use of atmospheric air at varying atmospheric pressure levels for medical purposes. He said that this treatment approach was one of the most significant developments in contemporary medicine and expressed surprise that England was ignoring it [8].

In the latter stages of World War I, Kansas-born physician Orval J. Cunningham built a hyperbaric chamber in Lawrence, Kansas, back in the United States. At the facility, he provided care to those affected by the Spanish influenza pandemic that decimated North America. Cunningham made the hypothesis that the higher mortality rates of people living at higher elevations were caused by atmospheric pressure or barometric factors after noticing that people in valleys fared better than those in the highlands. He observed that patients on HBO, especially those who were unconscious and cyanotic, recovered quite well. All patients were evacuated successfully, but the insulation burned, and a fire started in 1923 as a result of heat from open gas burners warming the chambers throughout the winter. In a different incident, a mechanical failure resulted in a complete loss of pressure inside the chamber, which killed all of the patients. Cunningham's enthusiasm for hyperbaric air did not diminish, either. He kept treating diseases, including syphilis, hypertension, diabetes mellitus, and cancer, all of which he thought were caused by anaerobic infections. Cunningham invested a million dollars in 1928 to build the biggest hyperbaric chamber in the world outside of Cleveland, Ohio, on the shores of Lake Erie, with the financial backing of roller bearing manufacturer and mogul Henry H. Timken. This "Steel Ball Hospital," also called "Cunningham's Sanitarium," was a 900-ton steel spherical with 60 rooms within that stood five stories tall. It had a 64-foot circumference. This skyscraper had 12 floors with all the amenities of a five-star hotel. Cunningham's treatments were growing in popularity, and as a result, the Bureau of Investigation of the American Medical Association urged the doctor to provide evidence to support his claims regarding the effectiveness of hyperbaric therapy. Cunningham's refusal to cooperate with the AMA and release the information led to accusations that he was a quack and a charlatan. The chamber was dismantled in 1937 and sold for scrap during World War II.

1.3 Hyperbaric Oxygen Therapy

Joseph Priestly's discovery of oxygen in 1775 was a groundbreaking scientific achievement [9]. Prior to this discovery, the nature of air and its composition were not well understood. Priestly's discovery not only revealed the existence of oxygen as a distinct gas but also laid the foundation for our understanding of the role of oxygen in supporting life and the potential therapeutic applications of oxygen. This discovery was a significant milestone in the history of hyperbaric oxygen therapy, as it provided the fundamental knowledge needed to explore the effects of oxygen at different pressures.

Lavoisier and Seguin were prominent scientists in the late eighteenth century who conducted extensive research on the properties of oxygen. Their reports in 1789 on the harmful effects of oxygen [9] were instrumental in shaping an early understanding of the risks associated with its use. They observed that exposure to high concentrations of oxygen could lead to oxidative stress, tissue damage, and even death. For example, they found that prolonged exposure to oxygen can cause lung inflammation and damage, as well as oxidative damage to other organs and tissues. These findings raised concerns about the safety of hyperbaric oxygen therapy and contributed to its discouragement in medical practice.

Beddoes and Watt's book was groundbreaking in its exploration of the medical applications of oxygen. At the time of its publication in 1796, there was a limited understanding of the therapeutic benefits of oxygen for various medical conditions. Beddoes and Watt not only compiled existing knowledge on oxygen therapy but also conducted their own experiments and documented their findings. This comprehensive approach not only expanded the scientific understanding of oxygen therapy but also provided evidence for its potential efficacy. Their work laid the foundation for further research and development in the field, including the subsequent establishment of hyperbaric oxygen therapy. In 1878, Bert, the pioneer of pressure physiology, established the scientific basis for oxygen toxicity and suggested normobaric oxygen for decompression sickness but not hyperbaric oxygen. Bert's findings built upon the knowledge established by Beddoes and Watt, expanding our understanding of the effects of oxygen and suggesting specific applications for medical conditions such as decompression sickness.

In a groundbreaking experiment in 1895, Haldane placed a mouse in an oxygen-filled jar at 2 ATA and observed that the mouse did not exhibit symptoms of carbon monoxide toxicity. This experiment provided crucial evidence that, under high-pressure conditions, the harmful effects of carbon monoxide can be mitigated. This finding further supported the exploration of hyperbaric oxygen therapy as a potential treatment for various medical conditions, highlighting the potential of pressurized oxygen environments to improve patient outcomes.

A South American is credited with developing the first application of hyperbaric oxygen therapy, though his contributions are still mainly disregarded to this day. In 1934, the Brazilian Academy of Sciences paid tribute to Madam Curie, who had just passed away, with a special conference. Speaking at the gathering was Brazilian doctor Álvaro Osório de Almeida, who studied under Curie and grew to be close to her. His talks on hyperbaric oxygen-induced central nervous system toxicity were very interesting to the audience because they discussed the research he did on this topic before using hyperbaric oxygen to treat cancer patients. He conducted extensive experiments to investigate the effects of hyperbaric oxygen on the brain and nervous system, and his findings shed light on the potential risks and limitations of hyperbaric oxygen therapy. For example, he demonstrated that prolonged exposure to high-pressure oxygen can lead to oxidative damage in the brain, resulting in neurological symptoms and cognitive impairments.

Dr. Álvaro Osório de Almeida's research on hyperbaric oxygen therapy had a significant impact on clinical practice. His findings on the potential risks and limitations of prolonged exposure to high-pressure oxygen led to the development of safety guidelines for hyperbaric oxygen therapy. For instance, his research prompted medical professionals to monitor patients' oxygen levels closely during treatment to avoid oxidative damage to the brain. Additionally, his work influenced the establishment of recommended treatment durations and pressure levels to minimize the risk of neurological symptoms and cognitive impairments.

Boerema, a renowned medical practitioner from the Netherlands, is widely regarded as the "father of modern hyperbaric medicine." In 1956, he made a groundbreaking advancement in the field by performing cardiac surgery in a hyperbaric chamber. This marked the first scientifically based therapeutic approach that utilized hyperbaric oxygen. Boerema's innovative technique proved successful in treating children with congenital cardiac disorders such as pulmonic stenosis, transposition of the great vessels, and tetralogy of Fallot. His use of hyperbaric oxygen led to the development of the concept of "life without blood," which proposed the possibility of the human body obtaining all the necessary oxygen without relying on red blood cells or hemoglobin.

In 1961, Willem Hendrik Brummelkamp et al. published an article on the use of hyperbaric oxygen in the treatment of clostridial gas gangrene [10]. In 1962, Smith and Sharp reported the successful treatment of carbon monoxide poisoning with hyperbaric oxygen [11].

In the early 1960s, Illingworth conducted a groundbreaking study in the United Kingdom that demonstrated the effectiveness of HBO therapy for limb artery blockage [9]. This study showed that HBO can improve blood flow and alleviate symptoms in patients with this condition. Building on Illingworth's findings, Perrins conducted a study in 1965, also in the United Kingdom, that provided evidence for the use of HBO therapy in treating osteomyelitis, a serious bone infection [12]. The following year, in 1966, Saltzman et al. conducted a study in the United States that further demonstrated the efficacy of HBO therapy, this time in stroke patients [9]. The study showed that HBO can improve neurological outcomes and enhance recovery in stroke patients. In the early 1970s, Lamm utilized HBO to treat abrupt deafness, Boschetty and Cernoch used HBO for multiple sclerosis, and Thurston demonstrated that HBO lowers mortality in myocardial infarction in a study published in 1973.

Since its introduction, hyperbaric oxygen therapy has undergone significant changes in its indications. As research and clinical experience have accumulated, the understanding of the therapy's benefits and limitations has improved. The establishment of the Undersea and Hyperbaric Medical Society in 1986 marked a significant milestone in the history of hyperbaric oxygen therapy. This society serves as the primary source of scientific information for diving and hyperbaric medicine physiology worldwide. It has played a crucial role in advancing the field, providing valuable research, guidelines, and standards for practitioners. The society's contributions have helped shape the indications for hyperbaric oxygen therapy over the years, leading to expanded usage and improved patient outcomes. Currently, there are 14 indications approved by the Undersea and Hyperbaric Medical Society for the use of hyperbaric oxygen therapy. These indications cover a wide range of conditions, including decompression sickness, carbon monoxide poisoning, gas gangrene, and diabetic foot ulcers. Other approved indications include radiation injuries, crush injuries, and non-healing wounds. The expanding list of indications highlights the growing recognition of hyperbaric oxygen therapy as an effective treatment option in various medical scenarios.

In conclusion, the history of diving and hyperbaric medicine is a testament to the human drive for exploration and the development of innovative medical treatments. From ancient breath-holding dives to the advancements in hyperbaric therapy, these fields have made significant contributions to our understanding of the underwater world and the treatment of various conditions. By appreciating their historical context and ongoing advancements, we can continue to harness the potential of diving and hyperbaric medicine to improve human health.

References

1. Bevan J. Diving bells through the centuries. South Pacific Underw Med Soc J [Internet]. 1999 [cited 2023 Dec 28];29(1). Available from: http://archive.rubicon-foundation.org/5991
2. Pseudo-Callisthenes, Stoneman R. The Greek Alexander romance. Penguin Books; 1991. Book 2, chapter 38
3. Eliav J. Guglielmo's secret: the enigma of the first diving bell used in underwater archaeology. Int J Hist Eng Technol. 2015;85(1):60–9.
4. Acott C. A brief history of diving and decompression illness. South Pacific Underw Med Soc J [Internet]. 1999 [cited 2023 Dec 28];29(2). Available from: http://archive.rubicon-foundation.org/6004
5. Krishnamurti C. We are IntechOpen, the world's leading publisher of Open Access books Built by scientists, for scientists TOP 1%. In: Historical [Internet]. 2016, p. 13. Available from: https://www.intechopen.com/books/advanced-biometric-technologies/liveness-detection-in-biometrics
6. Gill AL, Bell CNA. Hyperbaric oxygen: its uses, mechanisms of action and outcomes. QJM An Int J Med [Internet]. 2004 [cited 2023 Dec 28];97(7):385–95. Available from: https://doi.org/10.1093/qjmed/hch074.
7. About the UHMS - Undersea & hyperbaric medical society [Internet]. [cited 2023 Dec 28]. Available from: https://www.uhms.org/about-the-uhms.html
8. Thom SR. Carbon monoxide pathophysiology and treatment. Physiology and medicine of hyperbaric oxygen. Therapy. 2008:321–47.
9. Jain KK. Textbook of hyperbaric medicine; 2017.
10. Brummelkamp WH, Boerema I, Hoogendyk L. Treatment of clostridial infections with hyperbaric oxygen drenching. A report on 26 cases. Lancet (London, England) [Internet]. u [cited 2023 Dec 28];1(7275):235–8. Available from: https://pubmed.ncbi.nlm.nih.gov/14016240/
11. Sluijter ME. The treatment of carbon monoxide poisoning by administration of oxygen at high atmospheric pressure. Prog Brain Res. 1967;24(C):123–82.
12. Slack WK, Thomas DA, Perrins D. Hyperbaric oxygenation chronic osteomyelitis. Lancet (London, England) [Internet]. 1965 [cited 2023 Dec 28];1(7395):1093–4. Available from: https://pubmed.ncbi.nlm.nih.gov/14283767/

Chapter 2
Physical and Physiological Aspects of Hyperbaric Oxygen Therapy

Rasanee Wanigasuriya and Ahsina Jahan Lopa

2.1 Introduction

Hyperbaric oxygen therapy (HBOT) is a treatment modality in which 100% oxygen is applied at a higher atmospheric pressure via a pressurized chamber [1–3]. The basic understanding of the physical and physiological principles of HBOT is essential for effective management of the different medical conditions for which HBOT is used.

2.2 Physics of HBOT

2.2.1 Units of Pressure in HBOT

Pressure exerted by the earth's atmosphere is defined as atmospheric pressure. The international standardized units of pressure are kilopascals (kPa) and bar. In the field of HBOT, units such as atmospheres (atm), atmospheres absolute (ATA), millimeters of mercury (mmHg), feet of sea water (fsw), kilograms per square centimeter (kg/cm^2), pounds per square inch (psi) are still being used. The atmospheric pressure at sea level is 1 atm and is equal to 1 ATA, 101.3 kPa, 1.013 bar, 760 mmHg (Torr), 33 fsw, 14.69 psi, and 1.033 kg/cm^2.

R. Wanigasuriya (✉)
Colombo South Teaching Hospital, Colombo, Sri Lanka

A. J. Lopa
Department of ICU and Emergency, Brahmanbaria ICU Specialized Hospital, Brahmanbaria, Bangladesh

A. G. D'Almeida, J. Hidalgo (eds.), *Evidence-Based Hyperbaric Medicine*,
https://doi.org/10.1007/978-3-032-06346-5_2

Gauge pressure is the pressure difference between the chamber pressure and the atmospheric pressure and is calibrated to read as zero at sea level pressure. Therefore, the absolute pressure (ATA) would be the gauge pressure + atmospheric pressure. HBOT usually uses an absolute pressure of 1.5–3.0 ATA [3].

2.2.2 *Application of Ideal Gas Laws in HBOT*

Atmospheric air has a composition of nitrogen (78.08%), oxygen (20.94%), carbon dioxide (0.04%), and traces of other gases. These gases follow the ideal gas laws [1, 4].

2.2.2.1 Boyle's Law

According to Boyle's law, at a constant temperature, the volume (V) of a given mass of gas is inversely proportional to the absolute pressure (P). Therefore, at a constant temperature, when the pressure is increased in the hyperbaric chamber, the volume of gas in air-filled cavities will reduce. This is applicable during embolic phenomena such as decompression sickness, where HBOT reduces the size of nitrogen bubbles. In contrast, during chamber decompression, complications such as middle ear rupture and pneumothorax can happen due to expansion of air spaces.

2.2.2.2 Gay–Lussac's Law

At a constant volume, Gay–Lussac's law states that the absolute pressure of a mass of gas is directly proportional to absolute temperature (T). The rigid-walled hyperbaric chamber used for HBOT has a constant volume, and during compression, the temperature increases within the chamber and decreases during decompression. During rapid compression, an adiabatic (no heat exchange from outside) compression occurs, and the ambient gas heats up. When the temperature cools with time, the pressure in the hyperbaric chamber can drop, for which adjustments have to be made to keep pressure at therapeutic levels inside the chamber.

2.2.2.3 Charles Law

Boyle's law and Gay-Lussac's law, in combination with Charles' law (which states that, at a constant pressure, the volume of a given mass of gas is directly proportional to the absolute temperature), together form the Ideal Gas law, which shows that PV/T = constant. It explains that, in HBOT, changes in one component in this equation will cause corresponding changes in one or other components.

2.2.2.4 Dalton's Law

In HBOT, the hyperbaric oxygen chamber is pressurized by either medical-grade oxygen where the patient directly breathes pressurized 100% oxygen or pressurized by compressing atmospheric air where the patient breathes 100% oxygen via a specialized hood or a mask. As explained by Dalton's law, the total pressure exerted by a mixture of gases is equal to the sum of the partial pressures of each gas component. Partial pressure is calculated by multiplying the absolute pressure by the proportion in volume of a single component in the gas mixture.

At atmospheric pressure of 1 atm or 760 mmHg, the room air partial pressure of oxygen (pO_2) would be (760) × (21/100) = 160 mmHg (21.33 KPa). In a hyperbaric chamber with room air at a pressure of 3 ATA or 2280 mmHg, the pO_2 would be 478 mmHg (63.72 kPa). This verifies that the use of hyperbaric air is similar to supplying oxygen via a non-rebreathing face mask and does not serve the purpose of hyperbaric oxygen treatment, and hence the use of separate 100% oxygen via mask/hood. In comparison, the use of 100% oxygen at 3 ATA, the pO_2 would be 2280 mmHg (303.97 kPa), causing increased risk of oxygen toxicity. Therefore, the use of atmospheric air is cost effective and has reduced risk of oxygen toxicity to the health care workers who attend patients in multiplace chambers.

2.2.2.5 Henry's Law

When a gas is exposed to a liquid, the gas molecules dissolve in the liquid. According to Henry's law, at a constant temperature, the mass/volume of gas dissolved is proportionate to the partial pressure of that gas. The concentration of a gas dissolved depends on the partial pressure and the solubility coefficient, which changes according to the fluid type and temperature. In HBOT, higher partial pressure increases the solubility of gases. When considering oxygen, higher pressures increase the dissolved oxygen content in blood, which contributes to the therapeutic effect as described below in the section on physiological aspects of HBOT.

2.3 Physiology of HBOT

2.3.1 Physiological Effects of HBOT on Oxygen Transport

Oxygen is transported from the atmosphere to the cellular level via a pressure gradient, which is called the oxygen cascade [5]. HBOT provides a higher partial pressure of oxygen throughout the oxygen cascade.

2.3.1.1 Atmospheric to Alveolar Oxygen Transport

The atmospheric partial pressure of oxygen is 160 mmHg (21 kPa) at sea level. When water vapor is added within the airways, the barometric pressure reduces by 47 mmHg (6.26 kPa). This causes the inspired air partial pressure of oxygen (p_IO_2) calculated as FiO2 × (P_{atm}—P_{H2O}) to be about 150 mmHg (19.99 kPa). At the alveolar level, the alveolar partial pressure of oxygen (p_AO2) can be calculated by the ideal alveolar gas equation [5]:

$$p_AO_2 = (p_IO_2) - (pCO_2 / R)$$

This can be further elaborated as

$$p_AO_2 = F_IO_2 (P_{atm} - P_{H2O}) - (pCO_2 / R)$$

where F_IO_2 is the fractional concentration of inspired oxygen, P_{atm} is the barometric pressure, P_{H2O} is the water vapor pressure, pCO_2 is the partial pressure of CO_2, and R is the respiratory quotient with a value of 0.8.

The calculated p_AO_2 = 0.21(760 − 47) − (40/0.8) = 100 mmHg (13.3 kPa). If breathing 100% oxygen, the p_AO_2 is 663 mmHg (88.4 kPa). This equation is applicable to hyperbaric conditions within the HBOT therapeutic range. For example, at a barometric pressure of 2 ATA, 100% oxygen could provide a higher p_AO_2 of 1423 mmHg (189.7 kPa).

2.3.1.2 Alveolar to Pulmonary Capillary Oxygen Transport

The alveolar capillary membrane (ACM) provides a barrier between the alveolar air space and the pulmonary capillary blood. Fick's law of diffusion states the factors that determine gas transfer via a membrane.

- Rate of diffusion = (diffusion coefficient × partial pressure difference × diffusion area) / diffusion thickness.

Therefore, the higher the partial pressure difference, the higher the rate of diffusion. The difference between p_AO_2 (100 mmHg) and pulmonary mixed venous oxygen pvO_2 (40 mmHg) causes the diffusion of oxygen to pulmonary capillaries. HBOT creates a high-pressure gradient across the ACM and thereby facilitates an increased rate of diffusion of oxygen.

2.3.1.3 Pulmonary Capillary to Arterial Oxygen Transport

Oxygen is transported to tissues mainly bound to hemoglobin (Hb) within red blood cells (RBCs) (97%) and the rest as dissolved oxygen in plasma (3%) [6]. When the diffused oxygen enters the pulmonary capillaries, about one-third of the distance along the capillary, the Hb gets 100% saturated with oxygen, and the capillary partial pressure of oxygen (p_CO_2) builds up and reaches the end-capillary p_CO_2 level of 100 mmHg (13.33 kPa). As a result, oxygen transfer is considered to be perfusion-limited when the ACM is normal. Due to the normal ventilation/perfusion scatter and physiological shunts, venous admixture occurs, and this leads to a slight reduction in the arterial partial pressure of oxygen (paO_2) to about 97 mmHg (12.93 kPa) and the arterial blood oxygen saturation to about 97% [6]. In HBOT, a high paO_2 value can be achieved, facilitating a higher-pressure gradient at the tissue capillary level.

Additionally, an important effect of HBOT is the ability to increase the oxygen diffusion radius of capillaries, and therefore, in conditions like tissue edema, the oxygenation to tissues is preserved [7].

2.3.1.4 Tissues Oxygen Transport

At the tissue level, oxygen enters the tissues from capillaries via passive diffusion across a pressure gradient, leading to a tissue pO_2 value of about 20–40 mmHg (2.66–5.33 kPa) [2]. It is reached at equilibrium between tissue oxygen uptake and the cellular oxygen consumption. Therefore, factors such as tissue oxygen delivery (DO_2), changes in the oxygen dissociation curve (ODC), microcirculatory changes, tissue metabolism, and subsequent oxygen consumption (VO_2) and cellular mitochondrial activity play a role in the final tissue pO_2 (described in Sect. 2.3.1.5). Once the tissues extract oxygen, the venous oxygen saturation and partial pressure reduce. The venous blood draining from the superior and inferior vena cava mixes in the right side of the heart, and this confluence in the pulmonary artery is called mixed venous blood. It has a partial pressure of oxygen (pvO_2) of 40 mmHg (5.33 kPa) and the Hb saturation of 75%.

2.3.1.5 Cellular Oxygen Transport

The final step in the oxygen cascade is the cells, where oxygen diffuses into the cytoplasm across the cell membrane. The mitochondria are the major site of oxygen utilization for oxidative phosphorylation and the generation of ATP (adenosine triphosphate), which is the universal energy substrate within the cell. Within a range of extracellular pO_2 of 10–40 mmHg (1.33–5.33 kPa), the intracellular pO_2 is kept constant by autoregulation [3]. The exact intracellular oxygen pO_2 is difficult to measure, but experimental data using microelectrodes estimates it to be about 1–10 mmHg (0.13–1.33 kPa) [8]. HBOT provides an adequate tissue pO_2 value even in states of hypovolemia and low perfusion.

2.3.2 *Effect of HBOT on Factors Which Affect Tissue Oxygenation*

2.3.2.1 Oxygen Delivery

The global DO_2 to tissues is calculated by multiplying the arterial oxygen content by the cardiac output. HBOT increases the delivered oxygen to the tissues.

Cardiac Output

The normal cardiac output at rest is about 5–6 L/min [6]. An increased metabolic demand triggers an increase in cardiac output to increase the DO_2 to tissues. In exercise, cardiac output increases by fivefold to supply the increased demand of the skeletal muscles [6]. The effects of HBOT on the cardiovascular system are described in Sect. 2.3.3.1.

Oxygen Content

The oxygen content in blood is calculated by adding the oxygen bound to Hb to dissolved oxygen. The oxygen-carrying capacity of 1 g of Hb in vivo is considered as 1.34 ml when it is 100% saturated with oxygen. In a person with an arterial Hb concentration of 15 g/dl, and arterial oxygen saturation of 97%, the bound oxygen content would be $1.34 \times 15 \times 97/100 = 19.5$ ml/dl. As per Henry's law, the dissolved oxygen content is the solubility coefficient × partial pressure ($0.003 \times paO_2$) and gives a value of 0.29 ml/dl. The total oxygen content in arterial blood is 19.8 ml/dl. The venous oxygen content would be $(1.34 \times 15 \times 75/100) + (0.003 \times 40) = 19.5$ ml/dl with a venous Hb saturation of 75% and pvO_2 of 40 mmHg. Thus, the tissues extract about 4.6 ml/dl (≈5 ml/dl) of oxygen.

In HBOT, the Hb molecules become 100% saturated, and thereafter the arterial oxygen tension (p_aO_2) increases with a large amount of dissolved oxygen. With HBOT of 100% oxygen at 3 ATA, the dissolved oxygen content can increase to about 6.8 ml/dl [3]. In this condition, the tissue oxygen demand is met directly by the dissolved oxygen content alone without utilizing the bound oxygen. The extraction of dissolved oxygen leads to a large pressure drop along the capillaries, sometimes as large as 1900 mmHg when breathing 100% oxygen at 3 atm. HBOT is capable of increasing DO_2 in conditions of stress like shocked states with high oxygen consumption.

2.3.2.2 Oxygen Dissociation Curve

The sigmoid-shaped ODC illustrates the relationship of the Hb saturation or content with the partial pressure of oxygen at equilibrium. At the pulmonary level, the flat part of the curve favors the binding of oxygen to Hb. When arterial blood reaches the tissue capillaries, the lower oxygen tension in tissues facilitates the release of oxygen from Hb as depicted in the steep part of the ODC. Factors that shift the ODC cause changes in the amount of oxygen dissociated to the tissues.

In conditions like carbon monoxide toxicity, the Hb-bound oxygen content reduces due to the higher affinity of CO to Hb with increased carboxy-Hb (COHb) formation. In addition, the ODC shifts to the left, which reduces the tissue oxygen release. As a treatment modality for CO toxicity, HBOT increases the pO_2, which facilitates CO dissociation from Hb and increases the dissolved fraction, leading to adequate tissue oxygenation. The half-life for dissociation of COHb with 100% O_2 at sea level is 90 minutes, but at 2 ATA, it is reduced to 35 minutes [9].

Increased 2,3 DPG, pCO_2, temperature, and acidity cause the ODC to shift to the right. The CO_2 produced by tissue metabolism is carried in venous blood mostly dissolved as bicarbonate, but 20% is bound to Hb. With venous Hb being 100% saturated in HBOT, there is a rise in partial pressure of CO_2, and pH becomes slightly acidotic. Therefore, in the venous circulation, the ODC shifts to the right with increased oxygen release.

2.3.2.3 Microcirculation

The microcirculation plays an important role in regulating the blood flow to the tissues. It is autoregulated by locally released substances, and during periods of increased demand like exercise, there is local vasodilation and an increase in capillary blood flow to the tissues. The effects of HBOT on the microvasculature are described in Sect. 3.1.

2.3.2.4 Oxygen Consumption

The oxygen demand depends on the tissue metabolic rate, and thus, the oxygen extraction can vary depending on the type of tissue. For example, the cardiac tissue oxygen extraction is ten times higher than the skin oxygen extraction. The total body oxygen consumption (VO_2) is the sum of oxygen extraction by all organs. It is calculated by multiplying cardiac output by the difference between arterial and mixed venous oxygen contents. The normal oxygen consumption is about 250 ml/min in an average-built man. In situations of high metabolic demand like exercise, the skeletal muscle oxygen consumption increases, leading to a reduction in the mixed venous oxygen content. Usually, at rest and exercise, the VO_2 is independent of DO_2 [10]. But when the DO_2 falls to a critical level like in hemorrhage and sepsis, the VO_2 falls to match the DO_2, leading to a supply–demand dependence [11]. The evidence for the effects of HBOT on VO_2 is rare, while one study done on critically ill patients concluded that hyperbaric hyperoxia does not seem to increase VO_2 despite an increase in DO_2 [12].

2.3.3 Effects of HBOT on Organ Systems

The effects of HBOT on different organ systems may vary with the absolute pressure used, the duration of exposure, and the patient's underlying comorbidities.

2.3.3.1 Cardiovascular System

HBOT causes changes in both macrovascular and microvascular parameters.

Macrovascular Changes of HBOT

HBOT mainly causes bradycardia, an increase in mean arterial pressure, and a slight lowering of the cardiac output [13, 14]. Bradycardia is found to be mediated by either myocardial depression or by a baroreceptor-mediated reflex vagal stimulation [14–16]. The reduction in cardiac output is thought to be due mainly to bradycardia rather than due to a reduction in stroke volume. Hyperoxia-induced vasoconstriction can increase the systemic vascular resistance, which leads to an initial increase in arterial blood pressure. Later, due to baroreceptor activation, there is a reduction in the sympathetic outflow, leading to a reduction in mean arterial pressure [14, 17].

Microvascular Changes of HBOT

HBOT affects the microvasculature by causing local vasoconstriction due to hyperoxia-induced vascular smooth muscle contraction [2]. It is a protective mechanism against free radical formation and tissue injury. Compared to catecholamine-induced vasoconstriction, it does not seem to cause a reduction in DO_2 because even with low blood flow rates, the high pO_2 is adequate in providing the required oxygen. Concomitantly, it causes a reduction in tissue edema, which is useful in conditions such as compartment syndrome and even cerebral edema.

2.3.3.2 Nervous System

HBOT-induced hyperoxia causes cerebral vasoconstriction and a reduction in the cerebral blood flow [18, 19]. The mechanism is thought to be related to the changes in cerebral nitric oxide (NO) levels. Hyperoxia leads to an increase in oxygen free radicals (superoxide anions), which oppose the vasodilatory action of nitric oxide. This results in a reduction in cerebral blood flow, which does not seem to show any adverse effects in healthy individuals with barometric pressures less than 3 ATA. However, it is thought to be advantageous for ischemic cerebral tissues by reducing cerebral edema. The impact of HBOT on intracranial pressure (ICP) was studied in an animal study, which showed a reduction in ICP when carbon dioxide (CO_2) and arterial pressure were held constant [18]. While another animal study showed that HBOT resulted in increased brain tissue pO_2 levels but did not seem to have an effect on ICP or on lactate production [7]. Prolonged exposure to hyperbaric oxygen with higher ATA values leads to oxygen toxicity and convulsions.

2.3.3.3 Respiratory System

HBOT leads to an increased density of inspired gases, resulting in a high airway resistance during inspiration and expiration. Although the effects are negligible in healthy humans with a barometric pressure of <3 ATA, in patients with chronic obstructive lung pathology, this might lead to increased work of breathing and even dynamic hyperinflation [20]. HBOT-induced hyperoxia depresses the response of the carotid bodies to CO_2 and may cause a respiratory depression. HBOT in multiple sessions seems to have no clinically significant effect on forced expiratory volume in 1 second (FEV_1), forced vital capacity (FVC), or FEV_1/FVC ratio [21]. In HBOT, there is evidence of developing pulmonary histopathological changes such as alveolar edema, peribronchial mononuclear cell infiltration, and thickening of the alveolar and vessel wall due to oxygen toxicity with prolonged exposure [22]. However, a recent study done on mice showed that HBOT has partial reversal effects for bleomycin-induced lung fibrosis [23].

2.3.3.4 Hematological System

There is evidence that HBOT leads to an increase in the deformability of the RBCs [24]. Increased RBC deformability causes a reduction in blood viscosity so that the RBCs can pass through the small tissue capillaries easily. There is conflicting data on the effect of platelets with HBOT, but most studies show that HBOT reduces platelet aggregation [25, 26]. During HBOT, these changes improve the blood flow to tissues and improve the tissue oxygenation, which is useful in wound healing and the restoration function of neutrophils and macrophages, leading to improved host defense against invading pathogens [27].

2.4 Conclusion

HBOT has several important physical and physiological effects, such as the improvement in gas transport and tissue oxygenation, the compression of gas-filled cavities/compartments, and the hyperoxia-induced vasoconstriction. It is generally considered safe when used within a range of 1.5–3.0 ATA at a safe duration.

References

1. Neuman TS, Thom SR. Physiology and medicine of hyperbaric oxygen therapy. Philadelphia, PA: Saunders, Elsevier; 2008.
2. Daniel M. Part I, Physical and pathophysiological bases of hyperbaric oxygen therapy. In: Handbook on hyperbaric medicine. Netherland, NL: Springer; 2006. p. 15–161.
3. Jain KK. Chapter 2, Physical, physiological, and biochemical aspects of hyperbaric oxygenation. In: Textbook of hyperbaric medicine. 6th ed. Switzerland, CH: Springer; 2017. p. 11–22.
4. Parbrook GD, Davis PD, Kenny GNC. Basic physics and measurements in anaesthesia. 4th ed. Oxford, GB: Butterworth-Heinemann; 1995.
5. West JB. West's respiratory physiology. Philadelphia, PA: Lippincott Williams and Wilkins; 2008.
6. Barrett KE, Barman SM, Boitano S, Brooks HL. Ganong's review of medical physiology. 24th ed. New York, NY: McGraw-Hill Companies; 2012.
7. Van Hulst RA, Haitsma JJ, Klein J, Lachmann B. Oxygen tension under hyperbaric conditions in healthy pig brain. Clin Physiol Funct Imaging. 2003;23(3):143–8.
8. Dmitriev RI, Papkovsky DB. Optical probes and techniques for O2 measurement in live cells and tissue. Cell Mol Life Sci. 2012;69:2025–39.
9. Pace N, Strajman E, Walker EL. Acceleration of carbon monoxide elimination in man by high pressure oxygen. Science. 1950;11:652–4.
10. Kohzuki H, Sakata S, Ohga Y, Misawa H, Kishi T, Takashi M. Increase in O2 delivery with hyperoxia does not increase O2 uptake in tetanically contracting muscle. Jpn J Physiol. 2000;50(1):157–9.
11. Schlichtig R. Oxygen delivery and consumption in critical illness. In: Civetta JM, Taylor RW, Kirby RR, editors. Critical Care. Philadelphia: Lippincott-Raven; 1997. p. 337–42.
12. Mathieu D. Effets hémodynamiques et microcirculatoires de l'oxygénothérapie hyperbare (Thèse). Université de Lille II; 1994.
13. Kenmure AC, Murdoch WR, Hutton I, Cameron JV. Hemodynamic effects of oxygen at 1 and 2 ATA pressure in healthy subjects. J Appl Physiol. 1972;32:223–6.
14. Demchenko IT, Zhilyaev SY, Moskvin AN, Krivchenko AI, Piantadosi CA, Allen BW. Baroreflex-mediated cardiovascular responses to hyperbaric oxygen. J Appl Physiol. 2013;115:819–28.
15. Fagraeus L. Cardiorespiratory and metabolic functions during exercise in the hyperbaric environment. Acta Physiol Scand. 1974;414:1–40.
16. Doubt TJ, Evans DE. Effects of hyperbaric oxygen exposure at 31.3 ATA on spontaneously beating cat hearts. J Appl Physiol. 1983;55:139–45.
17. Dooley JW, Mehm WJ. Non-invasive assessment of the vasoconstrictive effects of hyperoxygenation. J Hyperbaric Med. 1989;4:177–87.
18. Miller JD, Ledingham IM, Jennett WB. Effects of hyperbaric oxygen on intracranial pressure and cerebral blood flow in experimental cerebral oedema. J Neurol Neurosurg Psychiatry. 1970;33:745–55.

19. Demchenko IT, Oury TD, Crapo JD, Piantadosi CA. Regulation of the brain's vascular responses to oxygen. Circ Res. 2002;91:1031–7.
20. Calvet JH, Louis B, Giry P, et al. Effect of gas density variations on respiratory input impedance in humans. Respir Physiol. 1996;104:241–50.
21. Hadanny A, Zubari T, Tamir-Adler L, et al. Hyperbaric oxygen therapy effects on pulmonary functions: a prospective cohort study. BMC Pulm Med. 2019;19:148.
22. Oruç M, Esen B, Taylan M, Nergis Y, Şahin A. The role of duration of hyperbaric oxygen therapy on lung injury: an experimental study lung injury and hyperbaric oxygen therapy. Turk Thorac J. 2018;19(2):61–5.
23. Yuan Y, Li Y, Qiao G, Zhou Y, Xu Z, Hill C, Jiang Z, Wang Y. Hyperbaric oxygen ameliorates bleomycin-induced pulmonary fibrosis in mice. Front Mol Biosci. 2021;8:675437. https://doi.org/10.3389/fmolb.2021.675437.
24. Mathieu D, Coget JM, Vinckier L, Saulnier F, Durocher A, Wattel F. Filtrabilité érythrocitaire et oxygénothérapie hyperbare. Med Sup Hyp. 1984;3:100–4.
25. Widiyanti P, Suryohudoyo P. The role of hyperbaric oxygen to platelet aggregation in noninsulin-dependent diabetes mellitus (NIDDM). J Basic Clin Physiol Pharmacol. 2021;32(4):617–21.
26. Ersöz G, Ocakçioğlu B, Baştuğ M, Fiçicilar H, Yavuzer S. Platelet aggregation and release function in hyperbaric oxygenation. J Undersea Hyperb Med Soc. 1998;25(4):229–32.
27. Bai Q, Gao Q, Hu F, Zheng C, Sun N, Chen W, Liu J, Zhang Y, Wu X, Lu T. Reoxygenation modulates the adverse effects of hypoxia on wound repair. Int J Mol Sci. 2022;23:15832.

Chapter 3
Toxic Effect of Hyperbaric Breathing Gas Mixture

Ahsina Jahan Lopa and Payel Bose

3.1 Introduction

Modern therapeutic use of hyperbaric oxygen (HBO_2) in clinical medicine began in the 1950s [1]. Boerema, a Dutch surgeon, in conjunction with the Royal Dutch Navy, was the first physician to "drench" the tissue of a patient with increased partial pressure of oxygen (PO_2) with the use of a hyperbaric chamber [2]. Through his work and subsequent experiments, HBO_2 has been shown to have positive effects in treating wounds [3], and as a treatment for carbon monoxide (CO) toxicity [4]. In 1977, Blue Cross/Blue Shield accepted a report from the Undersea Medical Society (now Undersea and Hyperbaric Medical Society (UHMS)) on hyperbaric oxygenation, which resulted in a list of disorders for which hyperbaric treatment should be considered.

HBOT is a therapeutic modality that exposes the body to 100% inspired oxygen (O2) at ambient pressures greater than one atmosphere. Therapeutic administration of supplemental O2 generally refers to increasing the fractional inspired O2 (FIo2). Without the use of a hyperbaric chamber, FIo2 equals the partial pressure of inspired O_2 (PIo2). This limits the range of PIo2 from 0.21 ATA [FIo2 5 21% at one atmosphere of absolute pressure (ATA)] to 1.0 ATA (FIo2 5100% at 1 ATA); 1 ATA equals one atmosphere of pressure at sea level.

Hyperbaric chambers increase ambient pressure, allowing the PIo2 to exceed 1 ATA.

Hyperbaric oxygen therapy (HBOT) involves breathing 100% oxygen intermittently in a chamber (either mono- or multiplace chamber) at a pressure greater than

A. J. Lopa
Department of ICU and Emergency, Brahmanbaria ICU Specialized Hospital, Brahmanbaria, Bangladesh

P. Bose (✉)
Critical Care Medicine, Medica Superspecialty Hospital, Kolkata, West Bengal, India

A. G. D'Almeida, J. Hidalgo (eds.), *Evidence-Based Hyperbaric Medicine*,
https://doi.org/10.1007/978-3-032-06346-5_3

1 atmosphere absolute (1 ATA). The chamber pressurization should be at least 1.4 ATA according to the UHMS. The pressures used in clinical therapies vary between 2 and 3 ATA. Therapy sessions are 90–120 min daily.

3.2 Clinical Uses

HBOT has been gaining increased attention in the popular press and among scientific researchers.

The majority of clinical uses for HBOT derive their benefit from the increased PO_2 that HBOT provides. The increased PO_2 delivered throughout the body causes reactive oxidative species (ROS) that promote wound healing and post-ischemic tissue survival [5].

Hydrostatic effects of HBOT that affect bubble size are beneficial for illnesses such as decompression sickness [6]. Recompression and hyperbaric oxygen (HBO) are used in the treatment for diving-related diseases such as decompression sickness and arterial gas embolism. For a long time, HBO has also been shown to be effective in carbon monoxide poisoning and anaerobic infections. More recently, HBO has been shown to have supplementary effects in the treatment of other disorders characterized by local ischemia. An increase in local oxygen supply due to an increased gradient for diffusion is achieved by increasing the partial pressure of oxygen (PO_2) in inspired gas. This results in local stimulation of fibroblast proliferation and collagen synthesis, angiogenesis, and enhanced granulocyte function and peroxidase activity in ischemic tissue. In this way, HBO treatment is an effective adjunct in the treatment of osteoradionecrosis, chronic osteomyelitis, diabetic leg ulcers, and radiation-induced proctitis and cystitis.

3.3 Toxicity Related to HBOT

The potential risks and risk–benefit ratio of hyperbaric oxygen have often been underemphasized in therapeutic trials. The side effects are often mild and reversible but can be severe and life-threatening. In general, if pressures do not exceed 300 kPa and the length of treatment is less than 120 min, HBOT is safe. Overall, severe central nervous system (CNS) symptoms occur in 1–2% of treated patients, symptomatic reversible barotrauma in 15–20%, pulmonary symptoms in 15–20%, and reversible optic symptoms in up to 20% of patients.

Fire Hazard is the most common and fatal complication. Besides, there are general features such as claustrophobia, reversible myopia, fatigue, headache, and vomiting. Reversible myopia, due to oxygen toxicity on the lens, can last for weeks or months. Features of barotrauma associated with HBOT are lung damage, sinus damage, and ruptured middle ear. Risks of HBOT also include decompression illness such as decompression sickness, pneumothorax, and gas emboli. A suggested carcinogenic effect of hyperbaric oxygen has not been substantiated in extensive studies.

The toxic nature of O_2 is often underappreciated. There are side effects of the hydrostatic and oxidative changes that HBOT creates, including HBO_2 seizures [7]. Determining mechanisms of HBO_2 toxicity and its ability to cause seizures has been an effort of researchers in the hopes of maximizing the potential benefits of HBO_2T while minimizing its risks.

Both patients and hyperbaric medical attendants are routinely exposed to the hyperbaric environment (although attendants do not routinely breathe HBO_2) and are therefore exposed to an increased risk of O_2 toxicity. There are special populations outside of medicine who are also routinely exposed to HBO_2, including military, commercial, and recreational divers, and subterranean workers [8].

The risk of O_2 toxicity is increased when the ratio of O_2 to inert gas is raised in the hopes of minimizing deleterious gas effects. Combat divers use pure O_2 via a rebreather apparatus for clandestine purposes (to avoid bubbles) [9]. High PO_2 greatly increases the risk of O_2 toxicity even at shallow depths, but it also purges nitrogen from a diver's body.

O_2 toxicity in humans can be categorized into two major types: low pressure or chronic O_2 toxicity, such as pulmonary toxicity, nonspecific cellular toxicity, organ damage, and erythrocyte hemolysis, and high pressure or acute O_2 toxicity, most commonly associated with CNS O_2 toxicity [10].

Chronic toxicity tends to occur when the PO_2 exceeds 0.5 ATA for extended periods of time. People may be most familiar with retinal manifestations of O_2 toxicity resulting in blindness of premature neonates. Prolonged exposure to elevated PO_2, whether increased concentrations of oxygen inspired at atmospheric pressure or low concentrations of inspired oxygen at high ambient pressures, places humans at risk for pulmonary oxygen toxicity [11]. It is characterized by a decrease in pulmonary function, chest tightness, exertional dyspnea, and cough. Moderate to severe cases can involve pulmonary edema, hemorrhage, or death.

3.4 Pulmonary Oxygen Toxicity

Pulmonary oxygen toxicity is well characterized with respect to changes in vital capacity in response to continuous exposures to partial pressures of oxygen >50 kPa. The concept of units pulmonary toxic dose (UPTD), as introduced by CLARK and LAMBERTSEN [12], is widely used for calculating acceptable oxygen exposure under different conditions, such as in diving procedures and treatment tables for diving-related disease. Less is known about changes in other lung function variables, in particular in response to exposure to low levels of hyperoxia. It has also been shown that this effect is attenuated by intermittent exposure to up to the same cumulative dose of oxygen [13], and tolerance to the oxidative stress develops. In a study with continuous exposure to a PO_2 of 40–50 kPa for 28 days, as in a deep saturation dive, where no changes in vital capacity were expected or found, there was a decrease in the forced expiratory flow rates at low lung volumes and in *T*L,CO.

The reduction in the flow rates was linear, as judged from the daily measurements during the exposure [14], and persisted up to 3 years after the exposure [15], There was also a reduction in *T*L,CO of 10% after correction for changes in hemoglobin concentration, which was normalized 1 month after the exposure. In another study, in which no changes in vital capacity were predicted or found, with continuous exposure to a PO_2 of 300 kPa for 3.5 h [16], there were significant reductions in FEV1, and FEF25–75% of 5.9% and 11.8%, respectively, and a significant increase in phase III of the single-breath nitrogen washout test (δ-N_2). A reduction in small airways conductance may thus take place before changes in vital capacity are seen.

Exposure to hyperoxia reduces the stimulus for hemoglobin and red blood cell production, and, after saturation dives, a reduction in hemoglobin concentration of 5–8% is usually seen [17]. The reduction in *T*L,CO in this study could apparently be explained by the reduction in hemoglobin concentration. This could, however, be a statistical coincidence since the variance in *T*L,CO,corr is larger than in *T*L,CO because of the additional variance caused by measurement error of hemoglobin concentration. The changes in *T*L,CO are small, however, and, as in saturation dives, normalized 1 month after the exposure. Oxygen toxicity is attenuated when the exposure is intermittent, implying that a cumulative dose, which would have resulted in a reduction in vital capacity if given continuously, can be given intermittently without resulting in changes in vital capacity. This development of tolerance to hyperoxia has also been demonstrated in survival studies of animals exposed to hyperoxia [18] and in cell cultures where there is stimulation to increased synthesis of antioxidant enzymes [19]. These enzymes are essential in the detoxification of oxygen radicals. With the HBO treatment protocols in common use, the daily exposure is equivalent to 275 UPTD, which is not expected to give changes in vital capacity, and the exposure is interrupted by two periods of breathing air for 5 min. The cumulative exposure over approximately 5 days of treatment, 1425 UPTD, will give a mean reduction in vital capacity of 10% if given continuously. Over a 3-week HBO treatment period, changes in vital capacity are still not seen. The susceptibility to oxidative stress and induction of defense mechanisms may be very different in healthy subjects than in patients who have this treatment for some underlying disease, which may already stress defense mechanisms.

In conclusion, the reduction in pulmonary function after 3 weeks of hyperbaric oxygen treatment is not considered to be of any clinical significance unless repeated treatment series are considered or pulmonary function is reduced before treatment. If so, the risk of pulmonary barotrauma has to be considered as a contraindication for hyperbaric oxygen treatment in addition to the risk of a further reduction in lung function.

3.5 HBOT and Neurotoxicity

The risk of CNS O_2 toxicity is a function of both PO_2 and exposure time, directly proportional to both: the greater the PO_2, the greater the risk of HBO_2 seizure [20]. While the onset of seizures is usually in the vicinity of 2–3 ATA, the pressure at onset may be significantly lowered by coexisting conditions such as immersion, exercise, and respiratory acidosis due to moderate CO_2 retention. 1.9 ATA is a noticeable threshold for increased risk. Even at lower PO_2, HBO_2 seizures can occur, particularly when combined with inert gases or carbon monoxide (CO)0.9,52 The most dramatic manifestation of CNS O_2 toxicity is an HBO_2-induced seizure. Additional effects of CNS O_2 toxicity may also occur, including autonomic, motor, and cardiorespiratory signs and symptoms [21], such as bradycardia, hyperventilation, dyspnea, and altered cardiorespiratory neural reflexes.

CNS O_2 toxicity often presents acutely with little or no warning.

Common signs and symptoms of CNS O_2 toxicity are easily remembered using the mnemonic VENTID-C3 [22].

Visual symptoms: tunnel vision, blurred vision, or decreased peripheral vision
Ear symptoms: tinnitus, roaring, pulsing sounds, or perceived sounds not from an external stimulus
Nausea: often with vomiting and headache
Twitching/Tingling: of extremities, facial muscles
Irritability: or any change in mental status such as confusion, agitation, anxiety, or undue fatigue
Dizziness or clumsiness, loss of coordination
Convulsions and death

Unfortunately, many of these symptoms are not exclusive to O_2 toxicity, and CNS O_2 toxicity does not usually proceed through any predictable sequence of the above signs. Convulsions, the most serious effect of O_2 toxicity due to its fatal potential if left untreated, may occur without warning or other accompanying signs. O_2-induced seizures are characterized as generalized tonic–clonic seizures, though focal seizures may be the only neurological manifestation at times [1].

After an O_2 toxicity convulsion, the individual usually remembers clearly the events up to the moment when consciousness was lost, but remembers nothing of the convulsion itself and little of the post-ictal phase.

Convulsions unrelated to O_2 toxicity may also occur in HBO_2 environments and would present identically to an HBO_2-induced seizure. It is critical to differentiate seizures resulting from hyperbaric oxygen from other etiologies, such as hypoglycemia. A convulsion due to O_2 toxicity has little lasting effect, assuming that the O_2 pressure is immediately decreased; however, a hypoglycemic seizure unrecognized and untreated can be fatal.

Unlike other tonic–clonic seizures, such as those seen in epilepsy, the danger of hypoxia during breathholding in the tonic phase of an HBO_2-induced convulsion is minimized by the high PO_2 in the brain and tissues; the source of the toxicity helps minimize hypoxia in the tissue during the seizure. A greater danger is posed by decreasing pressure in a chamber too quickly, which could potentially lead to a gas embolism. Since it would be difficult to differentiate between a post-ictal individual and an unconscious victim suffering from a cerebral arterial gas embolism, those experiencing O_2-induced seizures in a hyperbaric chamber under pressure are generally kept at that same pressure until their convulsions cease. The PO_2 in such cases is diminished solely by altering the breathing gas mixture.

Patients suffering from O_2-induced seizures generally have full recoveries within 24 h with no lasting effects, and it is unclear whether there is increased susceptibility to future incidents of O_2 toxicity.

The primary treatment for an O_2-induced seizure is to lower the inspired PO_2. This is accomplished by decreasing ambient pressure, switching to a breathing mixture with a lower percentage of O_2, or both. Decreasing inspired PO_2 may not immediately reverse the effects of CNS O_2 toxicity and is not without risk. It is believed that the biochemical processes responsible for the toxicity remain in place for a period after the PO_2 has been decreased in the ambient or inspired atmosphere. The individual experiencing the toxicity is not considered clear from danger until several minutes have passed after the PO_2 has been decreased.

In practice, the risk of acute O_2 toxicity is often mitigated by interspersing short periods of air amid the pure O_2 therapy at increased pressure, commonly referred to as "air breaks." It is a logical measure, and some species such as insects have evolved discontinuous breathing in order to minimize risks of O_2 toxicity even at 1 ATA [23]. Some data supports the use of intermittent air breaks of 5–10 min to prolong HBO_2 exposure prior to the onset of seizures [24]. Yet, animal models demonstrate the possibility that the rapid decreases in PO_2 may actually instigate seizure activity while appearing to be beneficial in preventing pulmonary oxygen toxicity. While intermittent exposures may decrease symptoms of CNS toxicity, measured molecular activities maintain prebreak levels, adding further confusion to the mechanism and success of air breaks during HBO_2T.

Therefore, understanding the mechanisms leading to HBO_2 CNS toxicity can help to mitigate toxicity.

3.6 Mechanisms

Methods and models used to investigate the mechanisms of HBO_2 toxicity on the nervous system must attempt to isolate two interdependent variables:

1. Effects due to the increased ambient pressure on the CNS
2. Effects due to the increased PO_2.

The normobaric hyperoxic mouse brain slice model is a common research model. It is a less desirable model to study the effects of oxygen toxicity on neuronal activity, since most in vitro preparations of CNS tissue and cells use a 95% O_2 control level during preparation. Humans inspiring normobaric air have relatively low PO_2

in their brain, 35 mmHg or less, depending on the region [25]. Murine brains have even lower ranges of PO_2 in their brain, from 5 to 25 mmHg [26]. Direct investigation using hyperbaric oxygen is preferred.

The use of in vitro electrophysiological methods to investigate the cellular mechanisms of O_2 toxicity within a hyperbaric chamber has been limited by the challenges of working with or in a sealed pressure chamber and the mechanical disturbances experienced during tissue compression. Chamber design improvements have minimized these obstacles, allowing easier experimentation on animal models in ambient pressures around 5 ATA. Refinements in chamber design and using an ambient atmosphere of 100% helium have allowed intracellular experiments in rat brain slices. Electrophysiological studies on rat neurons have shown that increases in the PO_2 in cerebral tissue lead to increased ROS production, followed by increased cortical EEG activity, and finally result in the onset of an O_2-induced seizure activity [27].

Effects on the CNS attributed to increased hydrostatic pressure, such as high-pressure nervous syndrome, tend to occur at very high pressures, ranging from 15 to 70 ATA. This results from compression of cerebral spinal fluid, circulation, and extracellular and intracellular fluid compartments of the CNS.

Cellular mechanisms most likely involve synaptic and membrane dynamic responses to severe and fast changes in pressure. Therefore, there is little evidence to suggest that hydrostatic pressure plays a significant role in HBO_2 seizures, particularly at pressures involved with HBO_2T less than 3 ATA [28].

Oxidative stress plays a key role in the mechanism of O_2 toxicity. CNS O_2 toxicity is an acute exposure to an oxidative environment, disrupting neurological function. HBO_2T greatly increases oxygen tension in the brain. Molecular O_2 is a natural oxidative reagent in cellular biochemical pathways producing various free radicals. The mammalian CNS response to hyperoxia ranges from moderate, reversible changes in neural activity to violent seizures that may lead to irreversible motor deficits and death.

The body scavenges oxidizing substances through enzymatic antioxidants such as superoxide dismutase for superoxide anions, catalase for hydrogen peroxide, and nonenzymatic antioxidants such as reduced glutathione and vitamin E [5]. Glutathione is regenerated by reaction with nicotinamide adenine dinucleotide phosphate (NADPH). Therefore, sufficient levels of both glutathione and NADPH may be critical to defending against the increased levels of oxidants [29].

Superoxide catalyzes superoxide anions to O_2. Therefore, increased levels or activity of superoxide dismutase should decrease levels of ROS. However, in transgenic mice bred to overexpress human extracellular superoxide dismutase in the brain, inhibition of superoxide dismutase increased resistance to HBO_2 seizures, contrary to expectations. By inhibiting superoxide dismutase, the catalysis of superoxide into O_2 (an in vivo antioxidant mechanism) is blocked, allowing superoxide levels to rise unopposed during HBO_2 exposure. A fourfold decrease in seizures was measured in these mice pretreated with diethyldithiocarbonate, an inhibitor of human extracellular superoxide dismutase [30]. The mechanism of this counterintuitive result appears to be the interaction between superoxide and other HBO_2-induced reactants.

Gamma-aminobutyric acid (GABA) has long been correlated with HBO_2 seizures. Though GABA has been found to be lowered in mammalian neuronal synapses during HBO_2 seizures when exposed to HBO_2 in short intervals [31], there is evidence to suggest that the increased steady-state levels of GABA over longer intervals may be responsible for O_2-induced seizures. In experiments involving transgenic mice with an HBO_2-sensitivity phenotype, data suggests that the excitatory amino acids, such as aspartate and glutamate, play as important or more important roles in HBO_2 seizures than GABA [32].

Glutamate, an excitatory amino acid, is a potent, fast-acting neurotoxin in neuronal cultures. It has been shown to create morphological changes in mature cortical neurons within minutes of HBO_2 exposure, with neuronal degeneration occurring over the course of hours. Decreased glutamate metabolism during HBO_2 exposure sensitizes neural networks to HBO_2 seizures [33]. Conflicting evidence exists as to the degree of change in excitatory amino acids prior to and during HBO_2 seizures. Recent evidence suggests that O_2-induced seizures may result from an imbalance of excitatory and inhibitory synaptic neurotransmitters, glutamate and GABA, respectively. The imbalance results in a greater relative decrease in presynaptic release of GABA than of glutamate, which suggests that the relative increase of excitatory neurotransmitters with respect to inhibitory neurotransmitters may be a basic mechanism of HBO_2 seizures.

Extracellular mediators of physiological functions such as NO also play a role in HBO_2 seizures. NO leads to neurotoxicities resulting from excess glutamate stimulation in cultures of rat cortex, striatum, and hippocampus. NO activity appears to increase the ratio of excitatory to inhibitory neurotransmitters, which increases the probability of O_2 seizures [34]. Neurons containing nitric oxide synthase (NOS), widespread throughout the cortex, react to HBO_2 by increasing NO production [35]. In HBO_2 environments, NO acutely decreases cerebral blood flow but then increases regional cerebral blood flow after prolonged HBO_2 exposure preceding neuronal excitation [36]. NO has been associated with changes in cerebral blood flow and HBO_2 seizures [37].

A relationship exists between high pressures and glycine receptors, which indicates possible roles pressure plays on HBO_2 seizures. High pressures have no effect on the maximum response of the glycine receptor to glycine; however, the half maximal effective concentration of glycine to its receptor and pressure become directly proportional at pressures above 100 ATA.101 While this seems less likely to be correlated with seizures occurring at 2–3 ATA, typical of HBO_2T, it appears to be associated with high-pressure neurological syndrome at much greater depths. The fact that glycine receptors are linked to myoclonic activity in mammals raises suspicion that conformational alterations at pressures less than 100 ATA may still participate in hyperbaric seizures to some degree at lower pressures [38].

A long-standing question regarding hyperbaric oxygen seizures is whether certain regions of the CNS are more susceptible to HBO_2. Neuroanatomic studies have shown that centrally located regions of the brain are most affected by exposure to

HBO_2, including: the globus pallidus, substantia nigra, superior olivary nucleus, ventral cochlear nucleus, limbic structures, amygdala, and the spinal cord gray matter [39].

The anatomical localization of neuroactive agents and their effects may also explain the anatomical distribution of increased O_2 sensitization.

Acute exposure to HBO_2 results in an increased firing rate of specific neurons, particularly carbon dioxide (CO_2)/proton chemosensitive neurons, which are coupled via gap junctions and baroreceptors, in the cerebral and cerebella cortex that demonstrate a high sensitivity to HBO_2, chemical oxidants, and neurotransmitters [21].

Certain conditions heighten one's risk to CNS toxicity and HBO_2 seizures. Hypercapnia elevates the risk of O_2 toxicity [40]. Hypercapnic-induced intracellular acidosis makes cells more susceptible to ROS. CO_2 causes cerebral vasodilation, increases cerebral blood flow, and heightens CNS exposure to elevated PO_2. Neurons in the solitary complex are particularly susceptible to increased PCO_2 and PO_2, resulting in an increased rate of excitatory firing. Increased PCO_2 in HBO_2 environments may occur by:

1. A decrease in CO_2-carrying capacity of venous hemoglobin since venous hemoglobin may be saturated with O_2;
2. Alveolar hypoventilation and CO_2 retention;
3. CO_2-contamination due to inadequate scrubbing of recirculated breathing gas.

Exercise also increases the risk of CNS O_2 toxicity, likely related to increased cerebral blood flow and metabolic rate [41]. CO toxicity significantly increases the risk of HBO_2 seizures [42].

3.7 Management

Numerous prophylactic treatments for HBO_2-induced seizures have been shown to be effective through in vivo experiments involving rats and mice.

NO is an important mediator of CNS O_2 toxicity. Inhibition of NOS with nitroarginine showed similar prevention of CNS toxicity and O_2-induced seizures in both transgenic and nontransgenic mice [43].

Intraperitoneal administration of GABA proved effective in protecting rats from O_2-induced seizures. Since GABA does not cross the blood–brain barrier, the mechanism of its protection is speculated to be an osmotic effect drawing a metabolite of GABA out of the brain.

MK-801, an NMDA receptor antagonist, has been shown to prevent EEG spikes associated with O_2 toxicity and O_2-induced seizures [44].

Other substances such as disulfiram (Antabuse) [45] and antioxidants also appear to delay or diminish O_2 toxicity in the brain.

Additional agents that hasten the onset or increase the incidence of HBO_2 seizures include:

Adrenocortical hormones, epinephrine, hyperthermia, norepinephrine, thyroid hormones, vitamin E deficiency, brain-derived neurotrophic factor, misonidazole, pseudoephedrine, hyperglycemia, and phosphodiesterase-5 inhibitors.

Additional agents that delay the onset or attenuate HBO_2 seizures include:

N-nitro-L-arginine, daurisoline, acclimitization to hypoxia, antioxidants, chlorpromazine, reserpine, starvation ganglionic blocking drugs and anti-epileptics, glutathione, hypothermia, hypothyroidism, insulin, CoQ10 and carnitine, acetazolamide, excitatoryamino acid antagonists, aminooxyacetic acid, delta-sleep-inducing peptide, beta-carotene, vigabatrin, propionyl-L-carnitine, leukotriene and PAF inhibitors, carbamazepine, propranolol, caffeine, Dilantin, and lithium. Some agents that one would expect to affect HBO_2 seizures, such as allopurinol and pyridoxine, did not.

Agents that mitigate O_2-induced seizures may also negatively affect the therapeutic benefits of HBO_2T, thus adding to the complexity of the study. For example, any antioxidant that can effectively eliminate ROS during HBO_2T may eliminate their role in causing HBO_2 seizures, but it would also eliminate the benefits ROS play in promoting wound healing and post-ischemic tissue survival [5].

The advent of nanoscale devices allows for more precise delivery and investigation of mediators of O_2-induced seizures such as NO [46].

Normobaric models of the effects of HBO_2 would also open the door to the wide array of experimental tools that otherwise would not be feasible to perform in hyperbaric chambers. Finally, as data and proposed theories of O_2 toxicity increase, this area of research becomes primed for computational simulations. Current prediction models have shown that it is very difficult to build a prediction model for mild hyperoxia given the current data [47].

However, computational analysis and simulations of molecular signaling interactions might enable existing and otherwise conflicting theories to coexist within a new model for CNS O_2 toxicity. This would provide a physiologically based model with greater precision and accuracy. Models of complex biological systems such as T lymphocyte activation demonstrate the feasibility of this approach [48].

3.8 Ocular Oxygen Toxicity

HBOT exposes the eye to increased oxygen concentration and the risk of oxidative damage in susceptible individuals. A review of the literature found that, in addition to cataract, age-related macular degeneration, and keratoconus, there may be other ocular diseases for which the pathology involves reactive oxygen species and so for which exposure to HBOT-related oxidative stress could be significantly adverse [49]. For example, a patient with a ruptured retinal arterial macroaneurysm experienced acute development of severe macular edema 2 days after the seventh HBOT treatment. Yonekawa and coauthors [50] recommended that HBOT could be contraindicated for retinovascular diseases. The involvement of oxidative stress in glaucomatous pathology [51, 52] suggests that patients with glaucoma could be contraindicated for HBOT. Alternatively, depending on the strength of an indication for HBOT, this form of treatment for a patient with glaucoma may proceed cautiously with progressive monitoring for any adverse effects. Studies in rats found that aging is the most significant risk factor for the loss of retinal ganglion cells (RGCs) [53]. As the animal ages, there is an inherent loss of RGCs, and when the older eye is exposed to retinal ischemia/reperfusion stress, a greater percentage of the remaining cells degenerate. These findings suggest that ischemia/reperfusion injury may occur more frequently and/or to a greater extent in older patients attending for HBOT. IOP in healthy subjects was measured during experimental exposure to normal atmospheric pressure and at double normal pressure (2 bar). IOP fell by a mean of 1.25 mmHg during HBOT conditions [54]. IOP was reduced significantly by a mean of 1.85 mmHg during HBOT (2.5 bar) treatment for a variety of indications. That means IOP was found to be reduced slightly in these studies does not eliminate the possibility that IOP may have been elevated during HBOT in any individual subject without that finding influencing the statistical significance of the reported differences between the mean findings. It is not known if any glaucoma patients were included in these studies. The global prevalence of glaucoma has been estimated to be 3.4% for ages 40–80, with primary open-angle glaucoma being more likely in people with African ancestry and primary closed-angle glaucoma being more likely in people with Asian ancestry [55]. However, oxygen concentration in aqueous humor, and the risk of damage to trabecular meshwork cells may be greater if hyperbaric oxygen is delivered by a hood which exposes the anterior ocular surface to higher than normal oxygen levels [56]. Oronasal mask delivery of HBOT appears to be indicated in these cases.

3.9 Conclusion

The exact mechanism of O_2 toxicity remains a mystery. Prophylactic measures and treatment for CNS O_2 toxicity remain centered on limiting exposure to high PO_2. A better understanding of molecular mechanisms causing O_2 toxicity can lead to prophylactic therapies for consideration in clinical trials.

References

1. Kindwall EP, Whalen HT. Hyperbaric medicine practice. 2nd ed. Flagstaff, AZ: Best Publishing Company; 2004.
2. Boerema I, Kroll JA, Meijne NG, Lobin E, Kroom B, Huskies JW. High atmospheric pressure as an aid to cardiac surgery. Arch Chir Neerl. 1956;8:193–211.
3. Kranke P, Bennett MH, Martyn-St James M, Schnabel A, Debus SE, Weibel S. Hyperbaric oxygen therapy for chronic wounds. Cochrane Database Syst Rev. 2015;6:CD004123.

4. Nelson LS, Lewin NA, Howland MA, Hoffman RS, Goldfrank LR, Flomenbaum NE. Goldfrank's toxicologic emergencies. 9th ed. New York, NY: McGraw Hill; 2011.
5. Thom SR. Oxidative stress is fundamental to hyperbaric oxygen therapy. J Appl Physiol (1985). 2009;106(3):988–95.
6. Naval Sea Systems Command, United States Department of the Navy. Navy diving manual. 5th ed. Washington, DC: U.S. Government Printing Office; 2005.
7. Camporesi EM. Side effects of hyperbaric oxygen therapy. Undersea Hyperb Med. 2014;41(3):253–7.
8. Fock AW. Analysis of recreational closed-circuit rebreather deaths 1998–2010. Diving Hyperb Med. 2013;43:78–85.
9. Moskvin AN, Zhilyaev SY, Sharapov OI, Platonova TF, Gutsaeva DR, et al. Brain blood flow modulates the neurotoxic action of hyperbaric oxygen via neuronal and endothelial nitric oxide. Neurosci Behav Physiol. 2003;33(9):883–8.
10. Thomson L, Paton J. Oxygen toxicity. Paediatr Respir Rev. 2014;15(2):120–3.
11. Eynan M, Krinsky N, Biram A, Arieli Y, Arieli R. A comparison of factors involved in the development of central nervous system and pulmonaryoxygen toxicity in the rat. Brain Res. 2014;1574:77–83.
12. Clark JM, Lambertsen CJ. Pulmonary oxygen toxicity: a review. Pharmacol Rev. 1971;23:37–133.
13. Hendricks PL, Hall DA, Hunter WL Jr, Haley PJ. Extension of pulmonary oxygen tolerance in man at 2 ATA by intermittent oxygen exposure. J Appl Physiol. 1977;42:593–9.
14. Thorsen E, Segadal K, Reed JW, Elliott C, Gulsvik A, Hjelle JO. Contribution of hyperoxia to reduced pulmonary function after deep saturation dives. J Appl Physiol. 1993;75:657–62.
15. Thorsen E, Kambestad BK. Persistent small airways dysfunction after exposure to hyperoxia. J Appl Physiol. 1995;78:1421–4.
16. Clark JM, Jackson RM, Lambertsen CJ, Gelfand R, Hiller WDB, Unger M. Pulmonary function in men after oxygen breathing at 3.0 ATA for 35 h. J Appl Physiol. 1991;71:878–85.
17. Thorsen E, Segadal K, Myrseth E, Påsche A, Gulsvik A. Pulmonary mechanical function and diffusion capacity after deep saturation dives. Br J Ind Med. 1990;47:242–7.
18. Harabin AL, Survanashi SS, Weathersby PK, Hays JR, Homer LD. The modulation of oxygen toxicity by intermittent exposure. Toxicol Appl Pharmacol. 1988;93:298–311.
19. Harabin AL, Braisted JC, Flynn ET. Response of antioxidant enzymes to intermittent and continuous hyperbaric oxygen. J Appl Physiol. 1990;69:328–35.
20. Jenkinson SG. Oxygen toxicity. New Horiz. 1993;1(4):504–11.
21. Demchenko IT, Gasier HG, Zhilyaev SY, Moskvin AN, Krivchenko AI, et al. Baroreceptor afferents modulate brain excitation and influence susceptibility to toxic effects of hyperbaric oxygen. J Appl Physiol (1985). 2014;117(5):525–34.
22. Bitterman N. CNS oxygen toxicity. Undersea Hyperb Med. 2004;31(1):63–72.
23. Hetz SK, Bradley TJ. Insects breathe discontinuously to avoid oxygen toxicity. Nature. 2005;433(7025):516–9.
24. Chavko M, McCarron RM. Extension of brain tolerance to hyperbaric O2 by intermittent air breaks is related to the time of CBF increase. Brain Res. 2006;1084(1):196–201.
25. Carreau A, El Hafny-Rahbi B, Matejuk A, Grillon C, Kieda C. Why is the partial oxygen pressure of human tissues a crucial parameter? Small molecules and hypoxia. J Cell Mol Med. 2011;15(6):1239–53.
26. Zhang C, Belanger S, Pouliot P, Lesage F. Measurement of local partial pressure of oxygen in the brain tissue under normoxia and epilepsy with phosphorescence lifetime microscopy. PLoS One. 2015;10(8):e0135536.
27. Torbati D, Church DF, Keller JM, Pryor WA. Free radical generation in the brain precedes hyperbaric oxygen-induced convulsions. Free Radic Biol Med. 1992;13(2):101–6.
28. Daniels S. Cellular and neurophysiological effects of high ambient pressure. Undersea Hyperb Med. 2008;35(1):11–9.

29. Davis JC, Hunt TK, editors. Hyperbaric oxygen therapy. Bethesda, MD: Undersea Medical Society, Inc.; 1977.
30. Oury TD, Ho YS, Piantadosi CA, Crapo JD. Extracellular superoxide dismutase, nitric oxide, and central nervous system O2 toxicity. Proc Natl Acad Sci USA. 1992;89(20):9715–9.
31. Hori S. Study on hyperbaric oxygen-induced convulsion with particular reference to gamma-aminobutyric acid in synaptosomes. J Biochem. 1982;91(2):443–8.
32. Mialon P, Joanny P, Gibey R, Cann-Moisan C, Caroff J, et al. Amino acids and ammonia in the cerebral cortex, the corpus striatum and the brain stem of the mouse prior to the onset and after a seizure induced by hyperbaric oxygen. Brain Res. 1995;676(2):352–7.
33. Li Q, Guo M, Xu X, Xiao X, Xu W, et al. Rapid decrease of GAD 67 content before the convulsion induced by hyperbaric oxygen exposure. Neurochem Res. 2008;33(1):185–93.
34. Demchenko IT, Piantadosi CA. Nitric oxide amplifies the excitatory to inhibitory neurotransmitter imbalance accelerating oxygen seizures. Undersea Hyperb Med. 2006;33(3):169–74.
35. Allen BW, Demchenko IT, Piantadosi CA. Two faces of nitric oxide: implications for cellular mechanisms of oxygen toxicity. J Appl Physiol. 2009;106(2):662–7.
36. Gutsaeva DR, Moskvin AN, Zhiliaev SIu, Kostkin VB, Demchenko IT. [Nitric oxide and carbon dioxide in neurotoxicity induced by oxygen under pressure]. [Article in Russian]. Ross Fiziol Zh Im I M Sechenova. 2004; 90(4):428–36.
37. Sato T, Takeda Y, Hagioka S, Zhang S, Hirakawa M. Changes in nitric oxide production and cerebral blood flow before development of hyperbaric oxygen-induced seizures in rats. Brain Res. 2001;918(1–2):131–40.
38. Lynch JW. Molecular structure and function of the glycine receptor chloride channel. Physiol Rev. 2004;84(4):1051–95.
39. Vion-Dury J, LeGal La Salle G, Rougier I, Papy JJ. Effects of hyperbaric and hyperoxic conditions on amygdala-kindled seizures in rat. Exp Neurol. 1986;92(3):513–21.
40. Seidel R, Carroll C, Thompson D, Diem RG, Yeboah K, et al. Risk factors for oxygen toxicity seizures in hyperbaric oxygen therapy: case reports from multiple institutions. Undersea Hyperb Med. 2013;40(6):515–9.
41. Koch AE, Koch I, Kowalski J, Schipke JD, Winkler BE, et al. Physical exercise might influence the risk of oxygen-induced acute neurotoxicity. Undersea Hyperb Med. 2013;40(2):155–63.
42. Sanders RW, Katz KD, Suyama J, Akhtar J, O'Toole KS, et al. Seizure during hyperbaric oxygen therapy for carbon monoxide toxicity: a case series and five-year experience. J Emerg Med. 2012;42(4):e69–72.
43. Wang WJ, Ho XP, Yan YL, Yan TH, Li CL. Intrasynaptosomal free calcium and nitric oxide metabolism in central nervous system oxygen toxicity. Aviat Space Environ Med. 1998;69(6):551–5.
44. Demchenko IT, Boso AE, O'Neill TJ, Bennett PB, Piantadosi CA. Nitric oxide and cerebral blood flow responses to hyperbaric oxygen. J Appl Physiol (1985). 2000;88(4):1381–9.
45. Chavko M, Braisted JC, Harabin AL. Attenuation of brain hyperbaric oxygen toxicity by fasting is not related to ketosis. Undersea Hyperb Med. 1999;26(2):99–103.
46. Roche CJ, Dantsker D, Samuni U, Friedman JM. Nitrite reductase activity of sol-gel-encapsulated deoxyhemoglobin. Influence of quaternary and tertiary structure. J Biol Chem. 2006;281(48):36874–82. Epub 2006 Sep 19
47. Shykoff B. Incidence of CNS oxygen toxicity with mild hyperoxia: a literature and data review. Panama City, FL: Navy Experimental Dive Unit; 2013. TA 12-03 NEDU TR 13-03
48. Jacobi Medical Center Hyperbaric Treatments [Internet]. Bronx, NY: Jacobi Medical Center; 2015 [cited 2015 Dec 15]. Available from: http://www.jacobi-hyperbaric.com/html/hyperbaric-treatments.html.
49. McMonnies CW. Hyperbaric oxygen therapy and the possibility of ocular complications or contraindications. Clin Exp Optom. 2015;98:122–5.
50. Yonekawa Y, Hypes SM, Abbey AM, Williams GA, Wolfe JD. Exac-erbation of macular oedema associated with hyperbaric oxygentherapy. Clin Experiment Ophthalmol. 2016;44:625–6.

51. Weinreb RN, Aung T, Medeiros FA. The pathophysiology andtreatment of glaucoma: a review. JAMA. 2014;311:1901–11.
52. Chrysostomou V, Rezania F, Trounce IA, Crowston JG. Oxidativestress and mitochondrial dysfunction in glaucoma. Curr OpinPharmacol. 2013;13:12d–5d.
53. Kawai S-I, Vora S, Das S, Gachie E, Becker B, Neufeld AH. Mod-eling of risk factors for the degeneration of retinal ganglioncells after ischemia/reperfusion in rats: effects of age, caloricrestriction, diabetes, pigmentation, and glaucoma. FASEB J. 2016;15:1285–7.
54. Van de Veire S, Germonpre P, Renier C, Stalmans I, Zeyen T. Influences of atmospheric pressure and tempera-ture on intraocualar pressure. Invest Ophthalmol Vis Sci. 2008;49:5392–6.
55. Tham Y-C, Li X, Wong TY, Quigley HA, Aung T, Cheng C-Y. Globalprevalence of glaucoma and projections of glaucoma burdenthrough 2040. Ophthalmology. 2014;121:2081–90.
56. Sharifipour F, Idani E, Zamani M, Helmi T, Cheraghian B. Oxygentension in the aqueous humor of human eyes under differ-ent oxygenation conditions. J Ophthalmic Vis Res. 2013;8:119–25.

Chapter 4
Cardiovascular Changes During Hyperbaric Oxygen Therapy

Manoj K. Singh and Rajesh Mishra

4.1 Introduction

When human cells are exposed to a higher supply of oxygen at atmospheric pressure or higher than normal partial pressure of oxygen, hyperoxia sets in. Hyperbaric oxygen therapy (HBOT) is used for various medicinal and surgical disorders.

Hyperoxia-induced oxidative stress affects the central nervous system, lungs, and eyes, along with the DNA of isolated lymphocytes and leukocytes [1, 2]. Cardiovascular effects have also been described in animal experimental models and human studies [3, 4].

HBOT provides oxygen at 1.5–3 times higher than atmospheric pressure. Hyperoxygenation and high pressure have various physiological and mechanical changes in the cardiovascular system. Recently, there has been a lot of interest in the impact of HBOT on cerebral blood flow, heart rate, cardiac output, and heart rate in normal individuals and those with existing cardiac conditions [5, 6]. Scientifically increased oxygen delivery was postulated to be a beneficial tool in certain cerebrovascular diseases associated with hypoxia, viz., coronary artery disease, arterial insufficiencies of extremities, cerebrovascular insufficiency, and surgical methods needing circulation interruption.

Experimental studies done five decades back reveal that HBOT definitively increases delivery of oxygen to tissues in debt, but the oxygen storage effect cannot

M. K. Singh (✉)
Sr Consultant Chest and Critical Care, Zydus Hospital & Research Centre, Thaltej, Ahmedabad, Gujarat, India
e-mail: drmanojsingh@gmail.com

R. Mishra
Ahmedabad, Gujarat, India
e-mail: mishr.c@gmail.com

A. G. D'Almeida, J. Hidalgo (eds.), *Evidence-Based Hyperbaric Medicine*,
https://doi.org/10.1007/978-3-032-06346-5_4

be relied upon in cardiovascular diseases due to poor diffusion of gas through non-vascular routes [7].

4.2 Physiology

Most of the cardiovascular physiology is focused on HBOT responses linked to heart rate, blood pressure, cardiac output, and organ perfusion due to flow dynamics secondary to vasoconstriction, rhythm disturbances, and microcirculation.

The three basic stages that could be altered during oxygen transport are respiration, circulation, and cell oxygenation. The global macrocirculatory level takes the following components: supply reservoir (lung and tissues), pumps (right and left ventricles), and pipes (arteries and veins). During HBOT, hemodynamic changes will be reflected when the abovementioned parameters interact with microcirculatory levels during the therapy times, which can vary from 30 min to 2 h. After the central hemodynamic variables are discussed, the regional blood flow influences the oxygen transport.

Oxygen is finally presented to microcirculation. Biochemical and cardiovascular studies done by M Kozakiewicz on healthy subjects prove that HBOT decreases heart rate and increases the mean blood pressure, diastolic blood pressure, total peripheral resistance, and afterload within almost 1 h after hyperbaric exposure [8].

Majority of trials have focused on bradycardia due to HBOT. The main reason for the reduction in heart rate is due to stimulation of neurons in the dorsal motor neurons of the vagus and the nucleus solitarius [6]. This increase in parasympathetic activity leads to bradycardia. An additional pathway responsible for this phenomenon is nitrogen-dependent beta-blockade of the heart due to hyperoxia and increased pressure. Both oxygen-dependent and non-oxygen-dependent factors (decrease in sympathetic heart tone and circulatory catecholamines) are involved in bradycardia. Decreased sensitivity of chemoreceptors to CO_2 also causes bradycardia during hyperoxia [9]. The bradycardia occurring is physiologically well tolerated by a normal heart and should not be seen as oxygen toxicity. Even systemic effects lead to an increase in blood pressure due to HBOT and stimulate baroreceptor reflex, causing bradycardia.

The second most important physiological effect studied in HBOT is a decrease in systolic ejection volume and thus effective cardiac output. The clinical significance of such a phenomenon is not reported at the doses used to treat patients in real-life scenarios. This effect can be detrimental, however, in patients with dilated cardiomyopathies and coronary artery disease. A decrease in cardiac output can also be the effect to counterbalance the increase in oxygen content in the blood to maintain peripheral oxygen delivery. It is also the effect of an increase in preload due to the peripheral arterial vasoconstrictive effect and bradycardia related to HBOT. Hyperbaric hyperoxic conditions provide oxygen to areas of myocardium with low oxygen tension, allowing cells to maintain sufficient energy and physiological capability [10].

The effect of HBOT on charges of mean, systolic, and diastolic blood pressure is controversial; few studies have reported a rise in blood pressure related to systolic vasoconstriction [1, 8]. Due to multiple interplays of vasculature, mediators, and anatomical and physiological differences related to organ perfusion and regional circulation, the net effect of vasoconstriction on blood pressure is variable. In a recent report, Heyboer et al. evaluated 155 elective patients, for a total of 3147 HBOT sessions, and showed an increase in ABP after treatment in the range of 4–7 mmHg [11]. In their retrospective longitudinal cohort study, Simone Schiavo et al. examined 3291 elective HBOT sessions. Non-invasive ABP was recorded before and after each session. It was proven that those with pre-existing hypertension had an increase in systolic blood pressure by 16 mmHg post HBOT [12].

Regional blood flow is regulated by the cardiac output and functional/metabolic demand of the organ itself. Cerebral circulation is decreased, corresponding to a decrease in Cardiac output. There is also a secondary increase in cerebral blood flow related to an increase in cerebral PCO_2. The vasodilatory effect of PCO_2 countered the vasoconstricting effect of hyperoxia.

Coronary blood flow is proportionally reduced with decreased cardiac output. Renal flow is also reduced during HBOT. Hepatosplanchnic and muscular circulation are not affected [9].

4.3 Conclusion

Since the advent of Henshaws' Domicilium in 1662 and subsequently the Cunningham's Steel Ball Hospital in 1928, HBOT has been used in widespread diseases both as a primary and as an adjunctive therapy. It was after Borema (Father of Hyperbaric Medicine) in 1956, that its use for heart diseases was explored. HBOT entails full body exposure and breathing of 100% oxygen while inside a hyperbaric chamber pressurized to greater than sea level uses both Henry's and Boyle's law of diffusion. Apart from severe LV dysfunction, no other cardiovascular conditions are a contraindication for its application [13]. Hemodynamic changes discussed are minor and clinically safe for practical application in day-to-day patients. Pre-HBOT check of vital parameters should be a prerequisite for safe sessions. Multiplace chambers would be preferable in such at-risk patients for efficient monitoring of cardiovascular events. Acute use in cardiovascular disease is still a controversial subject due to various reasons [14]. The hemodynamic effects, both on a central and a microcirculatory level, induced by HBOT-induced pressure changes should be taken into consideration in every session.

References

1. Schipke JD, Muth T, Pepper C, Schneppendahl J, Hoffmanns M, Dreyer S. Hyperoxia and the cardiovascular system: experiences with hyperbaric oxygen therapy. Med Gas Res. 2022;12(4):153–7.
2. Brugniaux JV, Coombs GB, Barak OF, Dujic Z, Sekhon MS, Ainslie PN. Highs and lows of hyperoxia: physiological, performance, and clinical aspects. Am J Physiol Regul Integr Comp Physiol. 2018;315(1):R1–R27.

3. Williams DL. Oxidative stress and the eye. Vet Clin North Am Small Anim Pract. 2008;38(1):179–92. vii
4. Gröger M, Oter S, Simkova V, Bolten M, Koch A, Warninghoff V, Georgieff M, Muth CM, Speit G, Radermacher P. DNA damage after long-term repetitive hyperbaric oxygen exposure. J Appl Physiol (1985). 2009;106(1):311–5.
5. Hu X, Cheng S, Yin Y, Ning L, Xiang L, Zhou Y. The role of oxygen therapy in normoxemic acute coronary syndrome: a systematic review of randomized controlled trials. J Cardiovasc Nurs. 2018;33(6):559–67.
6. Goyal A, Chonis T, Bhyan P, Cooper JS. Hyperbaric cardiovascular effects. 2022 Sep 2. In: StatPearls [Internet]. Treasure Island, FL: StatPearls Publishing; 2023.
7. Saltzman HA. Hyperbaric oxygen in cardiovascular disease. Circulation. 1965;XXXI(3):454–62.
8. Kozakiewicz M, Slomko J, Buszko K, Sinkiewicz W, Klawe JJ, Tafil-Klawe M, Newton JL, Zalewski P. Acute biochemical, cardiovascular, and autonomic response to hyperbaric (4 atm) exposure in healthy subjects. Evid Based Complement Alternat Med. 2018;2018:5913176.
9. Mathieu D, Favory R, Collet F, Linke JC, Wattel F. Physiologic effects of hyperbaric oxygen on hemodynamics and microcirculation. In: Mathieu D, editor. Handbook on hyperbaric medicine. Dordrecht: Springer; 2006. p. 75–101.
10. Wunderlich T, Frey N, Kähler W, Lutz M, Radermacher P, Klapa S, Koch I, Tillmans F, Witte J, Koch A. Influence of hyperoxia on diastolic myocardial and arterial endothelial function. Undersea Hyperb Med. 2017;44(6):521–33.
11. Heyboer RM, Wojcik SM, Smith G, Santiago W. Effect of hyperbaric oxygen therapy on blood pressure in patients undergoing treatment. Undersea Hyperb Med. 2017;44(2):93–9.
12. Schiavo S, Djaiani C, DeBacker J, Albertini L, Santa Mina D, Buryk-Iggers S, De Moraes MV, Kanj M, Katznelson R. Magnitude and clinical predictors of blood pressure changes in patients undergoing hyperbaric oxygen therapy: a retrospective study. Int J Environ Res Public Health. 2020;17(20):7586.
13. Ortega MA, Fraile-Martinez O, García-Montero C, Callejón-Peláez E, Sáez MA, Álvarez-Mon MA, García-Honduvilla N, Monserrat J, Álvarez-Mon M, Bujan J, et al. A general overview on the hyperbaric oxygen therapy: applications, mechanisms and translational opportunities. Medicina. 2021;57:864.
14. Ellestad MH. Hyperbaric oxygen: its application in cardiology: a historical perspective and personal journey. Cardiol Rev. 2009;17(6):280–2.

Chapter 5
Hyperbaric Oxygen Therapy in Pregnancy

Safaa Hilal and Paola Perez

5.1 Introduction

Hyperbaric oxygen therapy (HBOT) involves administering oxygen at higher-than-normal atmospheric pressure, typically two to three times greater than at sea level. This increases the amount of oxygen dissolved in the bloodstream, promoting tissue oxygenation and enhancing wound healing [1].

In pregnant women, HBOT is generally contraindicated during the first trimester due to concerns about potential teratogenic effects. Additionally, there is limited data on the safety of HBOT during the later stages of pregnancy. The increased oxygen concentration and pressure could potentially lead to oxidative stress and free radical formation, which may adversely affect fetal development [2].

Furthermore, HBOT can induce vasoconstriction and alter placental blood flow dynamics, potentially compromising fetal oxygenation and nutrient delivery. This can pose risks of intrauterine growth restriction, fetal distress, and even miscarriage or preterm labor [3].

Although there are rare cases where HBOT may be indicated for life-threatening conditions in pregnant women, such as carbon monoxide poisoning or severe decompression illness, it should only be considered after careful risk–benefit analysis and under close medical supervision [4].

Overall, due to the limited safety data and potential risks to fetal development, HBOT is generally avoided during pregnancy unless necessary and performed under

S. Hilal (✉)
Menoufia University Egypt working at the University Hospital of Menoufia University, Shebin El-Koum, Egypt

P. Perez (✉)
Department of Anesthesiology, University of Miami/Jackson Health System, Miami, FL, USA
e-mail: Paola.perez@jhsmiami.org

A. G. D'Almeida, J. Hidalgo (eds.), *Evidence-Based Hyperbaric Medicine*,
https://doi.org/10.1007/978-3-032-06346-5_5

strict medical guidance. Pregnant women should always discuss the risks and benefits with their healthcare provider before undergoing any hyperbaric oxygen treatment [5].

5.2 Physiology of Pregnancy

While HBOT is generally considered a relative contraindication during pregnancy due to potential risks to the fetus, there are specific indications where the benefits may outweigh the risks. Here are some additional details and scientific information about these indications:

1. Carbon Monoxide Poisoning

Carbon monoxide (CO) poisoning poses significant risks to both the pregnant woman and the fetus due to its ability to bind tightly to hemoglobin, displacing oxygen, and, in turn, leading to tissue hypoxia. HBOT is indicated in cases of severe CO poisoning to rapidly eliminate CO from the bloodstream and tissues, thus preventing maternal and fetal hypoxia [6].

2. Gas Gangrene

Gas gangrene is a rare but potentially life-threatening condition caused by certain bacteria, such as *Clostridium perfringens*, which produce gas and toxins in infected tissues. In pregnant women with gas gangrene, HBOT may be indicated to control the infection, prevent tissue necrosis, and avoid maternal and fetal complications [7].

3. Decompression Sickness (DCS)

Although rare during pregnancy, DCS can occur in pregnant women engaged in activities such as scuba diving or working in high-pressure environments. HBOT is indicated in severe cases of DCS to accelerate the elimination of nitrogen bubbles from the bloodstream and tissues, thereby preventing further tissue damage and neurological complications While there is limited specific data on the use of HBOT for DCS in pregnant women, extrapolation from non-pregnant populations suggests that HBOT may be beneficial in selected cases [8].

It is crucial to emphasize that the decision to administer HBOT to a pregnant woman must be made on a case-by-case basis, considering the severity of the condition, potential risks, and available alternatives. Additionally, experienced healthcare providers in facilities equipped to manage obstetric emergencies should only administer HBOT. Close monitoring of both the mother and the fetus is essential during HBOT sessions to minimize potential risks and optimize outcomes [9].

5.3 Safety Considerations

Certainly, here are more specific and scientific details regarding the safety considerations of HBOT during pregnancy:

1. Fetal oxygen toxicity: HBOT involves breathing 100% oxygen at increased pressure, which can lead to oxidative stress and tissue damage, known as oxygen toxicity. This risk is of particular concern during pregnancy due to the potential for harm to the developing fetus [10].
2. Teratogenic effects: There is limited human data on the teratogenic effects of HBOT during pregnancy. However, animal studies have suggested a potential risk of birth defects when pregnant animals are exposed to hyperbaric conditions. These effects may vary depending on the timing and duration of exposure [11].
3. Placental gas embolism: There is a theoretical risk of gas embolism in the placenta or fetal circulation during HBOT, particularly during decompression [12].
4. Timing of exposure: The first trimester is considered the most vulnerable period for fetal development, including organogenesis. Therefore, HBOT is generally contraindicated during this critical period. If HBOT is deemed necessary later in pregnancy, it may be recommended after the completion of organogenesis to minimize potential risks to the fetus [13].
5. Maternal considerations: Pregnant women undergoing HBOT may experience physiological changes, such as increased maternal oxygen tension and decreased uterine blood flow. These changes could potentially impact fetal oxygenation and placental function. Close maternal monitoring is essential to ensure maternal safety and fetal well-being during HBOT sessions [14].

While HBOT may offer therapeutic benefits for certain conditions, its use during pregnancy carries significant potential risks to both the mother and the fetus. Therefore, careful consideration and consultation with obstetric and hyperbaric medicine specialists are essential to ensure the safest possible management for pregnant patients requiring oxygen therapy [15].

The Food and Drug Administration (FDA), confirming efficacy in the treatment of decompression sickness, warns of lack of evidence of efficacy and safety in the treatment of HIV, Alzheimer's disease, asthma, facial paralysis, traumatic brain injury, cerebral palsy, depression, myocardial infarction, hepatitis, migraine, multiple sclerosis, parkinsonism, spinal cord injuries, sports injuries, and stroke [16].

It is also indicated that the use of a hyperbaric chamber can cause mild unpleasant symptoms: sinus pain, ear pressure, and joint pain. Severe consequences are possible in the form of paralysis and air embolism. Many medical institutions use an experimental method of treating COVID-19 using hyperbaric oxygenation.

According to scientists from Tel Aviv University, HBOT increases the length of telomeres and reduces the immune aging of isolated blood cells. They found that, in elderly people, when pure oxygen is received in a hyperbaric pressure chamber, the length of telomeres increases by 20%, which, in their opinion, can be used as a way to combat aging [17, 18].

This assumption does not stand up to criticism, since the data can be interpreted in another way: "... as a protective reaction to powerful oxidative (oxygen) stress, the body ejected relatively young lymphocytes from the bone marrow depot" due to the activation of hematopoiesis active precursor cells. They have longer telomeres because they divide less. When blood is analyzed, a misleading impression is created that telomeres have lengthened. In fact, there was a massive death of old cells and the release of previously unused "sleeping cells" into the blood in response to stress [19].

The dynamics of the parameters of the pituitary-ovarian system and the thyroid status were studied before and after the treatment with hyperbaric oxygenation. The examined women with insufficiency of the luteal phase of the menstrual cycle and hypofunction of the thyroid gland were divided into two groups. The initial (before treatment) state of the thyroid gland was regarded as euthyroid in 20 and as hypothyroid in 21. When prescribing hyperbaric oxygenation, thyroid hormone replacement therapy was not carried out, which made it possible to judge the therapeutic effect of hyperbaric oxygenation and the effect of hyperbaric oxygen on the secretion and excretion of sex and thyroid hormones, gonadotropins [20, 21].

Interestingly, one promising alternative therapy in infertility from a female's perspective is oxygen therapy. Findings from various studies suggest that increased oxygen supply to reproductive tissues can positively impact conception chances.

The endometrium's quality, the mucous membrane lining of the uterus, plays a crucial role in conception and embryo implantation [22].

Interestingly, while HBOT was not initially designed specifically for fertility issues, its application has shown impressive results in enhancing fertility from a male's perspective as well. Empirical studies reveal that after undergoing 2 months of HBOT, there was a significant improvement in sperm motility and spermatogenesis, the sperm formation process. This suggests HBOT's potential in improving sperm quality, contributing to increased fertilization chances [23].

Fertility in both men and women can be influenced by various factors, including genetics, hormonal, environment, and lifestyle. However, field experiences indicate that HBOT can contribute positively to addressing infertility issues. By enhancing oxygen supply to reproductive tissues, tissue repair and regeneration processes can be optimized, increasing the chances of a successful pregnancy for couples trying to have children. To strengthen this argument, it is crucial for researchers to conduct more in-depth and comprehensive studies on HBOT's benefits in the fertility context, providing stronger empirical evidence and uncovering other potential benefits of this therapy [24–26].

Purpura fulminans (PF) is a rare and fatal complication of septic shock or diffuse intravascular coagulation, resulting in skin and soft tissue necrosis. PF can be caused by congenital or acquired protein C or protein S deficiency. The most common cause of PF in a neonate is sepsis. In a case report, involving an extremely low birth weight preterm infant, PF initially manifested as necrotic lesions on the right-hand fingers. After close examination was made, protein S deficiency was detected, as well as MTHFR (A1298C) and Factor V Leiden (R506Q) homozygous mutations. While being unresponsive to fresh frozen plasma and unfractionated heparin therapy, the standard treatment in such cases. Notably, the introduction of HBOT led to clinical improvement, representing, to our knowledge, one of the first, if not the first reported use of HBOT for PF in an extremely low birth weight preterm infant. This case highlights HBOT's potential adjunctive role in refractory neonatal PF, although its mechanisms and safety profile in this population warrant further investigation [27].

In conclusion, the utilization of HBOT in pregnancy and peripregnancy presents both promising benefits and critical safety considerations. While HBOT shows potential for addressing various maternal health concerns, including in cases of severe CO poisoning, and certain conditions like gas gangrene, its use must be judiciously weighed against potential fetal risks. While HBOT has been shown in some studies to increase telomere length and potentially enhance cellular function, these findings remain controversial and may reflect stress-induced shifts in circulating cells rather than true rejuvenation. Interestingly, emerging evidence suggests that HBOT may improve fertility outcomes in both males and females by enhancing oxygenation, reducing inflammation, and supporting gamete quality thereby indirectly increasing the likelihood of conception. However, these theoretical benefits must be balanced against the potential risks of oxidative stress to maternal and fetal tissues, which are particularly vulnerable during gestation. Reports such as the successful use of HBOT in a neonate with purpura fulminans underscore the therapy's potential as a life-saving intervention in select, refractory cases. As research continues to evolve in this field, clinicians must remain vigilant in assessing both the benefits and potential hazards of HBOT in order to ensure optimized safety for both mother and fetus.

References

1. Price VE, Ledingham DL, Krumpel A, Chan AK. Diagnosis and management of neonatal purpura fulminans. Semin Fetal Neonatal Med. 2011;16(6):318–22.
2. Findley T, Patel M, Chapman J, Brown D, Duncan AF. Acquired versus congenital neonatal purpura fulminans: a case report and literature review. J Pediatr Hematol Oncol. 2018;40(8):625–7.
3. Zenciroglu A, Ipek MS, Aydin M, Kara A, Okumus N, Kilic M. Purpura fulminans in a newborn infant with galactosemia. Eur J Pediatr. 2010;169(7):903–6.
4. Rosenthal E, Benderly A, Monies-Chass I, Fishman J, Levy J, Bialik V. Hyperbaric oxygenation in peripheral ischaemic lesions in infants. Arch Dis Child. 1985;60(4):372–4.
5. Wiebers J, Purdy I, Lieber M, Milisavljevic V. Hyperbaric oxygen in treatment of neonatal arterial thromboembolism of lower extremities. J Perinatol. 2006;26(12):777–9.
6. Millar DS, Allgrove J, Rodeck C, Kakkar VV, Cooper DN. A homozygous deletion/insertion mutation in the protein C (PROC) gene causing neonatal purpura fulminans: prenatal diagnosis in an at-risk pregnancy. Blood Coagul Fibrinolysis. 1994;5(4):647–9.
7. Barnes C, Newall F, Higgins S, Carden S, Monagle P. Perinatal management of patients at high risk of homozygous protein C deficiency. Thromb Haemost. 2002;88(2):370–1.

8. Zenciroglu A, Karagol BS, Ipek MS, Okumus N, Yarali N, Aydin M. Neonatal purpura fulminans secondary to group B streptococcal infection. Pediatr Hematol Oncol. 2010;27(8):620–5.
9. Nicolas L, Philip J, Larson S, Islam S, Lew JF, Glavin FL, et al. Severe neonatal purpura fulminans caused by staphy-lococcus aureus. Clin Pediatr (Phila). 2017;56(8):776–80.
10. Yusupaliev UA, Mukhamedov BI, Ibragimovan NS, Pyagai GB, Solmetova MN. Dermatology: not everything is as simple as it seems. Difficulties in diagnosis. Conference zone; 2023. p. 337–44. Retrieved from http://conferencezone.org/index.php/cz/article/view/978
11. Borisovich PG, Ibragimova NS. criteria for selecting therapy for patients with actinic keratosis. Conference zone; 2023. p. 156–61. Retrieved from http://conferencezone.org/index.php/cz/article/view/949
12. Borisovich PG, Ibragimova NS. The effectiveness of conservative methods of treatment of actinic keratosis. Conference zone; 2023. p. 150–5. Retrieved from http://conferencezone.org/index.php/cz/article/view/948
13. Pyagay GB, Yuldashev KA. Comparative analysis of the therapeutic efficacy of various methods of treatment of syphilis patients suffering from drug addiction News of dermatovenereology and reproductive health; 2005, No. 3–4, pp. 118–122.
14. Lapasov OA, Latipov II. Basal cell skin cancer. Historical aspects, current achievements and problems at the present stage. Cent Asian J Med Nat Sci. 2022;3(5):381–91. Retrieved from https://cajmns.centralasianstudies.org/index.php/CAJMNS/article/view/1109
15. Lapasov OA, Zaslavsky DV, Sidikov AA, Pyagay GB, Kozlova DV, Gunchenko IV. Basal cell skin cancer. Historical aspects, current achievements and problems at the present stage. Dermatovenereol Cosmetol. 2022;8(1):27–42. https://www.elibrary.ru/item.asp?id=48197950
16. Aleida G, Huppelschoten A, Noortje T, Peter FJ, van Bommel PFJ, Kremer J, Nelen W. Do infertile women and their partners have equal experiences with fertility care? Fertil Steril. 2013;99(3):832.
17. American Society for Reproductive Medicine. Hyperbaric oxygen and ovarian follicular stimulation for in vitro fertilization: a pilot study. Fertil Steril. 2005;83:226–8.
18. ASRM. Definitions of infertility and recurrent pregnancy loss: a committee opinion. Fertil Steril. 2013;99(1):63.
19. ASRM. Endometriosis and infertility: a committee opinion. Fertil Steril. 2012;98:591–8.
20. Balen A, Jacobs H. Infertility in practice. Elsevier Science; 2003.
21. European Association of Urology (EAU). Guidelines on male infertility. EAU; 2010.
22. Feng J, Wang J, Zhang Y, Jia L, Zhang D, Zhang J, Han Y, Luo S. The efficacy of complementary and alternative medicine in the treatment of female infertility. Evid Based Complement Alternat Med. 2021;2021:6634309.
23. Harch PG, Andrews SR, Fogarty EF, Lucarini J, Van Meter KW. A phase I study of low-pressure hyperbaric oxygen therapy for blast-induced post-concussion syndrome and post-traumatic stress disorder. J Neurotrauma. 2019;29(S1):S-17–32.
24. Hiferi P, Perfitri I, Iaui P, Pogi. Konsensus penanganan infertilitas; 2013.
25. Jain KK. Textbook of hyperbaric medicine. 6th ed. Springer; 2017.
26. Kahyaoglu S. Does diagnostic laparoscopy have value in unexplained infertile couples? A review of the current literature. J Minim Invasive Surg Sci. 2012;4:124–8.
27. Yılmaza, Kayaa N, Meriçb R, Bayramlib Z, Örŏglud B, Celkanc TT, Vurala M, Perka Y. Department of Neonatology, Cerrahpasa Medical Faculty, Istanbul University, Istanbul, Turkey Department of Pediatrics, Cerrahpasa Medical Faculty, Istanbul University, Istanbul, Turkey Department of Pediatric Hematology and Oncology, Cerrahpasa Medical Faculty, Istanbul University, Istanbul, Turkey Istanbul Faculty of Medicine, Underwater and Hyperbaric Medicine Department, Istanbul University, Istanbul, Turkey.

Chapter 6
Safety in Hyperbaric Medicine

Paola Perez

6.1 Introduction to Hyperbaric Medicine

Hyperbaric medicine involves the therapeutic use of hyperbaric oxygen therapy (HBOT), where patients inhale 100% oxygen at elevated atmospheric pressures, typically ranging from around 1.5 atmospheres absolute (ATA) to as high as 3 ATA, within a hyperbaric chamber [1]. This medical treatment has many applications across various medical specialties, ranging from wound healing to treating carbon monoxide poisoning and decompression sickness.

To better understand the physiological basis of HBOT, HBOT exploits the principles of gas solubility and Boyle's law. That is, under increased atmospheric pressure, oxygen dissolves more readily in fluids, which include bodily fluids such as plasma, cerebrospinal fluid, and tissues. In turn, this greater oxygen solubility enhances tissue oxygenation, particularly in ischemic or hypoxic areas, leading to accelerated healing processes.

6.2 Applications of HBOT

HBOT is widely used in the management of chronic non-healing wounds, such as diabetic foot ulcers, radiation-induced tissue injuries, and refractory osteomyelitis [2]. The improved oxygenation promotes angiogenesis, collagen synthesis, and antimicrobial activity, fostering wound repair mechanisms [3]. Additionally, HBOT serves a purpose when treating carbon monoxide poisoning, by displacing

P. Perez (✉)
Department of Anesthesiology, University of Miami/Jackson Health System,
Miami, FL, USA
e-mail: Paola.perez@jhsmiami.org

A. G. D'Almeida, J. Hidalgo (eds.), *Evidence-Based Hyperbaric Medicine*,
https://doi.org/10.1007/978-3-032-06346-5_6

carboxyhemoglobin and facilitating its elimination [4]. Early initiation of HBOT in carbon monoxide poisoning cases mitigates the risk of delayed neurological sequelae and reduces morbidity and mortality associated with severe poisoning [5]. Furthermore, individuals exposed to rapid decreases in ambient pressure such as divers during an ascent may develop a phenomenon called decompression sickness. This condition is characterized by the formation of inert gas bubbles, typically nitrogen, within tissues and the circulatory system, resulting in a spectrum of symptoms ranging from joint pain to strokes, contingent upon the displacement of these gas bubbles [6]. Similarly, in such cases, HBOT can facilitate bubble dissolution and promote tissue reperfusion, alleviating symptoms and preventing further complications [7]. These examples represent only a proportion of the diverse applications of hyperbaric oxygen treatment; many others exist beyond those listed.

6.3 Safety in Hyperbaric Medicine

When administered correctly, hyperbaric therapy ranks among the safest medical treatments available today. Nevertheless, ensuring patient safety is paramount during hyperbaric interventions, given its broad application usage across different specialties. This chapter addresses fundamental structural safety concerns, such as fire risk, the integrity of the hyperbaric unit, and gas handling practices. Additionally, it delves into patient-related considerations and preemptive measures for adverse events, including patient selection and anticipation of potential complications.

Fire safety is one of the most critical areas of concerns, with historical incidents highlighting the dangers. Fires in hyperbaric chambers have resulted in numerous fatalities worldwide, often ignited by prohibited items carried inside the chambers [8]. These items, ranging from certain types of clothing to electronics such as phones and even children's toys, have been identified as significant hazards [8]. Rigorous control of potential ignition sources with adherence to safety guidelines can prevent fire incidents from occurring. It is imperative to thoroughly review the list of prohibited items with patients prior to commencing treatments, and the placement of a prominently displayed flyer listing these items nearby can help ensure that inadvertent breaches are avoided. Additionally, the presence of firefighting equipment is essential to mitigate fire risks. Engaging local firefighters to conduct routine inspections, assessing for fire hazards, ensuring compliance with fire codes and regulations, and evaluating emergency preparedness measures can greatly enhance overall preparedness. All in all, the prohibition of flammable materials inside the chamber and regular equipment inspections are imperative to mitigate the risk of fire-related incidents.

Building upon this, the hazards in the hyperbaric unit are associated with its operating system and usage, including components such as pipes, bolts, compressor chambers, and gas storage. It is crucial that the hyperbaric chambers that are used clinically adhere to standards like those set by the American Society of Mechanical Engineers or their international equivalents [9]. Adherence to these standards ensures safety. It is equally important that any modifications to chambers are carried out by qualified personnel according to these standards. Instances have occurred where the use of incorrect bolts or materials violations that were used led to explosions, causing injuries or fatalities among patients and staff [9]. Therefore, hospitals should ensure that equipment is sourced from reputable sources, constructed with appropriate materials, and maintained to high standards to safeguard the well-being of patients and staff alike.

Regarding safe gas handling, incidents involving the wrong gas being administered to patients have had tragic consequences. Examples include fatal mix-ups in hospitals and nursing homes due to incorrect labeling or mishandling of gas cylinders [10]. Several instances exemplify the grave consequences of administering incorrect gases to patients in health care settings. To name one, there was an incident at a hospital, where two patients tragically lost their lives when an industrial-grade nitrogen cylinder was mistakenly connected to the oxygen system [10]. This incident highlights the critical importance of implementing thorough systems checks and protocols. For instance, rigorous labeling checks can significantly reduce the risk of administering incorrect gases to patients in healthcare facilities, thereby preventing potentially fatal errors. Gas analysis mechanisms play a crucial role in ensuring the delivery of the correct type and purity of gas by the manufacturer. Moreover, strict adherence to storage and inspection protocols is vital to prevent issues such as temperature fluctuations, rendering gas unusable or expired gas from being utilized. Additionally, securing cylinders effectively can mitigate the risk of injuries, as dropping a cylinder can pose serious dangers due to the potential for ricocheting. These measures represent essential preventive strategies that can safeguard both patients and healthcare professionals.

Shifting the focus to patient selection, patient selection plays a pivotal role in ensuring the safety and efficacy of HBOT. Comprehensive screening protocols should be implemented to identify individuals who may be at increased risk of adverse events. The one absolute contraindication to HBOT is untreated pneumothorax, as it can progress to a tension pneumothorax under such changes in pressures [11]. Other relative contraindications to HBOT, including seizure disorders, and certain chemotherapy regimens, such as doxorubicin and bleomycin, must be carefully evaluated [11]. Additionally, comprehensive evaluation of medical history and thorough physical examination are imperative to uncover underlying conditions that could predispose patients to complications during hyperbaric interventions. For instance, conditions like asthma, which carry a risk of pulmonary barotrauma, or a history of eye surgery, which may lead to air trapping and poten tial eye damage, should be identified and considered prior to treatment [11].

Considering the therapy's potential for adverse effects and possible sequelae, it is associated with a multitude of side effects, including barotrauma, oxygen toxicity, and claustrophobia. Barotrauma, resulting from pressure differentials between body cavities and the environment, poses a significant risk during hyperbaric exposures. The most common adverse events are barotrauma specifically to the middle ear and sinuses, presenting as otalgia or discomfort, which can affect up to 33% of patients and is a leading cause of therapy discontinuation [12]. Decompression safety is vital, requiring thorough training for all hyperbaric staff. To prevent decompression sickness, patients and, in certain cases, any accompanying staff attendants must undergo a controlled decompression process. This typically involves gradually releasing pressure from the chamber over a specified period, allowing the gases in the body to safely exit without forming bubbles. The duration and rate of decompression depend on various factors, including the treatment protocol, the pressure reached during the therapy session, and individual patient factors. Thus, it is important to plan for the right approach prior to the initiation of treatment to allow for a seamless session. Inadequate decompression procedures have led to severe injuries and fatalities in past incidents. For example, there was a case where a patient's hyperbaric treatment had to be modified and extended due to an error that was noted during the session, and when the time came for the decompression protocol, the nurse and patient decompressed, but not for a sufficient time, forgetting to consider the added time that was in the chamber [13]. Staff must be well-versed in decompression protocols to ensure patient and staff safety during treatments. Moreover, alternative approaches exist to reduce the likelihood of additional barotrauma occurrences. For instance, implementing effective equalization methods, such as employing Valsalva maneuvers, has been cited in the literature as a potential means to diminish the risk of barotrauma affecting organs historically susceptible to such damage, including the ears, sinuses, and lungs [13]. Therefore, careful patient selection, education, and prophylactic measures (e.g. pressure equalization techniques) are essential to minimize these adverse events.

Moreover, prolonged exposure to high partial pressures of oxygen can lead to oxygen toxicity, manifesting as pulmonary and central nervous system complications. This damage primarily occurs due to the production of reactive oxygen species , which are highly reactive molecules that cause oxidative stress, leading to cellular damage and inflammation. Monitoring of oxygen partial pressures within the chamber and adhering to recommended treatment protocols, such as air brakes and oxygen dose adjustments, are essential to minimize the risk of oxygen toxicity. Furthermore, claustrophobia affects approximately 2% of the general population, potentially leading to confinement anxiety within the hyperbaric chamber. Mild sedation can be advantageous for these patients to facilitate the continuation of hyperbaric oxygen treatment, with certain studies suggesting the efficacy of benzodiazepines such as midazolam [14]. Ancillary staff should be trained to deal with basic psychotherapeutic techniques associated with improving anxiety as well.

6.4 Emergency Preparedness

Despite stringent safety measures, unforeseen emergencies may arise during hyperbaric treatments, necessitating prompt intervention to ensure patient and personnel safety. Thus, emergency preparedness plans should be in place. These plans should be documented, prominently displayed in familiar areas, and routinely practiced by all staff members. Such measures are essential for ensuring smooth coordination and cooperation during emergencies. Additionally, trained medical personnel should be readily available to respond to medical emergencies within the hyperbaric facility. Advanced life support equipment and medications must be accessible to manage acute complications, such as those more common in the general population like seizures, and cardiac events, and or those more specific to the chamber like barotrauma. In cases of external emergencies, such as fires or structural damage, evacuation procedures specific to hyperbaric facilities should be established to ensure the safety of patients and staff.

6.5 Conclusion

In hyperbaric medicine, prioritizing safety is crucial to reduce the likelihood of negative incidents and optimize patient results. The chamber operator must possess a thorough understanding of potential accidents, methods to anticipate and avert these risks, and updated expertise to guarantee that the chamber and its equipment are operated safely and effectively. By implementing rigorous patient screening protocols, adhering to chamber safety precautions, and maintaining comprehensive emergency preparedness plans, clinicians can ensure the safe and effective delivery of hyperbaric interventions in clinical practice.

References

1. Moon RE, Camporesi EM. Clinical hyperbaric oxygen therapy: indications and results. Undersea Hyperb Med. 2014;41(2):69–78.
2. Mago V. Safety of hyperbaric medicine in clinical scenarios. Ann Afr Med. 2024;23(1):1–4. https://doi.org/10.4103/aam.aam_16_22.
3. Eggleton P, Bishop A, Smerdon G. Safety and efficacy of hyperbaric oxygen therapy in chronic wound management: current evidence. Chronic Wound Care Manage Res. 2015;2:81–93.
4. Rose JJ, Wang L, Xu Q, McTiernan CF, Shiva S, Tejero J, Gladwin MT. Carbon monoxide poisoning: pathogenesis, management, and future directions of therapy. Am J Respir Crit Care Med. 2017;195(5):596–606. https://doi.org/10.1164/rccm.201606-1275CI. Erratum in: Am J Respir Crit Care Med. 2017;196 (3):398–9
5. Ning K, Zhou YY, Zhang N, Sun XJ, Liu WW, Han CH. Neurocognitive sequelae after carbon monoxide poisoning and hyperbaric oxygen therapy. Med Gas Res. 2020;10(1):30–6. https://doi.org/10.4103/2045-9912.279981.
6. Vann RD, Butler FK, Mitchell SJ, Moon RE. Decompression illness. Lancet. 2011;377(9760):153–64. https://doi.org/10.1016/S0140-6736(10)61085-9.
7. Moon RE. Hyperbaric oxygen treatment for decompression sickness. Undersea Hyperb Med. 2014;41(2):151–7.
8. Sheffield PJ. Hyperbaric chamber fires: to what extent is the problem? In: Workman WT, editor. Hyperbaric facility safety: a practical guide. Flagstaff, AZ: Best Publishing; 1999. p. 487–94.
9. ASME PVHO Subcommittee on Medical Hyperbaric Systems. STP-PT-047 Principles of safety and performance for medical hyperbaric chambers: guidelines for regulatory submission. New York: ASME Standards Technology, LLC; 2011.
10. Pougnet R, Henckes A, Pougnet L, Cochard G, Dantec F, Dewitte JD, Loddé B. Occupational accidents among attendants inside hyperbaric chambers in France. Med Lav. 2015;106(1):17–22.

11. Gawdi R, Cooper JS. Hyperbaric contraindications. [Updated 2023 Apr 8]. In: StatPearls [Internet]. Treasure Island, FL: StatPearls Publishing; 2024.
12. Sheffield PJ, Sheffield RB. Safety first: in the hyperbaric environment; 2028. Hmpgloballearningnetwork.com. https://www.hmpgloballearningnetwork.com/site/twc/articles/safety-first-hyperbaric-environment.
13. Hyperbaric chamber nurse dies of decompression sickness; unit gets OK. Hosp Secur Saf Manage. 1992;13(5):3.
14. Lemaitre MD, et al. Sedation in hyperbaric oxygen therapy: a prospective randomized double-blind placebo-controlled trial. Undersea Hyperb Med. 2014;41(2):105–12.

Chapter 7
Evidence-Based Hyperbaric Medicine: Concepts and Clinical Application

Waruni Samaranayake and Anushka Mudalige

7.1 Introduction

Hyperbaric oxygen therapy (HBOT) is a therapeutic approach based on exposing patient to a pure concentrations of oxygen (O_2) in an augmented atmospheric pressure, which is provided in a hyperbaric chamber. The first ever literature on the use of hyperbaric medical therapy was in 1662 by Henshaw, a British physician. Since then, the popularity of HBOT has not grown much owing to the observation of possible O_2-derived adverse effects at 100% concentrations by Lavoisier and Seguin in 1789. In 1872, Paul Bert, who is considered the "Father of the hyperbaric physiology," described the physiological basis of pressurized air in humans and defined the neurotoxic effects of O_2 in the human body, which was subsequently named the Paul Bert effect [1]. Later, Lorrain Smith came up highlighting the pulmonary toxicity of O_2 [2]. Growing interest in the use of HBOT was observed when HBOT was used in the treatment of divers who suffered decompression sickness during World War II [3]. Since then, an increasing number of studies on this area were carried out, and at the beginning of the twenty-first century, a considerable number of units providing HBOT were established [4].

Currently, there are well-recognized and approved indications for HBOT, primarily in the areas requiring (a) wound healing acceleration and angiogenesis enhancement and (b) antimicrobial effects, in addition to its use in certain medical emergencies and illnesses [5]. In this chapter, we intend to highlight the concepts of

W. Samaranayake (✉)
Coronary Care Unit, Institute of Cardiology, National Hospital of Sri Lanka, Colombo, Sri Lanka
e-mail: warunis@gmail.com

A. Mudalige
Medical Intensive Care Unit, Colombo North Teaching Hospital, Ragama, Sri Lanka
e-mail: anushdilani@gmail.com

A. G. D'Almeida, J. Hidalgo (eds.), *Evidence-Based Hyperbaric Medicine*,
https://doi.org/10.1007/978-3-032-06346-5_7

HBOT and relevant clinical applications and potential implications for different approaches with the available evidence.

7.2 Role of Oxygen in Physiology and as a Therapeutic Agent in HBOT

Oxygen is the key to performing cellular aerobic respiration in mitochondria, leading to ATP synthesis, as it is the final electron acceptor in oxidative phosphorylation. Once oxygen is diffused to the bloodstream from the alveoli, O_2 is mostly bound to hemoglobin (Hb) in the erythrocytes, and to a lesser extent in the dissolved form, to be systemically distributed to tissues. At the tissue level, oxygen exchange takes place between the microcirculatory vessels and the rest of the tissues, owing to the different partial pressure of O_2 and the Hb oxygen saturation (SO_2) [6].

Inadequate O_2 at the tissue level (hypoxia) induces a cellular pathological stress, which induces the onset and progression of a spectrum of diseases [7]. Accordingly, O_2 is considered a therapeutic agent for patients undergoing different acute or chronic conditions [8, 9].

At present, clinical management of hypoxia is geared mainly by modulating the global hypoxemia. Oxygen delivery within the tissues targeting cellular hypoxia of specific tissues is still being studied [10]. Therefore, HBOT plays a pivotal role in managing certain conditions related to hypoxia by creating hyperoxemia and hyperoxia [11].

7.3 Principles of Hyperbaric Medicine

HBOT comprises the supply of pure oxygen under augmented pressure, and this facility could be provided in a monoplace (only for one patient) or multiplace (for several patients) chamber. Depending on the protocol, the estimated duration of a session varies from 1.5 to 2 hours and may be performed from one to three times daily up to a number of 20–60 therapeutic doses depending on the condition [12].

Usually, the utilized augmented pressure is between 2 and 3 atm. Occasionally, therapy has been successful with pressures of 1.5 atm in certain studies. As per UHMS, a chamber pressurized to a minimum of 2 atm is required for the currently recommended indications [13]. It seems that little benefit is obtained when more than 3 atm is used, except for the treatment of gas embolism [14]. In conditions where higher pressures of more than 2.8 atm are needed, which makes it difficult to breathe pure O_2, other gases such as helium, nitrogen, or ozone are being used.

The therapeutic basis of hyperbaric oxygenation stems from the following key factors:

1. Breathing 100% O_2 generates an increased positive pressure gradient, which facilitates diffusion of O_2 to hypoxic tissues from hyperoxemia.
2. Augmented pressures with 100% O_2 increase the dissolved O_2 concentration in the blood, raising the PaO_2 to levels (according to Henry's law) sufficient enough to oxygenate tissues.

Therefore, HBOT facilitates tissue oxygenation independent of the contribution from the Hb, enabling correction of hypoxia and treatment of wound healing, necrosis, or reperfusion injuries [15, 16].

3. Hyperoxemia facilitates the reduction in the size of gas/air bubbles in the blood as per Boyle-Mariotte law and Henry's law [3].

7.4 Therapeutic Indications for HBOT

The last European Consensus Conference on Hyperbaric Medicine held in 2016 emphasized the use of HBOT as a primary treatment method for certain conditions such as carbon monoxide (CO) poisoning) with a moderate to high degree of evidence and as a potential adjuvant to consider in conditions like diabetic foot with moderate evidence [17].

Currently approved indications for HBOT

- Air or gas embolism.

Acute thermal burn injury.
Carbon monoxide poisoning.
Carbon monoxide poisoning complicated by cyanide poisoning.
Central retinal artery occlusion.
Clostridial myositis and myonecrosis (gas gangrene).
Compromised grafts and flaps.
Crush injury, compartment syndrome, and other acute traumatic ischemia.
Decompression sickness.
Delayed radiation injury (soft tissue and bony necrosis).
Enhancement of healing in selected problem wounds.
Idiopathic sudden sensorineural hearing loss.
Intracranial abscess (ICA).
Necrotizing soft tissue infections.
Refractory osteomyelitis.
Severe anemia.

7.5 HBOT for Wound Healing Via Angiogenesis Enhancement

Exposure to 100% oxygen accelerates wound healing, as the regeneration of tissues needs oxygen. Therefore, HBOT has shown its use extensively in different types of wound management including microbial-infected wounds (e.g., Clostridial myonecrosis and Fournier's gangrene), traumatic wounds, thermal burns, skin grafts, radiation-induced wounds, and diabetic and vascular insufficiency ulcers [18]. HBOT has a major role in treating "Diabetic foot ulcers," as it has shown prominent angiogenesis while reducing inflammation helping to increase wound healing rate with lower occurrence of anaerobic infections and amputation rates evident by trials showing significant changes in inflammatory and tissue repairing parameters [19–22]. Therefore, adjuvant use of systemic HBOT in the wound healing of diabetic foot ulcers is well established [23, 24]. Even studies have demonstrated that the use of HBOT may be associated with improved six-year survival in patients with diabetic foot [25]. It is still necessary to define which group of patients may benefit most and are suitable for HBOT.

HBOT causes increased levels of vascular endothelial growth factor and interleukin-6, and lower levels of endothelin-1, which leads to activation of host wound resolution factors, angiogenesis, and vascular tone [26]. Vasculogenesis is promoted by the upregulation of nitric oxide with HBOT and is associated with a reduction in wound area [27].

The enhancing angiogenesis and wound healing by HBOT has been an adequate adjuvant treatment in a wide variety of conditions. Osteoradionecrosis after radiotherapy in oncological practice has been treated successfully with HBOT [28]. Radiation-induced hemorrhagic cystitis and proctitis are other conditions where HBOT is being investigated [29].

7.6 HBOT and the Antimicrobial Activity

Antimicrobial effects of HBOT are particularly useful in wound healing, as microbial infections are the most important cause of non-healing wounds [30]. HBOT is considered a non-conventional approach for non-healing wounds consisting in a modification of biophysical parameters in the wound microenvironment, breaking the bacterial biofilms [31].

HBOT upregulates hypoxia-inducible factors that induce the expression of nitric oxide synthases and virus-killing peptides (defensins and cathelicidins such as cathelin-related antimicrobial peptide) with consequent neutrophil and monocyte phagocytosis of the microbes [32–34].

The most significant use of the antimicrobial activity of HBOT is for necrotizing soft tissue infections , which comprises necrotizing fasciitis, Fournier's gangrene, and gas gangrene, which can lead to deterioration of patients to a critical level. An early and combined HBOT therapy may be crucial as a lifesaving and cost-effective therapy, particularly in the most critical patients [35]. HBOT is useful in anaerobic infections, as anaerobic bacteria are killed by a much higher amount of pressurized O_2 [36, 37].

For instance, the use of HBOT in the anaerobic *Clostridium perfringens* bacteria is especially recommended [38]. This bacterium produces several recognized toxins out of which alpha and theta are the main mediators. *Clostridium perfringens* growth is restricted at O_2 tensions up to 70 mmHg, and alpha-toxin production is halted at tensions of 250 mmHg, also achieving bacteriostasis and other antimicrobial effects. The anti-inflammatory potential of HBOT also aids in lessening tissue damage and infection expansion [39], also explained by a decrease in neutrophil activation, eviting rolling and accumulation of white blood cells, hence limiting the production of ROS by neutrophils and avoiding reperfusion injury [18]. Moreover, this is observed in in vitro studies, having been demonstrated the biofilm shrinkage ability with the significant decreases in cellular load of anaerobic bacteria and fungi after HBOT [37].

HBOT provides a therapeutic option in the management of ICA. Due to the high morbidity and mortality, along with the urgency of a non-invasive and effective method, HBOT has been proposed as a well-accepted adjunctive therapy for ICA, being regarded as a safe and tolerated method [40]. The main mechanisms by which HBOT represents an additional tool in the management of ICA reside in the impairment of the acidotic and hypoxic environment in ICAs due to the proper infection and the use of antibiotics [41].

Similarly, osteomyelitis is a chronic infection in the bone marrow frequently caused by bacteria or mycobacteria, which is a difficult condition to treat, as many antimicrobials do not penetrate bone properly. When osteomyelitis does not respond to the treatment or recurs after receiving the therapy, HBOT is a potential indication as it provides synergistic antibiotic activity while enhancing angiogenesis, leukocyte oxidative killing, and osteogenesis process [42, 43]. HBOT has also been proposed as a medical emergency treatment for mucormycosis, which is a fungal infection [44].

7.7 HBOT in Medical Emergencies

HBOT is an urgent indication in certain acute medical emergencies such as decompression sickness, air or gas embolism, acute arterial insufficiencies such as central retinal arterial occlusion (CRAO), crush injury, compartment syndrome, and acute traumatic ischemia, carbon monoxide/cyanide poisoning, and certain infections. In these conditions, there is a rapid and effective response of the tissues for HBOT, which could otherwise be life-threatening [44, 45]. Potential uses of HBOT in a wide range of urgent conditions at least might be considered as an important tool in medical emergencies.

Decompression illness (DCI) is a condition occurring due to the formation of bubbles from dissolved gas caused by a reduction in ambient pressure. This can be seen among aviators, divers, astronauts, compressed air workers, and sometimes iatrogenically. These bubbles cause mechanical disruption of tissues, blood flow occlusion, endothelial dysfunction, platelet activation, and capillary leakage [46]. Clinical manifestations range from mild as generalized fatigue to serious such as pulmonary edema, shock, and death [47]. HBOT, which is an adjuvant therapy in DCI , provides the opposite effects of the pathological mechanisms of DCIs, therefore exerting its therapeutic efficacy [48].

Apart from DCI, the occurrence of bubble formation in large arteries by air embolism during surgical interventions could be life-threatening. This is observed during lung biopsy, arterial catheterization, cardiopulmonary bypass, and neurosurgeries [49].

CRAO is an ophthalmological complication caused by a permanent occlusion of the central retinal artery, mostly due to an embolus, leading to sudden loss of vision in the affected eye [22]. Prognosis is poor, and HBOT is a robust indication for patients with CRAO, and many studies have shown promising results [50].

Crush injury, varying from mild contusions to life-threatening damage, can be effectively treated with HBOT, which treats hypoxia and promotes revascularization. [51]

Carbon monoxide (CO) poisoning results from inhalation of this gas and can be lethal and cause long-term problems, particularly cognitive and brain deficits. To address these problems, HBOT has been applied [52], which reduces neurological sequelae [53] and cognitive sequelae [54]. In general, normobaric oxygen is immediately used after CO poisoning until HBOT is available [55]. Indications for HBOT during poisoning are loss of consciousness, ischemic cardiac changes, neurological deficits, significant metabolic acidosis, or COHb greater than 25% [56]. In cyanide toxicity, HBOT, in combination with hydroxycobalamin, ameliorates mitochondrial oxidative phosphorylation [57, 58].

Severe anemias and idiopathic sudden sensorineural hearing are also indications for HBOT [44]. The reduction in oxygen delivery in anemia can be overcome by HBOT [59]. This could be especially important in patients who cannot be transfused for religion, immunologic reasons, or blood availability problems. In idiopathic sudden sensorineural hearing loss or acute acoustic trauma, HBOT, in addition to standard medical therapy, aids in recovery [60, 61].

There is evidence to say that HBOT can significantly improve symptoms and quality of life of patients affected by femoral head necrosis (ECHM recommendation type II level of evidence B) [62].

7.8 Potential and Translational Applications of HBOT

Advances in research have demonstrated the potential for HBOT to modulate systemic inflammatory responses in many clinical conditions [63–72].

7.8.1 *COVID-19*

This property of HBOT is the main reason for its recent use in severe COVID-19 illness and during recovery after SARS-CoV-2 infection. Clinical trials have demonstrated the potential of HBOT to overcome hypoxia by redirecting oxygen in the body. In addition, COVID-19 has been mainly an inflammation-driven process. HBOT has repeatedly shown the modulation of this inflammation, resulting in early recovery. The inflammatory cytokines in the serum of patients treated with HBOT have been low compared to patients who were not treated with HBOT. Cases of silent hypoxia, which are early and milder forms of COVID-19 [73], can result in fatal outcomes due to the hypoxia itself [74]. For efficient treatment to prevent fast hypoxia, mechanical ventilation, or even fatality [75, 76], HBOT has been suggested as adjuvant therapy with promising outcomes [77].

When comparing other illnesses like livedoid vasculopathy where HBOT is used, COVID-19 seems to have effects on the following systems in the body. Anti-inflammatory actions (decreased ICAM-1, proinflammatory cytokines, and neutrophil rolling), anticoagulant actions (boosted fibrinolysis and increased plasminogen activator), and tissue healing actions (increased fibroblasts and stem cells) [78]. Initial studies have demonstrated compared to normobaric oxygen supply, better empiric outcomes with potential uses of HBOT in COVID-19 [79]. Attenuation of the innate immune system and increasing hypoxia tolerance [80] too are believed to occur with HBOT. Most reports up to now have shown potential benefit in the relief of cytokine storm [81]. In a controlled trial, the safety and efficacy of HBOT for COVID-19 patients were successfully evaluated [82]. A preliminary study has shown rapid recovery from hypoxemia when treated with HBOT from the beginning of the treatment in patients with COVID-19 pneumonia [83]. Despite the repeated evidence of benefit, COVID-19 is not yet an accepted indication for HBOT, but this may be recommended for post-viral complications [84].

7.9 Cancer

Although not an approved indication [85], HBOT has shown some promising results in cancer treatment. Angiogenesis occurs as a response to HBOT. This is not seen in tumor cells, so by combining HBOT with other methods, it could act as a potential cure in certain types of cancer. A recent study demonstrated the effectiveness of using HBOT to prevent chemotherapy-induced neuropathy in vivo [86]. Also, in non-small cell lung cancer, a combination of chemotherapy with HBOT has shown promising results [87]. On the contrary, certain chemotherapeutic agents in combination with HBOT might lead to enhancement of cardiotoxicity, pulmonary toxicity, or impairment of wound healing [88]. Overall, the benefits of HBOT in cancer management are a potential field to keep on exploring [89].

Other potential uses of HBOT are erectile dysfunction [90–92], ischemic stroke [93, 94], brain injury, and fields like aging [95].

7.10 Adverse Effects and Contraindications of HBOT

Hyperoxia and the hyperbaric environment may not be suitable for all patients. Claustrophobia and barotrauma are common adverse effects that occur in both monoplace or multiplace chamber compression [96]. Pulmonary toxicity reflected by fibrosis of lung parenchyma has not been common after protocolization of hyperbaric oxygen [97]. Ocular adverse events, such as hyperbaric myopia, cataracts, keratoconus, or retinopathy of prematurity, are reported [98, 99].

There are certain conditions in which HBOT might be absolutely or relatively contraindicated. Untreated pneumothorax is an absolute contraindication [100]. Careful consideration should be given when applying HBOT for patients on chemotherapeutic agents, pacemaker or any type of implantable devices, pregnancy [101], risk of hypoglycemia [102], underlying chronic lung disease like obstructive pulmonary disease, asthma [100], and hypertension [103].

7.11 Future of HBOT

It is evident that HBOT is an effective method to induce hyperoxemia and hyperoxia independent of the level of Hb. Therefore, HBOT is effective in management of hypoxia- and hypoxemia-derived conditions such as infections, wound healing, immunity modulation, certain medical emergencies, and angiogenesis. Further studies should be encouraged to extend the possible uses of HBOT, considering individual benefits and risks. HBOT may be used more frequently in the future in the management of certain common clinical conditions more than anticipated.

References

1. Dejours P, Dejours S. The effects of barometric pressure according to Paul Bert: the question today. Int J Sports Med. 1992;13:S1–5.
2. Hedley-Whyte J. Pulmonary oxygen toxicity: investigation and mentoring. Ulst Med J. 2008;77:39–42.
3. Jones MW, Wyatt HA. Hyperbaric, physics. Treasure Island, FL: StatPearls Publishing; 2019.
4. Moon RE, Camporesi EM. Hyperbaric oxygen therapy: from the nineteenth to the twenty-first century. Respir Care Clin N Am. 1999;5:1–5.
5. Ortega MA. A general overview on the hyperbaric oxygen therapy: applications, mechanisms and translational opportunities. Medicina. 2021;57:864. https://doi.org/10.3390/medicina57090864. https://www.mdpi.com/journal/medicina

6. Pittman RN. Oxygen gradients in the microcirculation. Acta Physiol. 2011;202:311322.
7. Chen PS, Chiu WT, Hsu PL, Lin SC, Peng IC, Wang CY, Tsai SJ. Pathophysiological implications of hypoxia in human diseases. J Biomed Sci. 2020;27:63.
8. Daste T. The oxygen therapy. Prat Vet. 2013;20:30–2.
9. Lee JW, Ko J, Ju C, Eltzschig HK. Hypoxia signaling in human diseases and therapeutic targets. Exp Mol Med. 2019;51:1–13.
10. Macintyre NR. Tissue hypoxia: implications for the respiratory clinician. Respir Care. 2014;59(1590–1596):24.
11. Choudhury R. Hypoxia and hyperbaric oxygen therapy: a review. Int J Gen Med. 2018;11:431–42.
12. Lam G, Fontaine R, Ross FL, Chiu ES. Hyperbaric oxygen therapy: exploring the clinical evidence. Adv Ski Wound Care. 2017;30:181–90.
13. UHMS. Position statement: low-pressure fabric hyperbaric chambers title: low-pressure fabric hyperbaric chambers; 2017. https://www.uhms.org/images/PositionStatements/UHMS_Position_Statement_LP_chambers_revised.
14. Camporesi EM, Mascia MF, Thom SR. Physiological principles of hyperbaric oxygenation. In: Handbook on hyperbaric medicine. Milan, Italy: Springer; 1996. p. 35–58.
15. Leach RM, Rees PJ, Wilmshurst P. ABC of oxygen: hyperbaric oxygen therapy. Br Med J. 1998;317:1140–3.
16. Brugniaux JV, Coombs GB, Barak OF, Dujic Z, Sekhon MS, Ainslie PN. Highs and lows of hyperoxia: physiological, performance, and clinical aspects. Am J Physiol Regul Integr Comp Physiol. 2018;315:R1–R27.
17. Mathieu D, Marroni A, Kot J. Tenth European consensus conference on hyperbaric medicine: recommendations for accepted and non-accepted clinical indications and practice of hyperbaric oxygen treatment. Diving Hyperb Med. 2017;47:24–31. HBO Indications—Undersea & Hyperbaric Medical Society. Available online: https://www.uhms.org/resources/hbo-indications.html#
18. Bhutani S, Vishwanath G. Hyperbaric oxygen and wound healing. Indian J Plast Surg. 2012;45:316–24.
19. Dhamodharan U, Karan A, Sireesh D, Vaishnavi A, Somasundar A, Rajesh K, Ramkumar KM. Tissue-specific role of Nrf2 in the treatment of diabetic foot ulcers during hyperbaric oxygen therapy. Free Radic Biol Med. 2019;138:53–62.
20. Löndahl M, Katzman P, Nilsson A, Hammarlund C. Hyperbaric oxygen therapy facilitates healing of chronic foot ulcers in patients with diabetes. Diabetes Care. 2010;33:998–1003.
21. Salama SE, Eldeeb AE, Elbarbary AH, Abdelghany SE. Adjuvant hyperbaric oxygen therapy enhances healing of nonischemic diabetic foot ulcers compared with standard wound care alone. Int J Low Extrem Wounds. 2019;18:75–80.
22. Hayreh SS. Central retinal artery occlusion. Indian J Ophthalmol. 2018;66:1684–94. [CrossRef] [PubMed]
23. Sharma R, Sharma SK, Mudgal SK, Jelly P, Thakur K. Efficacy of hyperbaric oxygen therapy for diabetic foot ulcer, a systematic review and meta-analysis of controlled clinical trials. Sci Rep. 2021;11:2189.
24. Game FL, Apelqvist J, Attinger C, Hartemann A, Hinchliffe RJ, Löndahl M, Price PE, Jeffcoate WJ. Effectiveness of interventions to enhance healing of chronic ulcers of the foot in diabetes: a systematic review. Diabetes Metab Res Rev. 2016;32(Suppl. 1):154–68.
25. Londahl M, Fagher K, Nilson A, Katzman P. Hyperbaric oxygen therapy is associated with improved six-year survival in people with chronic diabetic foot ulcers. Diabetes. 2018;67:2225.
26. Sureda A, Batle JM, Martorell M, Capó X, Tejada S, Tur JA, Pons A. Antioxidant response of chronic wounds to hyperbaric oxygen therapy. PLoS One. 2016;11:e0163371.
27. Boykin JV, Baylis C. Hyperbaric oxygen therapy mediates increased nitric oxide production associated with wound healing. Adv Ski Wound Care. 2007;20:382–38964.

28. Davis DD, Hanley ME, Cooper JS. Osteoradionecrosis. Curr Otorhinolaryngol Rep. 2021;6:285–91.
29. Oliai C, Fisher B, Jani A, Wong M, Poli J, Brady LW, Komarnicky LT. Hyperbaric oxygen therapy for radiation-induced cystitis and proctitis. Int J Radiat Oncol Biol Phys. 2012;84:733–40.
30. Malone M, Bjarnsholt T, McBain AJ, James GA, Stoodley P, Leaper D, Tachi M, Schultz G, Swanson T, Wolcott RD. The prevalence of biofilms in chronic wounds: a systematic review and meta-analysis of published data. J Wound Care. 2017;26:20–5.
31. Kadam S, Shai S, Shahane A, Kaushik KS. Recent advances in non-conventional antimicrobial approaches for chronic wound biofilms: have we found the "chink in the armor"? Biomedicine. 2019;7:35.
32. Kósciuczuk EM, Lisowski P, Jarczak J, Strzałkowska N, Józwik A, Horbánczuk J, Krzyzewski J, Zwierzchowski L, Bagnicka E. Cathelicidins: family of antimicrobial peptides. A review. Mol Biol Rep. 2012;39:10957–70.
33. Peyssonnaux C, Datta V, Cramer T, Doedens A, Theodorakis EA, Gallo RL, Hurtado-Ziola N, Nizet V, Johnson R. S HIF-1 expression regulates the bactericidal capacity of phagocytes. J Clin Invest. 2005;115:1806–15.
34. Zarember KA, Malech HL. HIF-1alpha: a master regulator of innate host defenses? J Clin Invest. 2005;115:1702–4.
35. Shaw JJ, Psoinos CM, Emhoff TA, Shah SA, Santry H. Not just full of hot air: hyperbaric oxygen therapy increases survival in cases of necrotizing soft tissue infections. Surg Infect. 2014;15:328–35.
36. Nedrebø T, Bruun T, Skjåstad R, Holmaas G, Skrede S. Hyperbaric oxygen treatment in three cases of necrotizing infection of the neck. Infect Dis Rep. 2012;4:73–6.
37. Sanford NE, Wilkinson JE, Nguyen H, Diaz G, Wolcott R. Efficacy of hyperbaric oxygen therapy in bacterial biofilm eradication. J Wound Care. 2018;27:S20–8.
38. Gibson A, Davis FM. Hyperbaric oxygen therapy in the management of clostridium perfringens infections. N Z Med J. 1986;99:617–20.
39. Memar MY, Yekani M, Alizadeh N, Baghi HB. Hyperbaric oxygen therapy: antimicrobial mechanisms and clinical application for infections. Biomed Pharmacother. 2019;109:440–7.
40. Bartek J, Jakola AS, Skyrman S, Förander P, Alpkvist P, Schechtmann G, Glimåker M, Larsson A, Lind F, Mathiesen T. Hyperbaric oxygen therapy in spontaneous brain abscess patients: a population-based comparative cohort study. Acta Neurochir. 2016;158:1259–67.
41. Das MJ, Tommeraasen MA, Cooper JS. Hyperbaric evaluation and treatment of intracranial abscess. Treasure Island, FL: StatPearls Publishing; 2020.
42. Hanley ME, Hendriksen S, Cooper JS. Hyperbaric treatment of chronic refractory osteomyelitis. Treasure Island, FL: StatPearls Publishing; 2021.
43. Rose D. Hyperbaric oxygen therapy for chronic refractory osteomyelitis. Am Fam Physician. 2012;86:888–93.
44. Kirby JP. Hyperbaric oxygen therapy emergencies. Mol Med. 2019;116:180–3.
45. Leung JKS, Lam RPK. Hyperbaric oxygen therapy: its use in medical emergencies and its development in Hong Kong. Hong Kong Med J. 2018;24(2):191–9.
46. Cooper JS, Hanson KC. Decompression sickness (DCS, bends, caisson disease). Treasure Island, FL: StatPearls Publishing; 2019.
47. Gaudreault É, Gosselin J. Leukotriene B4 induces release of antimicrobial peptides in lungs of virally infected mice. J Immunol. 2008;180:6211–21. [CrossRef]
48. Moon RE. Adjunctive therapy for decompression illness: a review and update. Diving Hyperb Med. 2009;39:81–7.
49. Malik N, Claus PL, Illman JE, Kligerman SJ, Moynagh MR, Levin DL, Woodrum DA, Arani A, Arunachalam SP, Araoz PA. Air embolism: diagnosis and management. Future Cardiol. 2017;13(4):365–78.
50. Olson EA, Lentz K. Central retinal artery occlusion: a literature review and the rationale for hyperbaric oxygen therapy. Mol Med. 2016;113:53–7.

51. Nakamura H, Makiguchi T, Atomura D, Yamatsu Y, Shirabe K, Yokoo S. Changes in skin perfusion pressure after hyperbaric oxygen therapy following revascularization in patients with critical limb ischemia: a preliminary study. Int J Low Extrem Wounds. 2020;19(1):57–62.
52. Martani L, Cantadori L, Paganini M, Camporesi EM, Bosco G. Carbon monoxide intoxication: prehospital diagnosis and direct transfer to the hyperbaric chamber. Minerva Anestesiol. 2019;85:920–2.
53. Rose JJ, Nouraie M, Gauthier MC, Pizon AF, Saul MI, Donahoe MP, Gladwin MT. Clinical outcomes and mortality impact of hyperbaric oxygen therapy in patients with carbon monoxide poisoning. Crit Care Med. 2018;46:e649–55.
54. Weaver LK, Hopkins RO, Chan KJ, Churchill S, Elliott CG, Clemmer TP, Orme JF, Thomas FO, Morris AH. Hyperbaric oxygen for acute carbon monoxide poisoning. N Engl J Med. 2002;347:1057–67.
55. Hampson NB, Piantadosi CA, Thom SR, Weaver LK. Practice recommendations in the diagnosis, management, and prevention of carbon monoxide poisoning. Am J Respir Crit Care Med. 2012;186:1095–101.
56. Rose JJ, Wang L, Xu Q, McTiernan CF, Shiva S, Tejero J, Gladwin MT. Carbon monoxide poisoning: pathogenesis, management, and future directions of therapy. Am J Respir Crit Care Med. 2017;195:596–606.
57. Hanley ME, Murphy-Lavoie HM. Hyperbaric, cyanide toxicity. Treasure Island, FL: StatPearls Publishing; 2019.
58. Lawson-Smith P, Jansen EC, Hilsted L, Johnsen AH, Hyldegaard O. Effect of acute and delayed hyperbaric oxygen therapy on cyanide whole blood levels during acute cyanide intoxication. Undersea Hyperb Med. 2011;38:17–26.
59. Van Meter KW. The effect of hyperbaric oxygen on severe anemia. Undersea Hyperb Med. 2012;39:937–42.
60. Rhee TM, Hwang D, Lee JS, Park J, Lee JM. Addition of hyperbaric oxygen therapy vs. medical therapy alone for idiopathic sudden sensorineural hearing loss: a systematic review and meta-analysis. JAMA Otolaryngol Head Neck Surg. 2018;144:1153–61.
61. Bayoumy AB, de Ru JA. The use of hyperbaric oxygen therapy in acute hearing loss: a narrative review. Eur Arch Otorrinolaringol. 2019;276:1859–80.
62. Paderno E, Zanon V, Vezzani G, Giacon T, Bernasek T, Camporesi E, Bosco G. Evidence-supported HBO therapy in femoral head necrosis: a systematic review and meta-analysis. Int J Environ Res Public Health. 2021;18:2888. [CrossRef]
63. Brenner I, Shephard RJ, Shek PN. Immune function in hyperbaric environments, diving, and decompression. Undersea Hyperb Med. 1999;26:27–39.
64. Xu X, Yi H, Kato M, Suzuki H, Kobayashi S, Takahashi H, Nakashima I. Differential sensitivities to hyperbaric oxygen of lymphocyte subpopulations of normal and autoimmune mice. Immunol Lett. 1997;59:79–84. [CrossRef]
65. Saito K, Tanaka Y, Ota T, Eto S, Yamashita U. Suppressive effect of hyperbaric oxygenation on immune responses of normal and autoimmune mice. Clin Exp Immunol. 1991;86:322–7. [CrossRef]
66. Chen SY, Chen YC, Wang JK, Hsu HP, Ho PS, Chen YC, Sytwu HK. Early hyperbaric oxygen therapy attenuates disease severity in lupus-prone autoimmune (NZB NZW) F1 mice. Clin Immunol. 2003;108:103–10. [CrossRef]
67. Harnanik T, Soeroso J, Suryokusumo MG, Juliandhy T. Effects of hyperbaric oxygen on t helper 17/regulatory t polarization in antigen and collagen-induced arthritis: hypoxia-inducible factor-1 as a target. Oman Med J. 2020;35:e90.
68. Novak S, Drenjancevic I, Vukovic R, Kellermayer Z, Cosic A, Tolusic Levak M, Balogh P, Culo F, Mihalj M. Anti- inflammatory effects of hyperbaric oxygenation during DSS-induced colitis in BALB/c mice include changes in gene expression of HIF-1, proinflammatory cytokines, and antioxidative enzymes. Mediat Inflamm. 2016;2016:7141430.
69. Resanovic I, Gluvic Z, Zaric B, Sudar-Milovanovic E, Jovanovic A, Milacic D, Isakovic R, Isenovic ER. Early effects of hyperbaric oxygen on inducible nitric oxide synthase

activity/expression in lymphocytes of type 1 diabetes patients: a prospective pilot study. Int J Endocrinol. 2019;2019:2328505. [CrossRef] [PubMed].
70. Bellato E, Marini E, Castoldi F, Barbasetti N, Mattei L, Bonasia DE, Blonna D. Fibromyalgia syndrome: etiology, pathogenesis, diagnosis, and treatment. Pain Res Treat. 2012;2012:17.
71. Guggino G, Schinocca C, Lo Pizzo M, Di Liberto D, Garbo D, Raimondo S, Alessandro R, Brighina F, Ruscitti P, Giacomelli R, et al. T helper 1 response is correlated with widespread pain, fatigue, sleeping disorders and the quality of life in patients with fibromyalgia and is modulated by hyperbaric oxygen therapy. Clin Exp Rheumatol. 2019;37(Suppl. 116):81–9.
72. Woo J, Min JH, Lee YH, Roh HT. Effects of hyperbaric oxygen therapy on inflammation, oxidative/antioxidant balance, and muscle damage after acute exercise in normobaric, normoxic and hypobaric, hypoxic environments: a pilot study. Int J Environ Res Public Health. 2020;17:7377.
73. Chandra A, Chakraborty U, Pal J, Karmakar P. Silent hypoxia: a frequently overlooked clinical entity in patients with COVID-19. BMJ Case Rep. 2020;13:237207.
74. Álvarez-Mon M, Ortega MA, Gasulla Ó, Fortuny-Profitós J, Mazaira-Font FA, Saurina P, Monserrat J, Plana MN, Troncoso D, Moreno JS, et al. A predictive model and risk factors for case fatality of Covid-19. J Pers Med. 2021;11:36.
75. Oliaei S, SeyedAlinaghi S, Mehrtak M, Karimi A, Noori T, Mirzapour P, Shojaei A, Mohsseni Pour M, Mirghaderi SP, Alilou S, et al. The effects of hyperbaric oxygen therapy (HBOT) on coronavirus disease-2019 (COVID-19): a systematic review. Eur J Med Res. 2021;26:96. [CrossRef] [PubMed]
76. Paganini M, Bosco G, Perozzo FAG, Kohlscheen E, Sonda R, Bassetto F, Garetto G, Camporesi EM, Thom SR. The role of hyperbaric oxygen treatment for COVID-19: a review. Adv Exp Med Biol. 2021;1289:27–35.
77. De Maio A, Hightower LE. COVID-19, acute respiratory distress syndrome (ARDS), and hyperbaric oxygen therapy (HBOT): what is the link? Cell Stress Chaperones. 2020;25:717–20.
78. Criado PR, Miot HA, Pincelli TPH, Fabro AT. From dermatological conditions to COVID-19: reasoning for anticoagulation, suppression of inflammation, and hyperbaric oxygen therapy. Dermatol Ther. 2021;34:e14565.
79. Xiaoling Z, Xiaolan T, Yanchao T, Ruiyong C. The outcomes of hyperbaric oxygen therapy to retrieve hypoxemia of severe novel coronavirus pneumonia: first case report. Chin J Naut Med Hyperb Med. 2020;27:E001.
80. Kjellberg A, De Maio A, Lindholm P. Can hyperbaric oxygen safely serve as an anti-inflammatory treatment for COVID-19? Med Hypotheses. 2020;144:110224.
81. Senniappan K, Jeyabalan S, Rangappa P, Kanchi M. Hyperbaric oxygen therapy: can it be a novel supportive therapy in COVID-19? Indian J Anaesth. 2020;64:835–41.
82. Thibodeaux K, Speyrer M, Raza A, Yaakov R, Serena TE. Hyperbaric oxygen therapy in preventing mechanical ventilation in COVID-19 patients: a retrospective case series. J Wound Care. 2020;29:S4–8. [CrossRef]
83. Guo D, Pan S, Wang M, Guo Y. Hyperbaric oxygen therapy may be effective to improve hypoxemia in patients with severe COVID-2019 pneumonia: two case reports. Undersea Hyperb Med J Undersea Hyperb Med Soc Inc. 2020;47:181–7.
84. El Hawa AAA, Charipova K, Bekeny JC, Johnson-Arbor KK. The evolving use of hyperbaric oxygen therapy during the COVID-19 pandemic. J Wound Care. 2021;30:S8–S11.
85. Feldmeier J, Carl U, Hartmann K, Sminia P. Hyperbaric oxygen: does it promote growth or recurrence of malignancy? Undersea Hyperb Med. 2003;30:1–18.
86. Brewer AL, Shirachi DY, Quock RM, Craft RM. Effect of hyperbaric oxygen on chemotherapy-induced neuropathy in male and female rats. Behav Pharmacol. 2020;31:61–72.
87. Ohguri T, Imada H, Narisada H, Yahara K, Morioka T, Nakano K, Miyaguni Y, Korogi Y. Systemic chemotherapy using paclitaxel and carboplatin plus regional hyperthermia and hyperbaric oxygen treatment for non-small cell lung cancer with multiple pulmonary metastases: preliminary results. Int J Hyperth. 2009;25:160–7.

88. Baude J, Cooper JS. Hyperbaric contraindicated chemotherapeutic agents. Treasure Island, FL: StatPearls Publishing; 2020.
89. Ortega MA, Fraile-Martínez O, García-Montero C, Pekarek L, Guijarro LG, Castellanos AJ, Sanchez-Trujillo L, García-Honduvilla N, Álvarez-Mon M, Buján J, et al. Physical activity as an imperative support in breast cancer management. Cancer. 2021;13:55.
90. Chiles KA, Staff I, Johnson-Arbor K, Champagne A, McLaughlin T, Graydon RJ. A double-blind, randomized trial on the efficacy and safety of hyperbaric oxygenation therapy in the preservation of erectile function after radical prostatectomy. J Urol. 2018;199:805–11.
91. Cormier J, Theriot M. Patient diagnosed with chronic erectile dysfunction refractory to PDE 5 inhibitor therapy reports improvement in function after hyperbaric oxygen therapy. Undersea Hyperb Med. 2016;43:463–5.
92. Yuan J-B, Yang LY, Wang YH, Ding T, Chen TD, Lu Q. Hyperbaric oxygen therapy for recovery of erectile function after posterior urethral reconstruction. Int Urol Nephrol. 2011;43:755–61.
93. Liska GM, Lippert T, Russo E, Nieves N, Borlongan CV. A dual role for hyperbaric oxygen in stroke neuroprotection: preconditioning of the brain and tem cells. Cond Med. 2018;1:151–66.
94. Ding Z, Tong WC, Lu X-X, Peng H-P. Hyperbaric oxygen therapy in acute ischemic stroke: a review. Interv Neurol. 2014;2:201–11.
95. Hachmo Y, Hadanny A, Abu Hamed R, Daniel-Kotovsky M, Catalogna M, Fishlev G, Lang E, Polak N, Doenyas K, Friedman M, et al. Hyperbaric oxygen therapy increases telomere length and decreases immunosenescence in isolated blood cells: a prospective trial. Aging. 2020;12:22445–56.
96. Camporesi EM. Side effects of hyperbaric oxygen therapy. Undersea Hyperb Med. 2014;41:253–7.
97. Hadanny A, Zubari T, Tamir-Adler L, Bechor Y, Fishlev G, Lang E, Polak N, Bergan J, Friedman M, Efrati S. Hyperbaric oxygen therapy effects on pulmonary functions: a prospective cohort study. BMC Pulm Med. 2019;19:148.
98. Mcmonnies CW. Hyperbaric oxygen therapy and the possibility of ocular complications or contraindications. Clin Exp Optom. 2015;98:122–5.
99. Sola A, Chow L, Rogido M. Retinopathy of prematurity and oxygen therapy: a changing relationship. An Pediatr. 2005;62:48–63.
100. Gawdi R, Cooper JS. Hyperbaric contraindications. Treasure Island, FL: StatPearls Publishing; 2020.
101. Arslan A. Hyperbaric oxygen therapy in carbon monoxide poisoning in pregnancy: maternal and fetal outcome. Am J Emerg Med. 2021;43:41–5.
102. Stevens SL, Narr AJ, Claus PL, Millman MP, Steinkraus LW, Shields RC, Buchta WG, Haddon R, Wang Z, Murad MH. The incidence of hypoglycemia during HBO2 therapy: a retrospective review. Undersea Hyperb Med. 2015;42:191–6.
103. Al-Waili NS, Butler GJ, Beale J, Abdullah MS, Finkelstein M, Merrow M, Rivera R, Petrillo R, Carrey Z, Lee B, et al. Influences of hyperbaric oxygen on blood pressure, heart rate and blood glucose levels in patients with diabetes mellitus and hypertension. Arch Med Res. 2006;37:991–7. [CrossRef] 213. Weaver LK, Churchill S. Pulmonary edema associated with hyperbaric oxygen therapy. Chest 2001;120:1407–1409.

Chapter 8
Hyperbaric Oxygen Therapy in the Management of Gas Embolism

Ranajit Chatterjee and Lalit Gupta

8.1 Introduction

With advancement in modern medical science, various medical procedures, from surgeries to simple administering fluids through a tube or giving parenteral medicines, can accidentally entrap air into the blood vessels. This can lead to a serious problem called vascular air embolism (VAE). The small blood vessels in the lungs can usually handle a small amount of air, but excessive entrapment can cause serious complications ranging from a cough and chest pain to more serious issues such as a heart attack, stroke, or loss of consciousness [1]. This makes VAE a risky emergency situation. Specifically, arterial gas embolism (AGE) can lead to stroke by obstructing blood flow to the brain and myocardial ischemia by interfering with the blood supply to the heart. The symptoms of VAE are directly related to the amount and speed at which air enters the blood vessels. Detecting gas embolism involves maintaining a high level of clinical suspicion, especially in situations where there is a potential for gas entrainment. The onset of symptoms is typically rapid, emphasizing the need for early recognition and intervention in settings where gas embolism is likely to occur. To deal with these complications, the timely initiation of hyperbaric oxygen therapy (HBOT) has emerged as an ideal of hope in the management of gas embolism [2].

R. Chatterjee
Swami Dayanand Hospital, Delhi, India

L. Gupta (✉)
Department of Anaesthesia and Critical Care, Maulana Azad Medical College and Lok Nayak Hospital, New Delhi, India

A. G. D'Almeida, J. Hidalgo (eds.), *Evidence-Based Hyperbaric Medicine*,
https://doi.org/10.1007/978-3-032-06346-5_8

8.2 Pathophysiology of Gas Embolism

Gas embolism arises when bubbles of gas enter the arteries or veins, and its manifestations vary based on the type of embolism.

1. AGE, historically associated with submarine escape training, occurs during rapid ascent after breathing compressed gas at depth. AGE can also result from lung conditions such as bullous disease and asthma, as well as incidents such as blast injuries, mechanical ventilation, chest trauma, chest tube placement, and bronchoscopy. On the other hand, venous gas embolism (VGE) is a common consequence of compressed gas diving. While typically harmless, large volumes of VGE can lead to symptoms such as cough, difficulty breathing, and pulmonary edema. Additionally, VGE can enter the arterial circulation directly through abnormalities such as atrial septal defects or a patent foramen ovale [3, 4].
2. Gas embolism is not confined to diving scenarios; it can also result from various medical and surgical procedures (Table 8.1). Understanding these diverse causes is essential for recognizing and managing gas embolism effectively [5–13].

The severity of VGE depends on the rate and volume of gas introduction into the circulation, alongside the patient's position. If there is no right-to-left shunting, the venous gas embolus typically lodges in the pulmonary artery within the lungs, causing pulmonary artery hypertension. Venous air embolism incidents may give rise to both tachyarrhythmias and bradyarrhythmias [14].

In certain instances, the gas embolus may pass through the pulmonary artery, reaching the left heart and entering the systemic arterial circulation, leading to more severe consequences such as stroke—referred to as arterial gas embolus or paradoxical embolism. This is more evident in the presence of right-to-left shunts [5]. Various mechanisms contribute to the potential injuries caused by gas embolism, including the phenomenon known as intracardiac "vapor lock," which can lead to hypotension or acute circulatory arrest, as well as direct arterial occlusion. Interestingly, this effect seems to be contingent on the involvement of neutrophils and may be initiated by the endothelial damage induced by the bubbles. In the context of cerebral AGE, proposed mechanisms for this phenomenon encompass edema, bubble regrowth, and secondary thrombotic occlusion [15].

In most cases, small air volumes undergo breakdown in the capillary bed and get absorbed into the systemic circulation without significant repercussions. However, symptoms are typically observed when more than 5 ml/kg of air is introduced into the venous system, with complications even possible with as little as 20 ml of air [16]. A fatal dose for humans is estimated to be between 300 and 500 ml of gas introduced at a rate of 100 ml per second. Additionally, infusion rates of air exceeding 1.5 ml per kilogram per minute are linked to bradycardia and cardiovascular decompensation [17]. Remarkably, injecting as little as 1–2 ml of air into the central nervous system can be fatal, while a mere 0.5 ml of air introduced into the coronary arteries may initiate ventricular fibrillation.

Table 8.1 Possible causes of gas embolism with signs and symptoms

Cause	Etiology	Signs and symptoms
Diving-related (AGE)	Rapid ascent after compressed gas breathing	Cough, difficulty breathing, pulmonary edema
Diving-related (VGE)	Compressed gas diving	Typically harmless, but large volumes may lead to cough, difficulty breathing, and pulmonary edema
Lung conditions (AGE)	Bullous disease, asthma	Cough, difficulty breathing,
Trauma and medical procedures	Blast injuries, mechanical ventilation, chest trauma, chest tube placement, bronchoscopy	Varied, including respiratory distress and chest pain
Accidental intravenous air injection	Medical errors	Systemic air embolism symptoms, including altered mental status, chest pain, and shortness of breath
Cardiopulmonary bypass accidents	Cardiovascular surgeries	Variable, ranging from neurological deficits to cardiovascular collapse
Hemodialysis	Dialysis procedure	Nausea, dizziness, hypotension, and cardiovascular collapse
Central venous catheter issues	Insertion or disconnection problems	Respiratory distress, chest pain, and hypotension
Gastrointestinal endoscopy	Endoscopic procedures	Abdominal pain, difficulty breathing, and hypotension
Hydrogen peroxide exposure	Irrigation or ingestion	Oxygen toxicity symptoms, including seizures and respiratory distress
Arthroscopy	Joint procedures	Variable, including joint pain and respiratory distress
Cardiopulmonary resuscitation	CPR procedures	Systemic air embolism symptoms, including altered mental status and cardiovascular collapse
Percutaneous hepatic puncture	Liver procedures	Abdominal pain, difficulty breathing, and hypotension
Sexual activities	Certain practices (nonsurgical pneumoperitoneum)	Recurrent chest pain, dyspnea
Laparoscopy	Minimally invasive abdominal surgery	Abdominal pain, difficulty breathing, and hypotension
Transurethral surgery	Urological procedures	Variable, including urinary symptoms and respiratory distress
Vitrectomy	Eye surgeries	Vision changes, eye pain, and respiratory distress
Endoscopic vein harvesting	Vein harvesting procedures	Abdominal pain, difficulty breathing, and hypotension
Hysteroscopy	Uterine procedures	Variable, including pelvic pain and respiratory distress

(continued)

Table 8.1 (continued)

Cause	Etiology	Signs and symptoms
Caesarean sections	Surgical childbirth	Abdominal pain, difficulty breathing, and hypotension
Prostatectomies	Prostate surgeries	Variable, including urinary symptoms and respiratory distress
Spine surgeries	Spinal procedures	Variable, including neurological deficits and respiratory distress
Hip replacements	Joint replacement surgeries	Joint pain, difficulty breathing, and hypotension
Liver resections	Liver surgeries	Abdominal pain, difficulty breathing, and hypotension
Liver transplantations	Liver transplant surgeries	Variable, including abdominal pain and respiratory distress
Dental implant insertions	Dental procedures	Facial pain, difficulty breathing, and hypotension

8.3 Management of Gas Embolism

It is crucial to note that the management of gas embolism requires immediate and coordinated efforts, and the specific approach may vary based on the severity of symptoms, the underlying cause, and the available medical resources. Early recognition and timely intervention play a critical role in improving outcomes for individuals affected by gas embolism (Table 8.2) [18–21].

8.4 Hyperbaric Oxygen Therapy

HBOT has emerged as a well-established treatment for both diving-related and iatrogenic AGE over several years. While the positive effects of HBOT have not been conclusively demonstrated through randomized controlled trials, a wealth of case reports, case series, and solid mechanistic principles strongly support its efficacy in treating AGE [22–24].

The key mechanisms underlying the effectiveness of HBOT in AGE involve the manipulation of oxygen tension and ambient pressure. Elevated oxygen tension facilitates the resorption of nitrogen from gas bubbles, while increased ambient pressure, in accordance with Boyle's law, reduces the size of the bubbles. For instance, at a conventional HBOT treatment pressure of 282 kPa, the diameter of spherical gas bubbles is reduced to 82%, resulting in a 45% decrease in volume. This reduction allows for the passage of bubbles through the microcirculation, contributing to the resolution of embolic phenomena [25].

HBOT exerts its therapeutic impact through several mechanisms (Table 8.3).

Table 8.2 Management of gas embolism

Stage	Actions
Recognition of symptoms	Prompt recognition of symptoms related to gas embolism, such as chest pain, shortness of breath, neurological symptoms, and loss of consciousness, is crucial
Essential emergency care	1. Administer 100% oxygen: Provide the affected individual with pure oxygen to support respiratory function 2. Use a pulse oximeter to measure oxygen saturation levels in the blood 3. Establish Intravenous Access: Set up intravenous access for administering medications or fluids 4. Cardiac/Hemodynamic Monitoring: Monitor heart and circulatory parameters for any abnormalities (ECG, non-invasive hemodynamic monitoring) 5. Transfer the higher facility equipped to handle gas embolism cases
Transport to medical facility	
HBOT	1. Consultation with a hyperbaric/diving physician is essential 2. Transfer to a hyperbaric chamber for HBOT 3. HBOT involves breathing pure oxygen in a pressurized room or chamber, which helps reduce the size of gas bubbles and promotes the elimination of dissolved gases in the bloodstream
Ventilatory support	Provide ventilatory support if necessary to ensure adequate oxygenation.
Normalization of carbon dioxide and blood pressure	Achieve normocapnia (normal carbon dioxide levels) and normotension (normal blood pressure)
Medication	Administer intravenous lidocaine in specific cases to address arrhythmias Lidocaine has also been suggested to depress the rise in blood pressure and ICP in cases of cerebral AGE (CAE)
Special considerations for transportation	If transportation is necessary, especially in cases requiring air travel, adhere to guidelines that may include avoiding altitudes above 1000 ft to prevent exacerbation of gas embolism
Continuous monitoring	Continuously monitor the patient's vital signs, neurological status, and response to treatment
Multidisciplinary approach	Collaborate with a multidisciplinary team, including hyperbaric medicine specialists, to optimize the management of gas embolism

Table 8.3 Mechanism of HBOT

Mechanism	Description
1. Diminishing volume of intravascular bubbles	By enhancing ambient pressure, HBOT decreases the volume of intravascular bubbles
2. Denitrogenating of cerebral tissue	The increase in the partial pressure of oxygen supports the denitrogenating of cerebral tissue, reducing cerebral edema
3. Improving oxygenation of ischemic tissue	HBOT increases the partial pressure of dissolved oxygen in the blood, facilitating better oxygenation of ischemic tissue

8.5 Limitations of Using HBOT for Gas Embolism

While HBOT is beneficial in the treatment of gas embolism, it comes with certain limitations: [26–30]

1. HBOT is most effective when started within the initial 6 h after an insult. Its efficacy extends to both arterial and venous emboli. However, the efficacy of HBOT is affected due to its limited availability at primary centers, leading to delays in transportation and the potential loss of the golden treatment window.
2. HBOT has other limitations also, such as the necessity to transfer to specialized chambers (the pressure is typically elevated to approximately 250–280 kPa) and the capacity of these chambers to manage critically ill patients during therapy.
3. Some hyperbaric chambers may not be equipped to handle critically ill patients during therapy.
4. Establishing and maintaining hyperbaric facilities can be costly. This may limit the widespread availability of HBOT, particularly in health care settings with budgetary constraints.
5. Although rare, there can be side effects or complications associated with HBOT, including barotrauma, oxygen toxicity, and ear or sinus discomfort. These risks must be carefully weighed against the potential benefits.

8.6 Conclusion

HBOT stands out as a crucial and effective intervention in the management of gas embolism. Whether resulting from iatrogenic or diving-related causes, gas embolism poses a serious threat to patients, with potential for significant morbidity and mortality. HBOT's ability to address bubble dynamics, promote resorption, and optimize tissue oxygenation emphasizes its importance in the clinical setting. The therapy is most effective when initiated promptly, ideally within the first six hours after the insult. While there are limitations, such as the need for specialized chambers and considerations for critically ill patients, the potential benefits, especially when started early, outweigh these challenges. By understanding the underlying principles and practical considerations associated with HBOT, health care professionals can optimize the management of gas embolism and improve patient outcomes. Further research and ongoing clinical trials will continue to refine our understanding of HBOT's role in this complex medical condition.

References

1. Ho AM, Karmakar MK, Critchley LA, Tay BA. Vascular air embolism: lung injury and its pathophysiology also need to be considered. Anesthesiology. 2007;107(5):853. author reply 853–854

2. Hatling D, Hogset A, Guttormsen AB, Muller B. Iatrogenic cerebral gas embolism—a systematic review of case reports. Acta Anaesthesiol Scand. 2019;632:154–60.
3. Hampson NB, Moon RE. Arterial gas embolism breathing compressed air in 1.2 metres of water. Diving Hyperb Med. 2020;50(3):292294.
4. Vann RD, Butler FK, Mitchell SJ, Moon RE. Decompression illness. Lancet. 2011;377(9760):15364.
5. Jørgensen TB, Sørensen AM, Jansen EC. Iatrogenic systemic air embolism treated with hyperbaric oxygen therapy. Acta Anaesthesiol Scand. 2008;52(4):5668.
6. Bothma PA, Schlimp CJ. Iatrogenic cerebral gas embolism, pneumocephalus and the concept of retrograde cerebral venous gas embolism. Acta Anaesthesiol Scand. 2019;63(6):831.
7. Berlot G, Rinaldi A, Moscheni M, Ferluga M, Rossini P. Uncommon occurrences of air embolism: description of cases and review of the literature. Case Rep Crit Care. 2018;2018:5808390.
8. Hendriksen SM, Menth NL, Westgard BC, Cole JB, Walter JW, Masters TC, Logue CJ. Hyperbaric oxygen therapy for the prevention of arterial gas embolism in food grade hydrogen peroxide ingestion. Am J Emerg Med. 2017;35(5):809.e5809.e8.
9. Malik N, Claus PL, Illman JE, Kligerman SJ, Moynagh MR, Levin DL, Woodrum DA, Arani A, Arunachalam SP, Araoz PA. Air embolism: diagnosis and management. Future Cardiol. 2017;13(4):365378.
10. Jacobs VR, Mundhenke C, Maass N, Hilpert F, Jonat W. Sexual activity as cause for nonsurgical pneumoperitoneum. JSLS. 2000;4(4):297300.
11. de Jong KIF, de Leeuw PW. Venous carbon dioxide embolism during laparoscopic cholecystectomy a literature review. Eur J Intern Med. 2019;60:912.
12. Muth CM, Shank ES. Gas embolism. N Engl J Med. 2000;342(7):476–82.
13. Austin LS, VanBeek C, Williams GR. Venous air embolism: an under-recognized and potentially catastrophic complication in orthopaedic surgery. J Shoulder Elbow Surg. 2013;22(10):1449–54.
14. Kerrigan MJ, Cooper JS. Venous gas embolism. StatPearls Publishing; 2022.
15. Nossum V, Hjelde A, Brubakk AO. Small amounts of venous gas embolism cause delayed impairment of endothelial function and increase polymorphonuclear neutrophil infiltration. Eur J Appl Physiol. 2002;86(3):20914.
16. Gordy S, Rowell S. Vascular air embolism. Int J Crit Illn Inj Sci. 2013;3(1):73–6.
17. Mirski MA, Lele AV, Fitzsimmons L, Toung TJ. Diagnosis and treatment of vascular air embolism. Anesthesiology. 2007;106:164–77.
18. van Hulst RA, Klein J, Lachmann B. Gas embolism: pathophysiology and treatment. Clin Physiol Funct Imaging. 2003;235:237–46.
19. Shaikh N, Ummunisa F. Acute management of vascular air embolism. J Emerg Trauma Shock. 2009;2(3):180–5.
20. Mitchell SJ, Pellet O, Gorman D. Cerebral protection by lidocaine during cardiothoracic operations. Ann Thorac Surg. 1999;67:1117–24.
21. Orebaugh SL. Venous air embolism: Clinical and experimental considerations. Crit. Care Med. 1992;20:1169–77.
22. Benson J, Adkinson C, Collier R. Hyperbaric oxygen therapy of iatrogenic cerebral arterial gas embolism. Undersea Hyperb Med. 2003;30(2):117–26.
23. Trytko BE, Bennett MH. Arterial gas embolism: a review of cases at Prince of Wales Hospital, Sydney, 1996 to 2006. AnaesthIntensive Care. 2008;36:60–4.
24. Moon R, Gorman D. Treatment of the decompression disorders. In: Brubank A, Neuman T, editors. Physiology and medicine of diving. 5th ed. London: Saunders; 2003. p. 600–50.
25. Gill AL, Bell CN. Hyperbaric oxygen: its uses, mechanisms of action and outcomes. QJM. 2004;97(7):385–95.
26. McCarthy CJ, Behravesh S, Naidu SG, Oklu R. Air embolism: diagnosis, clinical management and outcomes. Diagnostics. 2017;7:5.
27. Blanc P, Boussuges A, Henriette K, Sainty JM, Deleflie M. Iatrogenic cerebral air embolism: importance of an early hyperbaric oxygenation. Intensive Care Med. 2002;28(5):559–63.

28. Leach RM, Rees PJ, Wilmshurst P. Hyperbaric oxygen therapy. BMJ. 1998;317(7166):1140–3.
29. Kirby JP, Snyder J, Schuerer DJE, Peters JS, Bochicchio GV. Essentials of hyperbaric oxygen therapy: 2019 review. Mo Med. 2019;116(3):176–9.
30. Heyboer M 3rd, Sharma D, Santiago W, McCulloch N. Hyperbaric oxygen therapy: side effects defined and quantified. Adv Wound Care (New Rochelle). 2017;6(6):210–24.

Chapter 9
Recommended Indications: Carbon Monoxide Poisoning

Ahsan Ahmed, Chayan Bhattacharya, and Shreyans Agrawal

9.1 Introduction

Carbon monoxide (CO) is a colorless, odorless, imperceptible gas formed due to the incomplete combustion of any carbon-containing compound in a closed space and under restricted oxygen supply. Its presence in the environment is very difficult to detect due to its chemical and physical nature, even when present in significant concentrations, making it a leading cause of death in various accidents such as household fires, houseboat fires, being trapped in a car with running engines, and blocked exhaust pipes [1]. CO poisoning depends on the dose and duration of exposure.

Very commonly, closed space burn is associated with smoke inhalation injury and subsequent CO poisoning. Although CO poisoning cannot be pointed out as a single cause of death, 75% of deceased burn victims had significantly high concentrations of blood CO levels on presentation [2, 3].

A. Ahmed (✉)
Department of Anesthesiology, Critical Care and Emergency Services, KPC Medical College and Hospital, Kolkata, West Bengal, India

C. Bhattacharya
Department of Anaesthesia & Critical Care, In-charge Critical Care Unit, B R Singh Hospital, Eastern Railway, Kolkata, India

S. Agrawal
Intensive Care Unit, KPC Medical College and Hospital, Kolkata, West Bengal, India

A. G. D'Almeida, J. Hidalgo (eds.), *Evidence-Based Hyperbaric Medicine*,
https://doi.org/10.1007/978-3-032-06346-5_9

9.2 Pathophysiology of CO Poisoning and Its Effect on Various Organ Systems

Being a tasteless, colorless, odorless gas, CO remains undetectable by people. It is produced by incomplete combustion of hydrocarbons more so during closed space fire causing CO poisoning. The World Health Organization suggested a CO level greater than 6 PPM as toxic when there is prolonged exposure. Exposure to 10 PPM CO coincides with the approximate blood level of 2% COHb level, and a COHb level of more than 2% in non-smokers and 10% in smokers can produce symptoms [4, 5].

9.2.1 *Hemoglobin and CO Interaction*

CO has more than 200 times more affinity for heme moity than O_2. CO displaces oxygen from hemoglobin by occupying hemoglobin before oxygen can do the same due to its higher affinity, resulting in reduced oxygen-carrying capacity of hemoglobin in the presence of a significant amount of CO.

The hemoglobin remains in two allosteric states: T-state or tense state and relaxed state or R-state. T-state is a deoxygenated state with lesser affinity for oxygen, but as one molecule of oxygen attaches with hemoglobin in T-state, it gets converted to R-state and attracts more and more oxygen, but, at the tissue level, in the presence of CO_2, again hemoglobin gets converted to T-state and releases oxygen. But in the presence of CO, hemoglobin gets stabilized in the R-state and does not release oxygen at the tissue level, reducing tissue oxygen delivery [6]. Hemoglobin dissociation curve shifts to the left.

Besides hemoglobin, CO binds to other heme-containing proteins such as myoglobin in heart and skeletal muscles and cytochrome C oxidase at mitochondria. It denotes that CO poisoning exerts an effect on almost all systems of the body by reducing the availability of oxygen, by reducing cellular oxygenation and ATP production.

9.2.2 *CO and Mitochondria*

CO affects and targets cytochrome C oxidase present in the mitochondrial inner cell membrane and known as complex IV. The enzyme has a crucial role in cellular respiration by producing ATP. It competes with oxygen in binding to the active site of cytochrome C oxidase, which is the alpha 3 heme moiety, and shuts down oxidative phosphorylation, similar to the effects of both cyanide and nitric oxide. On the other hand, the rest of the enzymes continue to transport electrons to produce superoxide anions, increasing the oxidative stress to the tissue and damages the same.

Hence, lack of ATP production and oxidative stress in vital organs such as heart and brain depress their function in CO poisoning [7].

9.2.3 CO Poisoning, Oxidative Stress, and Platelet Function

As we have already understood that CO has got affinity for all heme-containing molecules, including myoglobin besides hemoglobin. Platelet surface hemoproteins also get occupied by the excess amount of CO and produce NO (nitric oxide), which, in turn, generates superoxide anions, causing oxidative stress and the generation of peroxynitrite. This peroxynitrite in low concentration prevents plate activation, but, in high concentration, as generated during CO poisoning, can activate platelets by thiol oxidation and a rise in intracellular Ca^{2+} concentration [7–9]. Platelet activation increases platelet neutrophil adhesion and, in turn, activates neutrophil by a complex mechanism through P-selectin, glycoprotein $\alpha_{IIb}\beta_3$, and platelet-activating factor, and neutrophil β_2 integrins [10].
Following adhesion of platelet and neutrophil, the neutrophil gest activated and degranulates. Following degranulation myeloperoxidase (MPO) gets released and oxidizes xanthine dehydrogenase to xanthine oxidase resulting in production of reactive oxygen species (ROS). These MPO and ROS will promote lipid peroxidation and microglial activation by triggering lymphocyte response. Thus, CO poisoning is associated with myocardial and delayed neurological sequelae. These effects continue even after the CO is removed from the body and are independent of COHb level [10].

9.3 Signs and Symptoms and Mechanism

Detection of CO poisoning depends on a high level of clinical suspicion. CO poisoning is suspected (1) when there is a history of suspected exposure; (2) symptoms consistent with CO poisoning; and (3) an elevated COHb level.

(1) When There Is a History of Suspected Exposure

CO is produced by the incomplete combustion of hydrocarbons. CO poisoning incidences increase during the winter months. Possible sources of CO exposure are gas furnaces, gas or kerosene space heaters, and kitchen stoves during the winter months, when used with inadequate ventilation [11]. Incidences increase when there is no electricity and people are using fuel-burning space heaters, stoves, and grills, which are meant for outdoor use only. Detailed history with soot/carbonaceous particles in sputum, singing of nasal hairs, perioral burn, hoarseness of voice, stridor, dyspnea, cyanosis, or cherry red colored nails all point toward a possibility of closed space burns and or smoke inhalation.

(2) Symptoms Consistent With CO Poisoning

The organ system mostly dependent on oxygen shows the most manifestations of CO poisoning, namely, the brain and the cardiovascular system [12].

Acute Poisoning
A dull, continuous, frontal headache is the most common symptom of CO poisoning [13]. Other symptoms are nausea, malaise, and fatigue, mimicking other common viral illnesses. With increasing exposure, other major symptoms such as tachycardia, hypotension, and other arrhythmias appear. Central nervous system symptoms include altered sensorium, confusion coma, delirium, gait abnormalities, coma, cardio or respiratory arrest, and death [14–16].

Less common symptoms are hyperglycemia, lactic acidosis, acute kidney injury, and visual or auditory disturbance.

Chronic Poisoning
Low level of chronic exposure may cause persistent headache, dementia, memory loss, worsening of hearing loss, atherosclerosis, and ischemic heart disease [17].

(3) Elevated COHb Level

Elevated COHb level confirms the diagnosis of CO exposure and its severity [18]. Normal pulse oximetry uses two different wavelengths of light to measure oxy and deoxy hemoglobin, but co-oximetry, which has been used routinely since 2005, uses eight different wavelengths of light to measure COHb, methemoglobin, and other species of hemoglobin. Use of co-oximetry at the site of accident can identify the elevated COHb level and CO exposure and can reduce the time for accurate diagnosis and initiation of management [19]. Diagnostic accuracy of co-oximetry in estimating COHb level in comparison to laboratory spectrophotometry is still debatable, and a study in 2013 had also shown that normal COHb level in co-oximetry cannot rule out CO poisoning and or exposure [18–20]. The ratio of COHb to Hb level around 5% does not show any significant symptoms. Heavy smokers show this level around 9% and symptomatic hospitalized patients usually have this level around 10–30% and in victims who already brought dead in hospital showed 30–90% of COHb level in their blood in postmortem examination [21, 22].

9.4 Clinical Manifestation

CO poisoning victims on their presentation showed the following symptoms in the following frequency [23].

Headache: 58%
Nausea: 33%
Dizziness: 29%
Drowsiness: 14%

Vomiting: 14%
Cough/choking: 6%
Confusion: 5%
Shortness of breath: 5%
Syncope: 5%
Throat or eye irritation, chest pain, and weakness: <5%

Among these presentations, cardiac and neurological manifestations are most significant, and early recognition and management may reduce the mortality and or delayed neurological or cardiac sequelae.

9.5 Cardiac Presentation

Myocardial injury is present in nearly one-third of patients of moderate to severe CO poisoning and is a predictor of mortality [24]. Multiple mechanisms are involved in the development of myocardial injury in CO poisoning, including global reduction in oxygen delivery, high oxygen demand due to tachycardia, endothelial injury, and production of ROS, production of NO-related vasoconstriction due to excess production of nitrite derivative, and reduction in mitochondrial oxidative phosphorylation. Myocardial infarction takes place even in the absence of coronary occlusion. Mitochondrial depression may cause a stunning effect, i.e., myocardial contractility reduction in the absence of coronary artery disease [15, 24, 25].

Moreover, CO excess also promotes arrhythmia by reducing mitochondrial oxidative phosphorylation and ATP production, resulting in an altered gradient of calcium in myocytes, making them sensitive to calcium, and CO excess also sensitizes myocardium to catecholamines. The excess production of NO also increases the inward late sodium current through the Nav 1.5 channel; this late sodium influx is proarrhythmogenic. The most common arrhythmia is QT prolongation, which can be treated by L-NAME, a novel NO synthetase inhibitor, and Ranolazine, a blocker of the Nav1.5 channel [26, 27].

9.6 Mechanism of Neurological Effect Acute and Delayed [28, 29]

Exposure to toxic levels of CO causes acute and delayed central nervous system changes. In the acute phase, reduced oxygen delivery and depressed mitochondrial oxidative phosphorylation will cause cerebral ischemia and anoxic brain injury, causing subtle changes in sensorium to coma and cardiorespiratory arrest and death. The same mechanism is also responsible for delayed cognitive dysfunction in survivors. Other important mechanisms for delayed cognitive dysfunction include oxidative stress, acidosis, ionic imbalance, excitotoxicity, and so on.

Reduction in mitochondrial oxidative phosphorylation results in a reduction in ATP production. In turn, reduced ATP levels will stimulate neurocellular lipid peroxidation and release of inhibitory neurotransmitter glutamate, which, on the other hand, activates *N*-methyl-D-aspartate receptors, enhancing cellular dysfunction and apoptosis.

9.7 Delayed Neurological Effect of CO Poisoning [18, 30–34]

Major concern for this CO poisoning is the late-onset cognitive and other neurological dysfunction. The effects appear within 2–40 days of poisoning. The chance of this delayed neurological effect is not predictable, but victims who are unconscious on presentation, with advanced age, and with pre-existing neurological abnormality and longer duration of exposure showed more delayed neurological effects. The effects include short-term or long-term memory loss, dementia, irritability, gait disturbance and Parkinsonism-like disorder, depression, and cortical blindness.

Most of the CO poisoning patients present with some sort of neurological symptoms, they undergo some sort neuroimaging in the form of CT scan and or MRI at the emergency, and the results are corroborative with symptoms.

CT findings include bilateral symmetric hypoattenuation in mild to moderate cases, but, in severe cases, hypoxia-resistant structures such as brainstem and cerebellum also get affected.

White matter hyperintensities and hippocampal atrophy are the most common MRI findings in the acute phase. MRI changes also involve the basal ganglia and thalamus. In the late stage, posthypoxic leukoencephalopathy diffuse post hypoxic leaucoencephalopathy (DPHL) is also evident in MRI due to inhibition of cellular oxidation, oxidative stress, and cellular apoptosis.

9.8 Management of CO Poisoning

The goal of management of CO poisoning is to eliminate CO from the body as early as possible to prevent long-term or short-term neurological sequelae. Before going into details of the management, the physiology of CO elimination from the body needs to be understood. CO gets eliminated through the lungs only after dissociation from COHb. The elimination half-life of CO is 320 minutes while inspiring room air containing 21% oxygen, and this half-life gets reduced to 50–100 minutes while the victim is inspiring 100% oxygen. This same half-life gets further reduced to 15–20 minutes when the victim is placed in a hyperbaric oxygen chamber with oxygen at 2–3 atmospheric pressure [36]. The basic goal is to increase the PO_2 as much as possible so that the dissolved fraction of oxygen increases and thus improves the tissue oxygenation and replaces CO from HB competitively [35, 36].

9.9 Management at the Site of Accident

Immediate management should be removal of the victim from the site of accident at earliest along with administration of 100% oxygen for possible CO exposure and probable poisoning. In case of household fire, concomitant cyanide poisoning should also be suspected, and a nontoxic antidote of cyanide like hydroxocobalamins should be administered with high flow oxygen therapy, though hydroxocobalamin significantly affects COHb measurement at the lab. Hence, the emergency physician must ask the transporting team whether hydroxocobalamin has already been administered en route or not.

9.9.1 Warning Signs of Severe Exposure to Be Identified

Signs and symptoms of severe poisoning are confusion, altered mental status, seizure, focal neurologic deficit, loss of consciousness, coma, chest pain, dyspnea, respiratory failure, and ventricular arrhythmia.

In the presence of severe symptoms and in case of inability to protect the airway or reduced respiratory efforts, placement of an invasive airway should be the first step. All monitors, including cardiac monitors, need to be attached to the ambulance itself. On-site COHb also needs to be measured at the site by co-oximetry.

9.9.1.1 Oxygen Administration at the Site

Providing 100% oxygen at the earliest is life saving and prevents long-term or short-term sequelae of CO poisoning. Oxygen can be provided through NIV (CPAP) with 5–12 cm H_2O can effectively reduce the half-life of CO [37]. High flow oxygen mask with reservoir bag with a flow of 15 L of oxygen flow or a mask with a demand valve with high flow can also be provided at the site of the incident.

9.9.1.2 Transport

After initial stabilization and taking care of the ABC patient is to be transported to the nearest emergency facility with the same oxygen support and monitoring of pulse oximetry, respiratory rate, ECG, and non-invasive blood pressure.

9.9.1.3 At the Emergency Department

There is a brief handover from the transport team, which includes duration of exposure, initial COHb level, oxygen administration process, and whether hydroxocobalamin has been administered or not.

9.9.1.4 Admission Criteria

Not all patients will come through the medical evacuation system; some victims may present themselves with nonspecific symptoms. Hence, importance of high level of suspicion for CO poisoning is emphasized here again.

Indication for admission:

(a) All symptomatic patients
(b) All patients on respiratory support
(c) Pregnant victims or children should be admitted even if asymptomatic.

Asymptomatic patients but exposed to CO and COHb levels less than 5% need not be admitted to the hospital.

9.9.1.5 Evaluation on Admission

- Again, at the emergency department, the COHb level is estimated by the spectrophotometric method to identify and quantify the level of CO burden in the body.
- Moreover, arterial blood gas, serum glucose level, cardiac enzymes including Troponin I, creatine phosphokinase muscle and brain, and last but not least ECG (12 leads) must be obtained on admission. Cardiac evaluation is most important in patients with positive ECG changes depicting ischemic changes or any other cardiac symptoms and a previous history of cardiac diseases.
- On admission, the patient must be examined neurologically. Mini-Mental State Examination needs to be done on admission, as chances of DNS (delayed neurological sequelae) can be predicted by neurological presentation on admission.
- *Measurement of pH and blood lactate level* is a very important investigation on admission and thereafter serially for depicting initial exposure and level of tissue hypoxia status and response to the treatment thereafter. Moreover, when, after adequate therapy, blood pH is not improving and or level below <7.2 along with elevated blood lactate level above 10 mmol/L, concomitant cyanide poisoning is very likely [37].
- When CO poisoning is suspected to be of suicidal in nature, concomitant other toxicology screening should also be done, including serum ethanol estimation [16].
- *Urine or serum pregnancy test*: In females of child-bearing age.
- *Chest radiograph:* Patients with dyspnea or hypoxia to evaluate for pulmonary edema.

9.9.1.6 Treatment at ER and on Admission

Providing highest possible concentration of oxygen is the key to the management of CO poisoning. There remains a controversy over the method of providing the highest possible concentration of oxygen between normobaric oxygen therapy and hyperbaric oxygen therapy (HBOT). Multiple studies have been conducted to find out the ideal method of providing oxygen in CO poisoning, but most of them failed to show any difference. However, a recent metanalysis by Wang W et al. [38] showed the positive effect of HBOT in preventing memory loss following severe CO poisoning.

- NBOT is provided to all patients of suspected CO poisoning through either non-rebreathing mask, CPAP, NIV, and high flow nasal oxygen therapy units.
- In case of patients with severe symptoms, management of airway breathing and circulation takes precedence, including intubation and invasive ventilation if not done already en route.
- Victims with suspected smoke inhalation injury with CO poisoning and showing severe symptoms like hemodynamic compromise, severe metabolic acidosis, and high blood lactate level with coma, seizures, or severely depressed neurological status must be provided with an antidote for cyanide poisoning [39, 40]. 70 mg/kg of hydroxocobalamin is given at the ER and can be repeated after 10–15 minutes if there is no clinical improvement.

9.9.1.7 HBOT in CO Poisoning

The European Committee on Hyperbaric Medicine [41] recommended that, in the following conditions, HBOT must be provided to the CO poisoning patients:

- Initial COHb level of more than 25%
- To all patients irrespective of COHb concentration, presenting with severely depressed neurological status, signs and symptoms of cardiac involvement, including elevated cardiac biomarkers and positive ECG changes, severe acidosis, and respiratory compromise
- To all pregnant women, irrespective of their COHb level

9.9.1.8 Mechanism of HBOT

According to Henry's law, the dissolved amount of an ideal gas in a solution is directly dependent on its partial pressure. At 1 ATA, the amount of dissolved oxygen is 0.3ml/dl, and at 3 ATA, this oxygen increases to 6 ml/dl, which is more than enough to meet the resting tissue oxygen demand even when the hemoglobin is not releasing oxygen in presence of CO. HBOT reduces the half-life of CO to 15–20 minutes from 320 minutes when breathing room air.

9.9.1.9 Regimen in Vogue [37]

- To be started within 6 hours of exposure.
- After 24 hours, the HBOT will not provide any significant advantage.

- The German Society for Diving and Hyperbaric Medicine (Gesellschaft für Tauch- und Überdruckmedizin, GTÜMe.V.) [42] recommends that either 3 ATA pressure for 90 minutes breathing oxygen, followed by gradual decompression (TS 300/90 regimen) or 2.4 ATA pressure for 90 minutes breathing oxygen (TS 240/90 regimen).

9.10 Difficulties of HBOT

- The HBOT facility is not widely available. Hence, before referral, the risk–benefit ratio must be weighted.
- Inside the HBOT chamber, emergency decompression takes time; hence, only hemodynamically stable patients without any airway issues are taken for HBOT. Patients with dysrhythmia are also not considered, as a defibrillator cannot be used inside the HBOT chamber.

9.11 Complications [16, 43]

Most encountered complications are

- Barotrauma
- Claustrophobia
- Seizure
- Pulmonary edema

9.12 Controversies

- The American College of Emergency Physicians clinical guidelines committee did not give blanket indication in favor of HBOT in CO poisoning [44].
- National Institute for Health Care Excellence also advocated for 100% oxygen through non re-breathing mask (NRBM) with reservoir and did not recommend HBOT due to lack of evidence [45].
- On the contrary, the Undersea and Hyperbaric Medical Society has recommended for HBOT in certain cases.

Hence, the HBOT may have some role in the management of CO poisoning but without a compelling rationale.

9.13 Extracorporeal Membrane Oxygenator

Very unstable patient not suitable for HBOT can be initially rescued with an extracorporeal membrane oxygenator.

9.14 Other Therapies Under Trial

- *Erythropoietin:* Initial studies showed some positive results in preventing neurological sequelae in animal and human models, as evidenced by reduced levels of S-100β—a glial-specific protein expressed mainly in matured astrocytes, and an increase in serum levels indicates acute neuronal damage [46, 47]. But, a recent study on the role of erythropoietin in stroke patients showed higher mortality in the erythropoietin arm; hence, its use is not encouraged [48].
- *Hydrogen-rich saline,* an antioxidant, nimodipine, granulocyte colony-stimulating factor, edaravone, and fructose di phosphate, all are under trial for their beneficial effects on neuronal protection following hypoxic brain injury [49–53].

9.15 Conclusion

In managing CO poisoning, a high level of suspicion is required to prevent delay in diagnosis and management. The goal of management is to prevent and or treat acute or delayed neurological sequelae and cardiac morbidity. Providing the highest possible oxygen concentration to the victims at the earliest is the cornerstone of management. HBOT has its role in specific cases, but, due to conflicting outcomes of various trials, the acceptability of this safe and effective therapy is yet to be established. Hence, a multicentric prospective trial with a larger cohort is warranted. Various governments must encourage and help to come up with more and more HBOT facilities in their country.

References

1. Goldfrank L, Flomenbaum N, Lewin N, Howland MA, Hoffman R, Nelson L. Carbon monoxide. In: Goldfrank's toxicologic emergencies. (7th ed.). ed. New York: McGraw-Hill; 2002. p. 1689–704.
2. National Fire Protection Association Fatal effects of fire. 2011 March [accessed 24 Feb 2015]. Available from: http://www.nfpa.org/news-and-research/fire-statistics-and-reports/fire-statistics/demographics-and-victim-patterns/fatal-effects-of-fire

3. Centers for Disease Control and Prevention (CDC) Nonfatal residential fire-related injuries treated in emergency departments—United States, 2001. 2003;52:906–908.
4. Penney D, Benignus V, Kephalopoulos S, Kotzias D, Kleinman M, Verrier A.CarbonmonoxideWHO guidelines for indoor air quality: selected pollutants. 2010 [Accessed 3 June 2023]. Available from: http://www.ncbi.nlm.nih.gov/books/NBK138710/
5. Raub JA, Mathieu-Nolf M, Hampson NB, Thom SR. Carbon monoxide poisoning—a public health perspective. 2000;145:1–14.
6. Mihailescu MR, Russu IM. A signature of the T → R transition in human hemoglobin. Proc Natl Acad Sci U S A. 2001 Mar 27;98(7):3773-7. https://doi.org/10.1073/pnas.071493598. Epub 2001 Mar 20. PMID: 11259676; PMCID: PMC31128.
7. Rose JJ, Wang L, Xu Q, McTiernan CF, Shiva S, Tejero J, Gladwin MT. Carbon monoxide poisoning: pathogenesis, management, and future directions of therapy. Am J Respir Crit Care Med. 2017 Mar 1;195(5):596-606. https://doi.org/10.1164/rccm.201606-1275CI. Erratum in: Am J Respir Crit Care Med. 2017 Aug 1;196 (3):398-399. PMID: 27753502; PMCID: PMC5363978.
8. Ly LD, Xu S, Choi SK, Ha CM, Thoudam T, Cha SK, Wiederkehr A, Wollheim CB, Lee IK, Park KS. Oxidative stress and calcium dysregulation by palmitate in type 2 diabetes. Exp Mol Med. 2017;49(2):e291. https://doi.org/10.1038/emm.2016.157. PMID: 28154371; PMCID: PMC5336562
9. Brown AS, Moro MA, Masse JM, Cramer EM, Radomski M, Darley-Usmar V. Nitric oxide-dependent and independent effects on human platelets treated with peroxynitrite. Cardiovasc Res. 1998;40(2):380–8. https://doi.org/10.1016/s0008-6363(98)00182-5. PMID: 9893732
10. Thom SR, Bhopale VM, Han ST, Clark JM, Hardy KR. Intravascular neutrophil activation due to carbon monoxide poisoning. Am J Respir Crit Care Med. 2006 Dec 1;174(11):1239-48. https://doi.org/10.1164/rccm.200604-557OC. Epub 2006 Aug 24. PMID: 16931637; PMCID: PMC2648106.
11. Heckerling PS. Occult carbon monoxide poisoning: a cause of winter headache. Am J Emerg Med. 1987;5(3):201–4. https://doi.org/10.1016/0735-6757(87)90320-2. PMID: 3580051
12. Kao LW, Nañagas KA. Toxicity associated with carbon monoxide. Clin Lab Med. 2006;26(1):99–125. https://doi.org/10.1016/j.cll.2006.01.005. PMID 16567227
13. Hampson NB, Hampson LA. Characteristics of headache associated with acute carbon monoxide poisoning. Headache. 2002;42(3):220–3. https://doi.org/10.1046/j.1526-4610.2002.02055.x. PMID 11903546. S2CID 8773611
14. Choi IS. Carbon monoxide poisoning: systemic manifestations and complications. J Korean Med Sci. 2001;16(3):253–61. https://doi.org/10.3346/jkms.2001.16.3.253. PMC 3054741. PMID 11410684
15. Tritapepe L, Macchiarelli G, Rocco M, Scopinaro F, Schillaci O, Martuscelli E, Motta PM. Functional and ultrastructural evidence of myocardial stunning after acute carbon monoxide poisoning. Critical Care Med. 1998;26(4):797–801. https://doi.org/10.1097/00003246-199804000-00034. PMID 9559621
16. Weaver LK. Clinical practice. Carbon monoxide poisoning. New Engl J Med. 2009;360(12):1217–25. https://doi.org/10.1056/NEJMcp0808891. PMID 19297574
17. Ryan CM. Memory disturbances following chronic, low-level carbon monoxide exposure. Arch Clin Neuropsychol. 1990;5(1):59–67. https://doi.org/10.1016/0887-6177(90)90007-C. PMID 14589544
18. Hampson NB, Piantadosi CA, Thom SR, Weaver LK. Practice recommendations in the diagnosis, management, and prevention of carbon monoxide poisoning. Am J Respir Crit Care Med. 2012;186(11):1095–101. https://doi.org/10.1164/rccm.201207-1284CI. Epub 2012 Oct 18. PMID: 23087025
19. Hampson NB, Weaver LK. Noninvasive CO measurement by first responders. A suggested management algorithm. JEMS. 2006;31(5):S10–2. PMID: 16739272
20. Weaver LK, Churchill SK, Deru K, Cooney D. False positive rate of carbon monoxide saturation by pulse oximetry of emergency department patients. Respir Care. 2013;58(2):232–40. https://doi.org/10.4187/respcare.01744. PMID: 22782305

21. Sato K, Tamaki K, Hattori H, et al. Determination of total hemoglobin in forensic blood samples with special reference to carboxyhemoglobin analysis. For. Sci. Int. 1990;48:89–96.
22. Baselt R. Disposition of toxic drugs and chemicals in man. 8th ed. Foster City: Biomedical Publications; 2008. p. 237–41.
23. Shin M, Bronstein AC, Glidden E, Malone M, Chang A, Law R, Boehmer TK, Strosnider H, Yip F. Morbidity and Mortality of Unintentional Carbon Monoxide Poisoning: United States 2005 to 2018. Ann Emerg Med. 2023 Mar;81(3):309-317. https://doi.org/10.1016/j.annemergmed.2022.10.011. Epub 2022 Dec 28. PMID: 36585319; PMCID: PMC9975060.
24. Henry CR, Satran D, Lindgren B, Adkinson C, Nicholson CI, Henry TD. Myocardial injury and long-term mortality following moderate to severe carbon monoxide poisoning. JAMA. 2006;295(4):398–402. https://doi.org/10.1001/jama.295.4.398. PMID: 16434630
25. Dziewierz A, Ciszowski K, Gawlikowski T, Rakowski T, Kleczyński P, Surdacki A, Dudek D. Primary angioplasty in patient with ST-segment elevation myocardial infarction in the setting of intentional carbon monoxide poisoning. J Emerg Med. 2013;45(6):831–4. https://doi.org/10.1016/j.jemermed.2013.05.061. Epub 2013 Oct 2. PMID: 24094806
26. Dallas ML, Yang Z, Boyle JP, Boycott HE, Scragg JL, Milligan CJ, Elies J, Duke A, Thireau J, Reboul C, Richard S, Bernus O, Steele DS, Peers C. Carbon monoxide induces cardiac arrhythmia via induction of the late Na+ current. Am J Respir Crit Care Med. 2012 Oct 1;186(7):648-56. https://doi.org/10.1164/rccm.201204-0688OC. Epub 2012 Jul 19. PMID: 22822026; PMCID: PMC3622900.
27. Macmillan CS, Wildsmith JA, Hamilton WF. Reversible increase in QT dispersion during carbon monoxide poisoning. Acta Anaesthesiol Scand. 2001;45(3):396–7. https://doi.org/10.1034/j.1399-6576.2001.045003396.x. PMID: 11207481
28. Doyle KP, Simon RP, Stenzel-Poore MP. Mechanisms of ischemic brain damage. Neuropharmacology. 2008 Sep;55(3):310-8. https://doi.org/10.1016/j.neuropharm.2008.01.005. Epub 2008 Jan 25. PMID: 18308346; PMCID: PMC2603601.
29. Piantadosi CA, Zhang J, Levin ED, Folz RJ, Schmechel DE. Apoptosis and delayed neuronal damage after carbon monoxide poisoning in the rat. Exp Neurol. 1997;147(1):103–14. https://doi.org/10.1006/exnr.1997.6584. PMID: 9294407
30. Roohi F, Kula RW, Mehta N. Twenty-nine years after carbon monoxide intoxication. Clin Neurol Neurosurg. 2001;103(2):92–5. https://doi.org/10.1016/s0303-8467(01)00119-6. PMID: 11516551
31. Hopkins RO, Weaver LK. Cognitive outcomes 6 years after acute carbon monoxide poisoning. Undersea Hyperb Med. 2008;35:258.
32. Mimura K, Harada M, Sumiyoshi S, Tohya G, Takagi M, Fujita E, Takata A, Tatetsu S. Long-term follow-up study on sequelae of carbon monoxide poisoning; serial investigation 33 years after poisoning. Seishin Shinkeigaku Zasshi. 1999;101(7):592-618. Japanese. PMID: 10502996.
33. O'Donnell P, Buxton PJ, Pitkin A, Jarvis LJ. The magnetic resonance imaging appearances of the brain in acute carbon monoxide poisoning. Clin Radiol. 2000;55(4):273–80. https://doi.org/10.1053/crad.1999.0369. PMID: 10767186
34. Shprecher D, Mehta L. The syndrome of delayed post-hypoxic leukoencephalopathy. Neuro Rehabil. 2010;26(1):65–72. PMID: 20166270; PMCID: PMC2835522
35. Weaver LK, Howe S, Hopkins R, Chan KJ. Carboxyhemoglobin half-life in carbon monoxide-poisoned patients treated with 100% oxygen at atmospheric pressure. Chest. 2000;117(3):801–8. https://doi.org/10.1378/chest.117.3.801. PMID: 10713010
36. Köhler A, Zoll FM, Ploner T, Hammer A, Joannidis M, Tilg H, Finkenstedt A, Hartig F. Oxygenation performance of different non-invasive devices for treatment of decompression illness and carbon monoxide poisoning. Front Physiol. 2022;26(13):885898. https://doi.org/10.3389/fphys.2022.885898. PMID: 35557974; PMCID: PMC9090223
37. Jüttner B, Busch HJ, Callies A, Dormann H, Janisch T, Kaiser G, Körner-Göbel H, Kluba K, Kluge S, Leidel BA, Müller O, Naser J, Pohl C, Reiter K, Schneider D, Staps E, Welslau W, Wißuwa H, Wöbker G, Muche-Borowski C. S2k guideline diagnosis and treatment of car-

bon monoxide poisoning. Ger. Med Sci. 2021;19:19:Doc13. https://doi.org/10.3205/000300. PMID: 34867135; PMCID: PMC8607608
38. Wang W, Cheng J, Zhang J, Wang K. Effect of hyperbaric oxygen on neurologic sequelae and all-cause mortality in patients with carbon monoxide poisoning: a meta-analysis of randomized controlled trials. Med Sci Monit. 2019;13(25):7684–93. https://doi.org/10.12659/MSM.917065. PMID: 31606731; PMCID: PMC6807531
39. Weaver LK, Valentine KJ, Hopkins RO. Carbon monoxide poisoning: risk factors for cognitive sequelae and the role of hyperbaric oxygen. Am J Respir Crit Care Med. 2007;176(5):491–7. https://doi.org/10.1164/rccm.200701-026OC. Epub 2007 May 11. PMID: 17496229
40. Vogel SN, Sultan TR, Ten Eyck RP. Cyanide poisoning. Clin Toxicol. 1981;18(3):367–83. https://doi.org/10.3109/15563658108990043. PMID: 7016420
41. Mathieu D, Marroni A, Kot J. Tenth European Consensus Conference on Hyperbaric Medicine: recommendations for accepted and non-accepted clinical indications and practice of hyperbaric oxygen treatment. Diving Hyperb Med. 2017 Mar;47(1):24-32. https://doi.org/10.28920/dhm47.1.24-32. Erratum in: Diving Hyperb Med. 2017 Jun;47(2):131-132. PMID: 28357821; PMCID: PMC6147240.
42. Almeling M, Welslau W. Hyperbare Sauerstofftherapie–Qualitätsstandards, Gesellschaft für Tauch-und Überdruckmedizin (GTÜM) eV. 2nd ed. Kiel: Archimedes; 1996.
43. Sanders RW, Katz KD, Suyama J, Akhtar J, O'Toole KS, Corll D, Ladenburger RN. Seizure during hyperbaric oxygen therapy for carbon monoxide toxicity: a case series and five-year experience. J Emerg Med. 2012;42(4):e69–72. https://doi.org/10.1016/j.jemermed.2008.12.017. Epub 2009 Apr 15. PMID: 19372022
44. Wolf SJ, Lavonas EJ, Sloan EP, Jagoda AS. American College of Emergency Physicians. Clinical policy: Critical issues in the management of adult patients presenting to the emergency department with acute carbon monoxide poisoning. Ann Emerg Med. 2008;51(2):138–52. https://doi.org/10.1016/j.annemergmed.2007.10.012. PMID: 18206551
45. National Institute for Health and Care Excellence (NICE) Clinical Knowledge Summaries: Carbon Monoxide Poisoning.
46. Shahsavand S, Mohammadpour AH, Rezaee R, Behravan E, Sakhtianchi R, Moallem SA. Effect of Erythropoietin on Serum Brain-derived Biomarkers after Carbon Monoxide Poisoning in Rats. Iran J Basic. Med Sci. 2012;15(2):752–8. PMID: 23493953; PMCID: PMC3586885
47. Pang L, Bian M, Zang XX, Wu Y, Xu DH, Dong N, Wang ZH, Yan BL, Wang DW, Zhao HJ, Zhang N. Neuroprotective effects of erythropoietin in patients with carbon monoxide poisoning. J Biochem Mol Toxicol. 2013;27(5):266–71. https://doi.org/10.1002/jbt.21484. Epub 2013 Apr 3. PMID: 23554277
48. Kumral A, Genc S, Kutluk K, Ozkan H. Safety concerns with the clinical use of erythropoietin in acute ischemic stroke. Stroke. 2010;41(7):e469. https://doi.org/10.1161/STROKEAHA.110.585943. Epub 2010 May 13. PMID: 20466989
49. Wang W, Tian L, Li Y, Wang X, Xia F, Li L, Li J, Zhang Z. Effects of hydrogen-rich saline on rats with acute carbon monoxide poisoning. J Emerg Med. 2013;44(1):107–15. https://doi.org/10.1016/j.jemermed.2012.01.065. Epub 2012 Aug 14. PMID: 22897968
50. Ghorbani M, Moallem S, Abnous K, Tabatabaee Yazdi SA, Movassaghi AR, Azizzadeh M, Mohamadpour AH. The effect of granulocyte colony-stimulating factor administration on carbon monoxide neurotoxicity in rats. Drug Chem Toxicol. 2013;36(1):102–8. https://doi.org/10.3109/01480545.2012.737802. PMID: 23167836
51. Yang J, Zhao X, Zhou Q, Jiang Q. Effects of nimodipine and fructose-1,6-diphosphate on cerebral damage in carbon monoxide poisoning mice. Chin Med J (Engl). 2003;116(12):1911–5. PMID: 14687483
52. Qingsong W, Yeming G, Xuechun L, Hongjuan L, Jing W. The free radical scavenger, edaravone, ameliorates delayed neuropsychological sequelae after acute carbon monoxide poisoning in rabbits. Undersea Hyperb Med. 2013;40(3):223–9. PMID: 23789557
53. Sun X, Xu H, Meng X, Qi J, Cui Y, Li Y, Zhang H, Xu L. Potential use of hyperoxygenated solution as a treatment strategy for carbon monoxide poisoning. PLoS One. 2013;8(12):e81779. https://doi.org/10.1371/journal.pone.0081779. PMID: 24312588; PMCID: PMC3847038

Chapter 10
Hyperbaric Oxygen Therapy in Necrotizing Soft Tissue Infections

Sulagna Bhattacharjee and Souvik Maitra

10.1 Introduction

Necrotizing soft tissue infections (NSTIs) encompass a wide spectrum of infections involving the epidermis, dermis, subcutaneous tissue, and muscle, clinically presenting as cellulitis, fasciitis, or myositis. It is also referred to as "flesh eating bug disease." NSTI is variably referred to as necrotizing fasciitis, Fournier's gangrene (FG), and gas gangrene or clostridial myonecrosis. Annual incidence varies substantially, with an estimated rate of 4/100,000 population in developed countries [1]. Although presentation can differ based on infectious etiology or anatomical site, the principles of diagnostic and therapeutic management remain similar. The clinical course is characterized by non-specific symptoms in the early phase, such as fever, tachycardia, swelling, pain, and erythema, followed by severe fulminant tissue necrosis with hemorrhagic bulla, crepitus, and foul-smelling discharge, progressing to sepsis with multiorgan failure. Mortality is high unless treated early. With a historically reported mortality to be as high as 76%, recent studies have reported mortality ranging from 16% to 34% [2, 3].

The initial introduction of pathogenic bacteria to the soft tissues occurs via trauma, surgery, or even spontaneously, followed by rapid bacterial proliferation and endotoxin release. This results in leukocyte platelet adhesion and aggregation, vascular occlusion, edema, and tissue necrosis. NSTIs can be broadly classified as follows:

(a) Necrotizing fascitis (NF) is a rapidly spreading infection (2–3 cm/hour) of the relatively poorly vascularized muscle fascia and the overlying subcutaneous fat,

S. Bhattacharjee (✉) · S. Maitra
Department of Anaesthesiology, Pain Medicine and Critical Care, All India Institute of Medical Sciences, New Delhi, India
e-mail: souvikmaitra@aiims.edu

A. G. D'Almeida, J. Hidalgo (eds.), *Evidence-Based Hyperbaric Medicine*,
https://doi.org/10.1007/978-3-032-06346-5_10

in contrast to the underlying muscle, which remains unaffected. The overlying skin may remain normal in the initial stages, with the development of skin anesthesia preceding skin necrosis. Incidence ranges from 0.3% to 15%/100,000 population. Microbiologically, NF can be classified as follows:

- Polymicrobial infections caused by both anaerobic and aerobic bacteria, typically in combination with an anaerobic (Bacteroides, Clostridium, or Peptostreptococcus), an Enterobacteriaceae (*Escherichia coli*, Klebsiella, etc.), and a facultative anaerobic streptococcus. NF of the perineum, occurring due to breach of gastrointestinal or urothelial mucosal integrity, is termed as FG . NF in the head and neck region can occur from a breach of the oropharyngeal membrane following surgery, instrumentation, or dental procedures.
- Monomicrobial infections due to Group A streptococci (GAS) can occur across all age groups and in patients without comorbidities.

(b) Necrotizing myositis is a rare infection of the skeletal muscles, caused by GAS or other beta-hemolytic streptococci. Another spectrum comprises the clostridial myonecrosis or gas gangrene, occurring commonly following trauma or rarely spontaneously.
(c) Necrotizing cellulitis, characterized by pain, swelling, and crepitus, is a relatively milder variant caused by clostridial or polymicrobial infections [4, 5].

Early diagnosis, along with early surgical debridement, use of appropriate broad-spectrum antibiotics, and supportive therapy form the cornerstones of management. Hyperbaric oxygen therapy (HBOT) has been commonly used as an adjunctive treatment for NSTI to reduce morbidity and mortality.

10.1.1 Mechanism of Action of HBOT

Infected necrotic tissue, edema, and blocked blood vessels result in local tissue hypoxia. Hyperbaric oxygen (HBO) is a form of treatment that delivers 100% oxygen at ambient pressures more than the atmospheric pressure. The mechanism of the benefit of HBOT in NSTI is multifactorial (Fig. 10.1) [2, 4].

1. Hyperoxia: At a pressure of 2 atmospheric absolute (ATA), dissolved oxygen partial pressure can increase by 17 times, muscle oxygen tension by eight times, and tissue oxygen tension by four times, with an increase in the effective diffusion range of oxygen. This salvages critically compromised ischemic areas.
2. Antimicrobial effect: Bacterial killing by direct effect on anaerobic bacteria through the generation of oxygen free radicals, and by potentiating the phagocytic activity of white blood cells.
3. Potentiation of antibiotic efficacy: Potentiates the action of antibiotics like aminoglycosides.

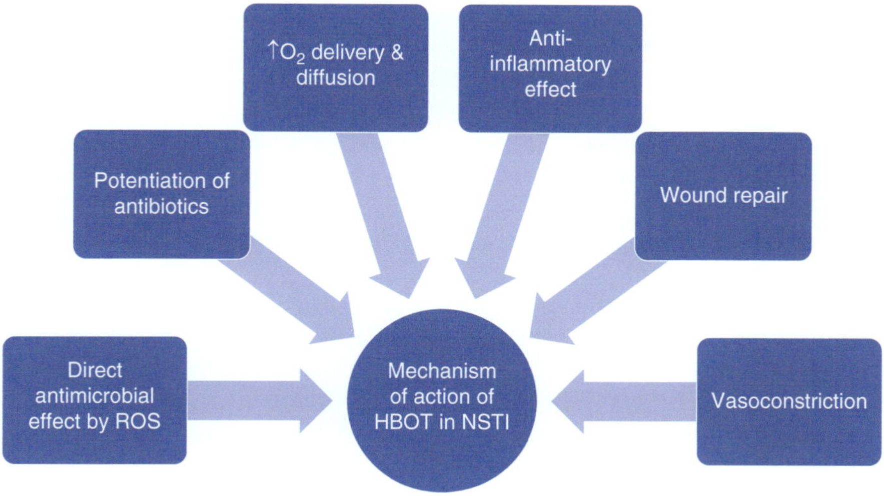

Fig. 10.1 Mechanism of action of HBOT in NSTI

4. Wound healing: Promotes growth of fibroblasts and angiogenesis, stimulating wound healing.
5. Anti-inflammatory action: HBO exhibits anti-inflammatory properties, by preventing endothelial damage and reducing ischemia reperfusion injury, reducing inflammatory cytokines, and stimulating the production of anti-inflammatory enzymes.
6. Vasoconstriction: Hyperoxic vasoconstriction reduces tissue edema and redistribution of blood to ischemic regions.

The most important application of the antimicrobial effect of HBOT is in NSTI . HBOT directly inhibits the growth of anaerobic bacteria like *Clostridium difficile* at tissue oxygen tension of 70 mmHg and inhibits production of its alpha toxin at 250 mmHg. Biofilm shrinkage for anaerobic bacteria and fungi has also been demonstrated with the use of HBOT. The anti-inflammatory effect of HBOT limits tissue damage beyond the infected sites and prevents reperfusion injury by reducing the production of reactive oxygen species by leukocytes [1].

As in hypoxia, hyperoxia too induces the generation of hypoxia inducible factor (HIF), which, in turn, activates multiple pathways involving production of reactive oxygen and nitrogen species, growth factors, activation of stem cells, neovascularization, and immunomodulation. This is referred to as the hyperoxic–hypoxic paradox. HIF induces production of nitric oxide (NO) synthases and other antimicrobial peptides like defensins, which enhance phagocytosis by neutrophils and macrophages [5, 6].

Reactive oxygen species exert a dose-dependent mode of effect on DNA damage, membrane lipid peroxidation, and protein denaturation, thereby inducing direct bactericidal effect on species lacking antioxidant pathways. Downregulation of inflammatory cytokines such as TNF-alpha, interleukin (IL)-1, and IL-6, transient reduction in CD4:CD8 ratio, and upregulation of anti-inflammatory cytokine IL-10 result in wound healing [7].

Hyperoxia can influence antibiotic efficacy, such as beta-lactams, aminoglycosides, and quinolones, whose action partly depends on the bacterial aerobic metabolism. The efficacy of vancomycin, teicoplanin, and linezolid has shown a significant increase when used in conjunction with HBOT for methicillin-resistant *Staphylococcus aureus*. HBOT has also been shown to be helpful in treating drug-resistant bugs like OXA-48-producing *Klebsiella pneumonia,* causing osteomyelitis [7].

The early use of HBOT in mice models of sepsis demonstrated improved survival within 1 hour of cecal ligation and puncture, as compared to no HBOT (52% vs. 13%). Multiple sessions of HBOT beyond 1 hour did not add to the survival benefit. The benefit was attributed to the reduction in systemic inflammatory response as evidenced by decreased expression of cytokines such as TNF alpha, IL-6, and IL-10 [8].

10.1.2 Recommendations

The 10th European Consensus Conference (2017) on Hyperbaric Medicine formulated consensus-agreed recommendations on the standard practice of hyperbaric medicine. Though the level of evidence is C (weak evidence based on uncontrolled studies), these recommendations are type 1, based on strong agreement among the experts [9].

- HBOT is recommended in the treatment of anaerobic or mixed bacterial infection.
- HBOT should be used for the treatment of NSTI in any location, especially perineal infection (FG).
- HBOT should be integrated with early optimum surgical intervention and broad-spectrum antibiotic therapy directed to treat the common anerobic and aerobic bacteria.

The National Health Service England specialized services clinical reference group, after a detailed review of available literature in 2018 for clinical commissioning policy on HBOT, found a scarcity of high-quality evidence and discrepancies among the studies, due to which they failed to arrive at a conclusion. Though HBOT may reduce mortality, it can also increase the duration of hospital stay and the cost of treatment. Therefore, they were unable to recommend this treatment for patients with NSTI [10].

10.1.3 *Dose of HBOT*

Though the precise dosing schedule of HBOT in NSTI varies from center to center, the common protocol involves application of HBOT with 100% oxygen at 2–3 ATA, for 60–120 minute sessions, twice within 24 hours, followed by one or two sessions daily thereafter, till there is no evidence of necrosis, or for a prolonged period depending on the response to treatment [1].

10.1.3.1 Evidence From Clinical Studies

Since Brummelkamp's report of successful application of hyperbaric oxygen at 3 ATA to treat anaerobic infections [11], HBOT has been used widely over the last 50 years for NSTI. The antimicrobial effect of HBOT has been used in several clinical scenarios, such as NSTI, surgical site infection, traumatic wounds, diabetic foot, and osteomyelitis. However, evidence in support of HBOT in NF is limited in the absence of randomized controlled trials.

One of the major studies that evaluated the role of HBOT in NSTI was published in 2012 as a large retrospective review of the nationwide inpatient sample of the US database involving 45,913 patients during the time period of 1988–2009. Patients who received HBOT had a lower mortality (4.5% vs. 9.4%, $p = 0.001$). After adjusting for confounders, HBOT was associated with a statistically significant lower risk of mortality, increased treatment cost, and increased duration of hospital stay, which was attributed to HBOT. No adverse effects were reported. Contrary to the popular belief, patients with clostridial myonecrosis did not appear to benefit from HBOT . However, this database review had several limitations, such as a lack of complete information on several important baseline clinical variables, such as time and adequacy of surgical debridement, extent of myonecrosis, use of appropriate antibiotics, baseline serum lactate level, disease severity scale, use of supportive therapy, dose of HBOT used, and so on [12].

Another important study published by Shaw et al. in 2014 included 1583 NSTI cases from the database of 14 HBOT-capable centers under the University Health Consortium, during the time period of 2008–2010. A total of 117 patents received HBOT. No difference in mortality, length of hospital stay, direct cost of treatment, or complications was found on univariate analysis across all (minor, moderate, severe) severity of illness (SOI) classes. However, the extreme SOI group showed reduced mortality (4% vs. 23%, $p = 0.01$), as well as complications (45% vs. 66%) with HBOT use, with no increased cost or hospital stay. Multivariable analysis revealed an increased risk of death in patients who did not receive HBOT during index hospitalization [13].

A single-center retrospective case–control study from an HBOT facility in Australia reported the outcome of HBOT use in 341 patients from 2002 to 2014, of whom 275 received HBOT. Polymicrobial infection was more common (50.7%) than monomicrobial Group A streptococcal infection (25.7%). The dose of HBOT was 90 minutes at 2.8 ATA, with two to three sessions on day 1, followed by two sessions on day 2, and daily as required thereafter. HBOT was significantly associated with a reduction in mortality when adjusted for disease severity and need for ICU care. This study also highlights that not just type 1, but type 2 NSTIs too can benefit from early application of HBOT [14].

Meanwhile, several small observational studies reported no benefit of HBOT in NSTI. In a retrospective analysis of 80 patients by Massey et al., HBOT did not appear to decrease in hospital mortality or amputation rate, even after adjusting for age, comorbidity, and disease severity [15]. Similarly, George et al. in 2009 reported no mortality benefit of HBOT, but rather an increased requirement of debridement in the HBOT group [16].

With the publication of several small and large studies on HBOT, a systematic review for the Cochrane database was attempted (2015). However, no high-quality randomized trials were found to support or refute the use of adjunctive HBOT in NSTI. HBOT was also found to be rarely associated with adverse effects. The authors highlighted the need for future multicentric randomized controlled studies [17]. A recent Danish population registry-based analysis (2023) reported that HBOT was associated with a significant reduction in mortality after propensity score matching. The benefit of HBOT was evident both in patients with or without septic shock and in patients with high SAPS II scores [18]. This study recruited more than 600 patients with NSTI, and more than 250 patients received HBOT.

In 2021, Hedetoft et al. published a systematic review and meta-analysis [1] of 21 retrospective studies involving more than 48,000 patients of NSTI, with 1237 patients receiving HBOT versus 47,507 patients treated without HBOT, which reported a possible survival advantage of HBOT over standard management with an odds ratio of 0.44 (95% CI 0.33–0.58). This was suggestive of a number needed of roughly 19 with HBOT to prevent 1 death from NSTI, as calculated from the odds ratio. Though the requirement of debridement was increased with HBOT, the requirement of amputation remained similar. However, only a small number of studies reported these outcomes. Complications such as sepsis, shock, myocardial infarction, and so on were similar, but the incidence of multiorgan dysfunction syndrome was reduced with the use of HBOT. Although this meta-analysis was PROSPERO registered and had a robust plan for statistical analysis, the results should be interpreted with caution. First, all the included studies in this review were retrospective in nature. Second, the indications, duration, and frequency of HBOT were different across the studies and incurred significant heterogeneity. Third, the duration of follow-up was also variable, and mostly, long-term follow-up data were unavailable. Fourth, though the review included a large number of patients, nearly 90% of the patients are from the large database review mentioned above. However, a sensitivity analysis excluding the largest study did not significantly affect the pooled estimate, implying that the result of this meta-analysis was not biased by the inclusion of this study. Finally, visual inspection of the funnel plot for mortality revealed the existence of possible publication bias in favor of HBOT.

Another recent meta-analysis of 23 retrospective studies [2], incorporating the recent publications, included data of more than 49,000 patients, of whom 1448 patients were treated with HBOT. It reported a significant reduction in mortality rate (with HBOT 10.6% and without HBOT 25.6%). The benefit from HBOT was evident in patients with FG and in other types of NSTIs. This meta-analysis also reported a higher requirement of surgical debridement in the HBOT group, but a similar rate of amputation. An interesting finding of the study was that the development os multi-organ dysfunction syndrome appeared to be less with the use of HBOT.

FG is one of the most serious manifestations of NSTIs, causing a high mortality ranging from 18% to 50%, with an average of 20–30%. A meta-analysis of 10 retrospective observational studies from 1998 to 2021, which investigated the effect of HBOT specifically in patients with FG, included around 650 patients, of whom 269 received HBOT. Patients with HBOT had a significantly lower mortality as compared to the non-HBOT group (odds ratio 0.29, 95% CI 0.12–0.69, $p = 0.005$). However, the requirement of surgical debridement and the length of hospital stay were not significantly different. As with the previous meta-analyses, this one too has serious drawbacks. Lack of standardization of other confounding factors such as adequacy of antibiotic therapy and use of other adjunctive therapy, high degree of heterogeneity in terms of baseline characteristics, intervention, and study end points limits the interpretation of its results to arrive at a definitive conclusion [19].

10.2 Conclusion

Evidence from the meta-analyses of nonrandomized studies involving large populations of patients with NSTIs shows that HBOT, as an adjunctive therapy, reduces the risk of dying, without causing any significant adverse event related to treatment. HBOT appears beneficial across type 1 or type 2 NSTIs, in different anatomical sites, and in both anerobic and aerobic infections, and across all SOI categories. Although the evidence is weak, data from uncontrolled studies are more likely to include patients from the full spectrum of clinical presentations, making the results more generalizable. Significant heterogeneity of the studies with respect to the treatment intervention, for example, the pressure applied, duration, and the number of HBOT sessions, limits the formulation of optimum dosing recommendations. Considering the rarity of the disease and limited availability of HBOT across health care facilities, high-quality randomized controlled trials need to be carefully designed to establish the dose and efficacy of HBOT in NSTIs.

References

1. Hedetoft M, Bennett MH, Hyldegaard O. Adjunctive hyperbaric oxygen treatment for necrotising soft-tissue infections: a systematic review and meta-analysis. Diving Hyperb Med. 2021;51(1):34–43.

2. Huang C, Zhong Y, Yue C, et al. The effect of hyperbaric oxygen therapy on the clinical outcomes of necrotizing soft tissue infections: a systematic review and meta-analysis. World J Emerg Surg. 2023;18:23.
3. Steiner T, Seiffart A, Schumann J, Bucher M. Hyperbaric oxygen therapy in necrotizing soft tissue infections: a retrospective study. Adv Exp Med Biol. 2018;1072:263–7.
4. Stevens DL, Baddour LM. Necrotizing soft tissue infections. Wessels MR & Edwards MS, ed. UpToDate. Waltham, MA: UpToDate Inc. https://www.uptodate.com. Accessed on 28 July 2023
5. Ortega MA, Fraile-Martinez O, García-Montero C, Callejón-Peláez E, Sáez MA, Álvarez-Mon MA, García-Honduvilla N, Monserrat J, Álvarez-Mon M, Bujan J, Canals ML. A general overview on the hyperbaric oxygen therapy: applications, mechanisms and translational opportunities. Medicina (Kaunas). 2021;57(9):864.
6. Hadanny A, Efrati S. The hyperoxic-hypoxic paradox. Biomolecules. 2020;10(6):958. https://doi.org/10.3390/biom10060958.
7. Memar MY, Yekani M, Alizadeh N, Baghi HB. Hyperbaric oxygen therapy: Antimicrobial mechanisms and clinical application for infections. Biomed Pharmacother. 2019;109:440–7.
8. Halbach JL, Prieto JM, Wang AW, Hawisher D, Cauvi DM, Reyes T, Okerblom J, Ramirez-Sanchez I, Villarreal F, Patel HH, Bickler SW, Perdrizet GA, De Maio A. Early hyperbaric oxygen therapy improves survival in a model of severe sepsis. Am J Physiol Regul Integr Comp Physiol. 2019;317(1):R160–8.
9. Mathieu D, Marroni A, Kot J. Tenth European Consensus Conference on Hyperbaric Medicine: recommendations for accepted and non-accepted clinical indications and practice of hyperbaric oxygen treatment. Diving Hyperb Med. 2017;47(1):24–32.
10. Clinical Commissioning Policy: Hyperbaric Oxygen Therapy for necrotising soft tissue infections (all ages). https://www.england.nhs.uk/wp-content/uploads/2018/07/hbot-for-necrotising-soft-tissue-infections-v2.pdf. Accessed on 28 July 2023
11. Brummelkamp WH, Hogendyk J, Boerema I. Treatment of anaerobic infections by drenching the tissue with oxygen under high atmospheric pressure. Surgery. 1961;49(3):299–302.
12. Soh CR, Pietrobon R, Freiberger JJ, Chew ST, Rajgor D, Gandhi M, Shah J, Moon RE. Hyperbaric oxygen therapy in necrotising soft tissue infections: a study of patients in the United States Nationwide Inpatient Sample. Intensive Care Med. 2012;38(7):1143–51.
13. Shaw JJ, Psoinos C, Emhoff TA, Shah SA, Santry HP. Not just full of hot air: hyperbaric oxygen therapy increases survival in cases of necrotizing soft tissue infections. Surg Infect (Larchmt). 2014;15(3):328–35.
14. Devaney B, Frawley G, Frawley L, Pilcher DV. Necrotising soft tissue infections: the effect of hyperbaric oxygen on mortality. Anaesth Intensive Care. 2015;43(6):685–92.
15. Massey PR, Sakran JV, Mills AM, Sarani B, Aufhauser DD Jr, Sims CA, Pascual JL, Kelz RR, Holena DN. Hyperbaric oxygen therapy in necrotizing soft tissue infections. J Surg Res. 2012;177(1):146–51.
16. George ME, Rueth NM, Skarda DE, Chipman JG, Quickel RR, Beilman GJ. Hyperbaric oxygen does not improve outcome in patients with necrotizing soft tissue infection. Surg Infect (Larchmt). 2009;10(1):21–8.
17. Levett DZ, Bennett MH, Millar I. Adjunctive hyperbaric oxygen for necrotizing fasciitis. CDSR. 2015; Issue 1. Art. No.: CD007937
18. Hedetoft M, Madsen MB, Hyldegaard O. Hyperbaric oxygen treatment in the management of necrotising soft-tissue infections: results from a Danish nationwide registry study. BMJ Open. 2023;13(2):e066117.
19. Raizandha MA, Hidayatullah F, Kloping YP, Rahman IA, Djatisoesanto W, Rizaldi F. The role of hyperbaric oxygen therapy in Fournier's Gangrene: A systematic review and meta-analysis of observational studies. Int Braz J Urol. 2022;48(5):771–81.

Chapter 11
Refractory Osteomyelitis

Ahsina Jahan Lopa and Srikant Behera

11.1 Introduction

The inflammation of bone and bone marrow due to infectious etiology is called osteomyelitis. This infection of bone and bone marrow may be caused by systemic blood infections, from the extension of the local infections, or due to a traumatic infection. Almost all microorganisms, including bacteria, viruses, fungi, and so on, can cause osteomyelitis. The most common organism responsible for osteomyelitis in adults is *Staphylococcus aureus*. The other common causative agents causing osteomyelitis are Salmonella, *Staphylococcus epidermidis*, *Pseudomonas aeruginosa*, *Serratia marcescens*, *Escherichia coli*, Bartonella, Mycobacteria, Candida, Cryptococcus, and so on [1]. Osteomyelitis is a difficult-to-treat condition in view of the paucity of the vascular supply and the limited penetration of antimicrobial agents into the bone. There is a high risk of morbidity and mortality in patients suffering from osteomyelitis particularly when the spine, skull, or sternum is affected. When there is persistence of infection in the bone and bone marrow characterized by the presence of microorganisms, sequestrum, inflammation, and so on, it is termed chronic osteomyelitis [2]. It commonly happens after a grossly contaminated complicated fracture, but also sometimes after prosthetic joint replacement, and fracture internal fixation surgery. Its management requires treatment with antibiotics for a long duration, staged surgeries, prolonged hospital stay, and high cost of therapy. Managing a case of chronic osteomyelitis continues to be a challenge for

A. J. Lopa
Department of ICU and Emergency, Brahmanbaria ICU Specialized Hospital, Brahmanbaria, Bangladesh

S. Behera (✉)
Department of General Medicine, All India Institute of Medical Sciences (AIIMS), Bhubaneswar, Odisha, India
e-mail: genmed_srikant@aiimsbhubaneswar.edu.in

A. G. D'Almeida, J. Hidalgo (eds.), *Evidence-Based Hyperbaric Medicine*,
https://doi.org/10.1007/978-3-032-06346-5_11

the treating team. It compromises the mobility, functional status, and independence, especially when it affects the young population in the productive age group [3].

11.2 Refractory Osteomyelitis

The acute osteomyelitis that did not respond to standard treatment modalities, and persists in spite of best accepted therapy, or the chronic osteomyelitis that persists or recurs even after the appropriate therapeutic interventions, is defined as refractory osteomyelitis. Usually, when patients suffering from osteomyelitis do not respond to appropriate therapeutic interventions for at least 4–6 weeks, they are referred to as having chronic refractory osteomyelitis. This leads to significant morbidity, mortality, as well as negatively affects the quality of life with pain and decreased functional status [4].

11.3 Epidemiology

The overall incidence of osteomyelitis is about 21.8 cases per 100,000 person-years. The incidence of osteomyelitis is higher in the male population as compared to females, but the exact cause is not known. The incidence of osteomyelitis increases with increasing age, the likely explanation for this being the increased prevalence of comorbid conditions such as diabetes mellitus and peripheral vascular disease [5, 6].

Almost half of the cases of osteomyelitis are from the infected post-traumatic complicated fractures. The other important causes that favor osteomyelitis are diabetic neuropathy, hematogenous spread of infections, and so on. Osteomyelitis is more common in patients with immunocompromised status, having uncontrolled diabetes, intravenous (IV) drug abusers, and so on. The incidence of osteomyelitis varies from 4% to 64% in cases of long-bone fractures and from 1% to 2% cases of prosthetic joint replacement surgery. The incidence rate of osteomyelitis is much higher in the range of 2–20% in the case of revision joint replacement surgery. The resolution rate of osteomyelitis with appropriate management varies from 35% to 100%, and the overall cure rate is in the range of 70–80%. The recurrence rate of osteomyelitis ranges from 20% to 30%. When the infection progresses or persists in spite of best possible medical and surgical interventions, this results in refractory osteomyelitis [1, 7–10].

11.4 Etiology

The most common organism causing osteomyelitis is *Staphylococcus aureus*. *Staphylococcus aureus* is responsible for about two-third of cases of osteomyelitis in adult patients. In pediatrics population, Streptococcus along with Staphylococcus infection contributes to the majority of cases of osteomyelitis. The other common organisms causing osteomyelitis are *Staphylococcus epidermidis*, *Enterococcus* spp., *Pseudomonas aeruginosa*, *Enterobacter* spp., *Mycobacterium* spp., anaerobes, fungi, and so on [1, 9, 11–16]. The osteomyelitis caused by methicillin-resistant staphylococcus aureus (MRSA) and multidrug-resistant (MDR) organisms is posing more and more challenges in the management of these cases [9]. Multiple organisms may be isolated from osteomyelitis caused by the contiguous spread of infection. In a large series of osteomyelitis cases, about 30% cases were found to have polymicrobial infection [16].

11.5 Pathophysiology

The pathophysiology of osteomyelitis starts when an infection affects the bone either from the hematogenous spread from a distant source, or a contiguous spread of infection from the surrounding tissue and joints, or directly by the inoculation of infection into the bone from trauma or surgery. In the pediatric population, osteomyelitis occurs commonly by hematogenous spread of infection, whereas osteomyelitis in young adults usually occurs by the spread of infection from contiguous structures, usually in the setting of trauma and trauma-related surgery. The contiguous spread of infection causing osteomyelitis may also follow the surgical procedure for an open fracture, including placement of prosthetics. The osteomyelitis in older patients is typically related to infected neuropathic/decubitus ulcers and prosthetic joint replacement surgery. The common site of osteomyelitis varies from pediatric to adult population, also from one etiology to another. In case of hematogenous spread of infection causing osteomyelitis, the long bones are usually affected in children, whereas the vertebra is commonly affected in adults. In patients with diabetes, osteomyelitis usually results from vascular insufficiency to the lower extremities, which contributes to impaired local immunity and skin healing, promoting the spread of infection. Also, the diabetic neuropathy predisposes to the formation of skin ulceration at pressure and trauma points, favoring the progression of osteomyelitis. Contiguous spread of infections causing osteomyelitis frequently develops following pressure sores, especially in the pressure-bearing points such as sacrum, buttock, hips, and heel. These decubitus ulcers are usually colonized by polymicrobial flora from the skin and gastrointestinal tract and microorganisms from these colonizations spread quickly to the underlying bone causing polymicrobial osteomyelitis. The polymicrobial osteomyelitis also occurs in cases of trauma, leading to infected, exposed skin, and soft tissue. Osteomyelitis can also occur by the direct inoculation of bacteria in case of open fractures, bone reconstructive surgery, or other orthopedic interventions [1, 17, 18].

Chronic osteomyelitis may result from inadequately or improperly treated acute osteomyelitis originating either from a hematogenous spread of infection or more commonly from a contiguous source of infection. There is an inflammatory obliteration of vasculature supplying the bones following acute osteomyelitis. If the infection is not managed promptly and adequately, inadequate blood supply along with cytokines (e.g., IL6, TNF, etc.) present at the site of infection leads to necrosis of bone. This results in the formation of sequestrum, and the sequestrum provides a base for the formation of the biofilm. The biofilm is developed in a step-wise manner: initially, there is adhesion of microorganisms to a surface (e.g., sequestrum, prosthesis, etc.), followed by multiplication of the microbes and then formation of an organized structure with a high density of microorganisms surrounded by a matrix formed by polysaccharides. Inside the biofilm, the microorganisms are protected from the host immune system as well as from the effect of antibiotics, stay inactive due to limited access to oxygen and nutrients, but these microorganisms remain as the persisters. The inflammatory cells along with the cytokines lead to further bone destruction of bone, and microorganisms propagate within the destroyed bone. There is also new bone formed from the intact periosteum and endosteum, and called as involucrum. There are many factors that help the progression of acute osteomyelitis to chronic and refractory osteomyelitis. The major factors responsible for chronic osteomyelitis are the presence of sequestrum, foreign bodies, for example, metal implants, virulent organisms, immunocompromised host status, and so on [11, 19, 20].

11.6 Classification

Osteomyelitis was classified by Waldvogel et al. on the basis of the presumed mechanism of infection into the bone either from the hematogenous spread or from the direct inoculation from the contiguous infected soft-tissue or from a chronic infected open wound. This system of classification does not help in any decision-making for treatment or for prognostication purposes, so it has very limited use in clinical practice [21]. The widely used classification system for osteomyelitis was proposed by Cierny et al. (Cierny-Mader Classification). This takes into consideration of [A] the extent of bone involvement (medullary osteomyelitis—disease confined to the medullary cavity of bone; superficial osteomyelitis—medullary canal and superficial part of cortex involved; localized osteomyelitis—involving both cortical and medullary bone but stable; and diffuse osteomyelitis—involving the entire thickness of the bone and results in structural instability); [B] the physiologic class of the patient (normal physiologic response—minimal or none, local or systemic factors; local impairment—cellulitis, prior trauma, surgery, presence of scar, or sinus; systemic factors—coexistent diseases such as diabetes, immunocompromise, vascular disease, hypoproteinemia; severe infection—severe systemic and local compromise);

and [C] systemic factors such as malnutrition, renal or hepatic failure, diabetes mellitus, chronic hypoxia, malignancy, extremes of age, immunosuppression or deficiency, and so on, and local factors such as chronic lymphedema, major-vessel compromise, small-vessel disease, vasculitis, venous stasis, extensive scarring, radiation fibrosis, neuropathy, tobacco abuse, and so on, affecting immune-system response, metabolism, and local vascularity [22]. This system of classification for osteomyelitis correlates with treatment as well as prognosis [23].

11.7 Clinical Features

In chronic refractory osteomyelitis, symptoms usually persist for a longer duration over a period of 4–6 weeks. There are varied presentations of osteomyelitis and no specific symptoms or signs to diagnose a case of chronic or refractory osteomyelitis. The patients with risk factors osteomyelitis such as uncontrolled diabetes, peripheral vascular disease, peripheral neuropathy, immunocompromised status, decubitus ulcers, history of open/compound fracture, post orthopedic prosthetic implantation, and so on who presents with deep or extensive non healing ulcers in spite of adequate therapy should be evaluated for chronic refractory osteomyelitis. The presenting features are fever, pain, swelling, redness, tenderness, and other signs of inflammation at the site of infection. Fever and other constitutional symptoms of infections may not be that prominent in a case of chronic refractory osteomyelitis. The other various manifestations are malaise, generalized weakness, chronic pain, chronic non-healing ulcer, tissue necrosis, persistent wound discharge, open wound, exposed bone, presence of a sinus tracts, and so on. These clinical features may be persistent or even occur recurrently after a period of quiescence [2, 24].

11.8 Laboratory Diagnosis

The diagnosis of chronic refractory osteomyelitis needs careful history taking along with laboratory and radiological investigations. All routine investigations along with markers of infection need to be done in all cases. The total leukocyte count may be within normal limits in a case of chronic refractory osteomyelitis. Renal function and liver function test must be done to check for any organ dysfunction as well as to see the effects of treatment (antibiotics) on these organs' function. The non-specific markers of inflammation such as C-reactive protein and erythrocyte sedimentation rate are usually raised, and it is very important to follow their trends to monitor the disease progression and the response to therapy. The nutritional status must be monitored with albumin and prealbumin levels at regular intervals. Blood sugar and diabetes status of the patient need to be strictly monitored as uncontrolled blood sugar promotes non-healing ulcer and a very important risk factor for chronic refractory osteomyelitis. Laboratory investigations for microbiological analysis are a very important and crucial step in the diagnosis of chronic refractory osteomyelitis. Samples for microbiological evaluation must be collected from dipper tissues, and if required, bone biopsy should be performed for sample collection. In all cases, the microbiological sample must be sent for Gram staining, ZN staining, and cultures, including anaerobic as well as aerobic bacteria, fungus, and mycobacteria. One must remember that negative growth in culture does not rule out chronic osteomyelitis. Another important point to note in regard to microbiological diagnosis of chronic refractory osteomyelitis is that some of the low-virulence organisms may require prolonged incubation time for growth in culture media and may even need special culture media for their growth. With the advancement of modern diagnostics, polymerase chain reaction can be used for early microbiological diagnosis of difficult cases [25–27].

11.9 Radiology in Diagnosis

Radiographic imaging is vital in diagnosis and evaluation of extent of disease in a case of chronic refractory osteomyelitis. The commonly advised radiological tests for diagnosis of chronic refractory osteomyelitis are plain radiographs, magnetic resonance imaging (MRI), and technetium-99-based bone scintigraphy. Though a plain radiograph is many often the initial imaging of choice, an accurate diagnosis requires a combination of various radiological techniques. In a plain X-ray, the periostitis/osteitis, sequestrum, and involucrum (ta layer of new bone formed about the sequestrum) can be noted. CT scan offers better multiplanar imaging and is able to clearly show the bone changes of chronic refractory osteomyelitis such as details of cortical involvement, medullary canal encroachment, discharging sinus, as well as helps in the detection of sequestrum by surrounding osseous changes, which is not visualized by a plain radiograph. Computed tomography (CT) scan also helps in taking a sample for microbiological investigations, for example, aspiration and biopsy. MRI is another helpful radiological investigation for the assessment of chronic refractory osteomyelitis. It is very good at detecting factors critical to making a therapeutic decision such as the extent of the disease, disease activity, vascularity of the lesion, as well as viability of the tissues. An ultrasound may also provide useful information in diagnosing a chronic refractory osteomyelitis by localizing soft-tissue abscesses, especially in the presence of metal implants, where a CT scan or MRI may not provide valuable information. Another important modality of investigating a case of chronic refractory osteomyelitis is nuclear imaging. Though nuclear medicine imaging techniques are more useful in acute osteomyelitis cases, cases of bone scintigraphy and leukocyte scintigraphy have been extensively used for the diagnosis of chronic refractory osteomyelitis. Positron-emission tomography has higher accuracy in confirming or ruling out chronic osteomyelitis compared to bone scintigraphy or MRI, and it is the most sensitive and specific modality for the diagnosis of chronic refractory osteomyelitis. Bone scintigraphy and leukocyte scintigraphy are also commonly used for the diagnosis of chronic refractory osteomyelitis [1, 28, 29].

11.10 Treatment

While managing a case of osteomyelitis, various factors need to be taken into consideration. The important factors to be considered are the disease pathogenesis, the anatomical stage of the disease, the causative microorganism, the particular surgical procedure performed, the use of prosthetics, and various local as well as systemic host factors. The goal of treatment in a case of chronic refractory osteomyelitis is to eradicate the infection completely, to preserve the soft-tissue envelope, to allow healing of the bone segment, and to keep the limb length and function maintained. The mainstay of treatment for osteomyelitis is appropriate and adequate antibiotic therapy along with timely and proper surgical debridement of the wound. For patients who do not respond to appropriate and adequate therapy for 4–6 weeks, the diagnosis of chronic refractory osteomyelitis is made. Treatment with hyperbaric oxygen (HBO_2) therapy is considered an adjuvant treatment modality for chronic refractory osteomyelitis cases. The treatment plan has to be individualized after assessing the extent of disease, microbiological study, and optimizing the patient's physiological status. As there are many issues to be dealt with simultaneously while managing a case of osteomyelitis, a multidisciplinary team effort is required for better management. The team members should include an orthopedic and reconstructive surgery specialist, an infectious disease expert, a nutritionist, a wound care specialist, a hyperbaric medicine specialist, and a psychologist to treat these cases effectively. The treatment plan has to be individualized after proper workup, thorough assessment of the disease extent, microbiological evaluation, and radiological/nuclear imaging along with optimization of the physiological condition of the patient [30].

11.11 Antibiotic Therapy

Along with the proper surgical debridement of necrotic tissue, the adequate and effective antibiotic therapy forms the mainstay of treatment in a case of chronic refractory osteomyelitis. Antibiotics play a vital role in the management plan of chronic refractory osteomyelitis. A well-designed course of properly selected antibiotics in an optimal dose for an adequate duration is required for the treatment of the infection in a case of chronic refractory osteomyelitis. The antibiotic therapy must be tailored to the culture and sensitivity report of the identified microorganism from the lesion. Also, the antimicrobial susceptibility pattern of the isolated organism as well as the pharmacokinetic and pharmacodynamics parameters of the antibiotics to be administered must be kept in mind while treating a case of chronic refractory osteomyelitis. The various challenges faced during the antibiotic treatment of a chronic refractory osteomyelitis are the presence of necrotic tissue, biofilm formation, and adverse local medium at the site of infection, making the drug less effective. The antibiotics must be effective against the identified microorganism, as well as must attain the desired concentration at the site of action of the osteomyelitis. The route of administration can be IV or oral, depending on the pharmacological property of the drug, but the achievement of the desired drug concentration at the site of infection is one of the most important factors deciding the effectiveness of antimicrobial therapy. If an effective targeted antibiotic can be administered via oral route and able to achieve therapeutic drug concentration at the site of infection, it will be the preferred drug as the treatment of chronic refractory osteomyelitis requires prolonged duration of therapy. Oral antibiotic therapy is simple, economical, and more convenient for patients; it also avoids risks associated with the use of an IV access. Another controversial issue regarding the antibiotic treatment of chronic refractory osteomyelitis is the duration of therapy. In general, it requires more than 4–6 weeks of antibiotic therapy, as even after adequate surgical debridement of the necrotic tissue, the infected bed may still remain contaminated. The local application of an antimicrobial agent can also be considered in the management of chronic refractory osteomyelitis. The local antibiotic delivery system has progressed to include the polymethyl methacrylate (PMMA) bone cement for local application of antibiotics. A heat-stable and soluble antibiotic is impregnated into PMMA cement, and this antibiotic impregnated bone cement is used to provide structural supports and fill up the gap in the bone defect, as well as supplies high concentrations of medication locally with minimal systemic effects. The most commonly used antibiotics in PMMA bone cement are Vancomycin, Gentamycin, and Tobramycin. The duration of antibiotic therapy must be individualized according to the clinical profile of the patient and clinical-radiological response to the therapy. The patient to kept in close follow-up after the completion of the antibiotic course [14, 30–32].

11.12 Surgical Management

Standard treatment of chronic refractory osteomyelitis involves adequate surgical management of infected or necrotic tissue along with appropriate antibiotic therapy. The essential steps in the surgical management of chronic refractory osteomyelitis include adequate debridement, management of dead space, soft-tissue coverage, skeletal stabilization, and treatment of skeletal defects. The adequate and aggressive surgical debridement of infected and devitalized tissue, removal of foreign material, and reconstruction of soft tissue and bone defects are the cornerstone of successful treatment of chronic osteomyelitis, of course, along with the appropriate antimicrobial therapy. The dead space created after debridement should be managed properly either by mobilization of local muscle, rotational muscle flap, or a free-muscle flap [25, 33]. For the construction of a well-vascularized soft-tissue envelope, microvascular free-muscle transfer is considered the gold standard, though other options like rotational muscle flaps are available. The microsurgical vascularization procedure can be done in a single-stage procedure or as a two-stage procedure [34, 35]. Skeletal stabilization is a very important step in the surgical management of chronic refractory osteomyelitis. It is required following excision of the devitalized bone, and the preferred method is the external fixation. Internal fixation can also be considered after control of infection [36]. The bone defects are filled up with either autogenous bone grafts (if less than 6 cm) or by using distraction osteogenesis using an Ilizarov ring fixator or vascularized bone graft typically taken from the fibula for larger defects [37].

11.13 HBO_2 Therapy

As the patient with chronic refractory osteomyelitis do not respond to appropriate therapeutic interventions for at least 4–6 weeks, and it is associated with significant morbidity, mortality, as well as compromised quality of life with pain and decreased functional status, it is important to provide all possible available therapeutic modalities to improve the patient's function and to reduce the pain. The available data shows that the use of HBO_2 therapy as an adjuvant therapy in the management of chronic refractory osteomyelitis to the standard of care surgical management and antibiotics therapy leads to better outcomes in terms of functional recovery and resolution of infection. To get the best results, HBO_2 is to be administered along with culture directed antibiotics and adequate surgical debridement. HBO_2 therapy is administered by providing 100% oxygen (O_2) at 2.5–3 atmospheres of pressure for 90–120 minutes per session. Usually, HBO_2 is given on a daily basis for a period of 4–6 weeks. Commonly, 20–40 HBO_2 sessions are required to get sustained therapeutic benefit. HBO_2 therapy is recommended by the Underwater and Hyperbaric Medicine Society as an adjunctive therapy for chronic refractory osteomyelitis. If there is no clinical response to the culture-directed antibiotics and HBO_2 therapy, then the management plan should be reviewed and additional surgical debridement, and or modification of the antibiotics regimen should be considered on priority. Subsequently, HBO_2 therapy can be reinitiated to get the maximum benefit of therapy and increased chances of recovery [4, 38]. There are many rational features behind using HBO_2 in the management of chronic refractory osteomyelitis. The O_2 tension is reduced at the site of osteomyelitis. As the neutrophils require tissue oxygen tensions of 30–40 mmHg to destroy bacteria by oxidative killing mechanisms, by raising the O_2 tension at the osteomyelitis lesion site to physiologic or supraphysiologic levels, leukocyte-mediated killing of aerobic organisms is returned to normal or above normal levels. The HBO_2 therapy also has a direct suppressive effect on anaerobic organisms, and as the anaerobes contributes to significant number of cases of chronic refractory osteomyelitis, this has an impressive effect on clinical outcome. The transport of antibiotics (e.g., aminoglycosides, cephalosporins, etc.) across the bacterial cell wall is oxygen-dependent and is inhibited in a hypoxic environment. Therefore, HBO_2 therapy may enhance transport and augment the antibiotic efficacy. The osteoclast function in removing necrotic bone is an oxygen-dependent function, and also, the osteogenesis process is enhanced by HBO_2 therapy. So, HBO_2 therapy provided an optimal environment for the proper functioning of the host machinery in the recovery process. As the demarcation between healthy and involved bone is not clear at the time of surgical debridement, enhancement of osteoclast activity improves the overall quality of debridement and reduces the chances that local infection to recur. Finally, HBO_2 therapy has been shown to be acutely effective in reducing tissue edema, lowering intra-compartmental pressures, and ameliorating the detrimental effects of inflammatory reactions. Also, HBO_2 therapy favors new collagen formation and capillary angiogenesis in the hypoxic bone and surrounding tissues. This provides sustained improvements in the arterial perfusion of previously hypoxic bone and surrounding soft tissue. HBO_2 reduces the susceptibility of these tissues to recurrent infection and subsequent tissue breakdown [4, 39–41].

There is lack of high-quality data as well as standard practice guidelines for the use of HBO_2 therapy in the management of refractory osteomyelitis. The use of HBO_2 is also limited by the cost, availability, and risks involved. However, the available literature suggests its great potential in the management of refractory osteomyelitis [39, 42]. A recent systematic review compiling treatment outcomes of over 450 patients with chronic refractory osteomyelitis found that more than 70% responded to the management when HBO_2 was added to the therapeutic regimen [43]. Other studies have also shown benefit of using HBO_2 in the management of refractory osteomyelitis [44–46]. So, HBO_2 therapy is a useful adjunct in the management of refractory osteomyelitis. However, additional studies would help to validate its efficacy in the future.

11.14 Conclusion

Management of refractory osteomyelitis is challenging, needs a highly coordinated, efficient, and dedicated team due to the complicated nature of disease pathophysiology, prolonged course of therapy, requirement of multiple surgical interventions, and targeted antibiotics in an optimized manner, along with nutrition and psychological support. Though the main line of management involves surgical intervention and culture-sensitive targeted antibiotic therapy, HBO_2 therapy can be considered as an adjuvant modality of management along with the standard of care.

References

1. Hatzenbuehler J, Pulling TJ. Diagnosis and management of osteomyelitis. Am Fam Physician. 2011;84:1027–33.

2. Mouzopoulos G, Kanakaris NK, Kontakis G, Obakponovwe O, Townsend R, Giannoudis PV. Management of bone infections in adults: the surgeon's and microbiologist's perspectives. Injury. 2011;42(Suppl 5):S18–23.
3. Masini BD, Waterman SM, Wenke JC, Owens BD, Hsu JR, Ficke JR. Resource utilization and disability outcome assessment of combat casualties from operation Iraqi freedom and operation enduring freedom. J Orthop Trauma. 2009;23:261–6.
4. Hart BB. Hyperbaric oxygen for refractory osteomyelitis. Undersea Hyperb Med. 2021 Third Quarter;48(3):297–321. PMID: 34390634.
5. Kremers HM, Nwojo ME, Ransom JE, Wood-Wentz CM, Melton LJ, Huddleston PM. Trends in the epidemiology of osteomyelitis: a population-based study, 1969 to 2009. J Bone Joint Surg Am. 2015;97(10):837–45.
6. Kurtz SM, Lau E, Schmier J, Ong KL, Zhao K, Parvizi J. Infection burden for hip and knee arthroplasty in the United States. J Arthroplast. 2008;23:984–91.
7. Schenker ML, Yannascoli S, Baldwin KD, Ahn J, Mehta S. Does timing of operative debridement affect infectious complications in open long fractures? A systematic review. J Bone Joint Surg Am. 2012;94:1057–64.
8. Lentino JR. Prosthetic joint infections: bane of orthopedists, challenge for infectious disease specialists. Clin Infect Dis. 2003;36:1157–61.
9. Tice AD, Hoaglund PA, Shoultz DA. Risk factors and treatment outcomes in osteomyelitis. J Antimicrob Chemother. 2003;51:1261–8.
10. Conterno LO, Turchi MD. Antibiotics for treating chronic osteomyelitis in adults. Cochrane Database Syst Rev. 2013;9:CD004439.
11. Ciampolini J, Harding KG. Pathophysiology of chronic bacterial osteomyelitis. Why do antibiotics fail so often? Postgrad Med J. 2000;76:479–83.
12. Lew DP, Waldvogel FA. Osteomyelitis. Lancet. 2004;364:369–79.
13. Lazzarini L, Lipsky BA, Mader JT. Antibiotic treatment of osteomyelitis: what have we learned from 30 years of clinical trials? Int J Infect Dis. 2005;9:127–38.
14. Calhoun JH, Manring MM. Adult osteomyelitis. Infect Dis Clin N Am. 2005;19:765–86.
15. Jorge LS, Chueire AG, Baptista AR. Osteomyelitis: a current challenge. Braz J Infect Dis. 2010;14:310–5.
16. Sheehy SH, Atkins BA, Bejon P, et al. The microbiology of chronic osteomyelitis: prevalence of resistance to common empirical antimicrobial regimens. J Infect. 2010;60:338–43.
17. Schmitt SK. Osteomyelitis. Infect Dis Clin N Am. 2017 Jun;31(2):325–38.
18. Lew DP, Waldvogel FA. Osteomyelitis. N Engl J Med. 1997;336(14):999–1007.
19. Gristina AG, Oga M, Webb LX, Hobgood CD. Adherent bacterial colonization in the pathogenesis of osteomyelitis. Science. 1985;228:990–3.
20. Zimmerli W, Moser C. Pathogenesis and treatment concepts of orthopaedic biofilm infections. FEMS Immunol Med Microbiol. 2012;65:158–68.
21. Waldvogel FA, Medoff G, Swartz MN. Osteomyelitis: a review of clinical features, therapeutic considerations and unusual aspects. N Engl J Med. 1970;282:198–206.
22. Cierny G 3rd, Mader JT, Pennick JJ. A clinical staging system for adult osteomyelitis. Clin Orthop Relat Res. 2003;414:7–24.
23. Bowen TR, Widmaier JC. Host classification predicts infection after open fracture. Clin Orthop Relat Res. 2005;433:205–11.
24. American Society of Plastic Surgeons. Evidence based clinical practice guideline: chronic wounds of the lower extremity. 2007. Available from: http://www.plasticsurgery.org/Documents/medical-professionals/health-policy/evidence-practice/Evidence-based-Clinical-PracticeGuideline-Chronic-Wounds-of-the-Lower-Extremity.pdf. Accessed 22 April 2015.
25. Lazzarini L, Mader JT, Calhoun JH. Osteomyelitis in long bones. J Bone Joint Surg Am 2004;86-A:2305–2318.
26. Forsberg JA, Potter BK, Cierny G 3rd, Webb L. Diagnosis and management of chronic infection. J Am Acad Orthop Surg. 2011;19(Suppl 1):S8–S19.

27. Perry CR, Pearson RL, Miller GA. Accuracy of cultures of material from swabbing of the superficial aspect of the wound and needle biopsy in the preoperative assessment of osteomyelitis. J Bone Joint Surg Am. 1991;73:745–9.
28. Pineda C, Espinosa R, Pena A. Radiographic imaging in osteomyelitis: the role of plain radiography, computed tomography, ultrasonography, magnetic resonance imaging and scintigraphy. Semin Plast Surg. 2009;23:80–9.
29. Termaat MF, Raijmakers PG, Scholtein HJ, Bakker FC, Patka P, Haarman HJ. The accuracy of diagnostic imaging for the assessment of chronic osteomyelitis: a systematic review and meta-analysis. J Bone Joint Surg Am. 2005;87:2464–71.
30. Pande K. Optimal management of chronic osteomyelitis: current perspectives. Orthop Res Rev. 2015;7:71–81.
31. Chang Y, Chen WC, Hsieh PH. In vitro activities of daptomycin-, vancomycin-, and teicoplanin-loaded polymethylmethacrylate against methicillin-susceptible, methicillin-resistant, and vancomycin-intermediate strains of *Staphylococcus aureus*. Antimicrob Agents Chemother. 2011;55:5480–4.
32. Hanssen AD, Spangehl MJ. Practical applications of antibiotic-loaded bone cement for treatment of infected joint replacements. Clin Orthop. 2004;427:79–85.
33. Verhelle N, Van Zele D, Liboutton L, Heymans O. How to deal with bone exposure and osteomyelitis: an overview. Acta Orthop Belg. 2003;69:481–94.
34. Rhomberg M, Frischhut B, Ninkovic M, Schwabegger AH. A singlestage operation in the treatment of chronic osteomyelitis of the lower extremity including reconstruction with free vascularized iliac bone graft and free-tissue transfer. Plast Reconstr Surg. 2003;111:2353–61.
35. Dinh P, Hutchinson BK, Zalavaras C, Stevanovic MV. Reconstruction of osteomyelitis defects. Semin Plast Surg. 2009;23:108–18.
36. Paley D, Herzenberg JE. Intramedullary infections treated with antibiotic cement rods: preliminary results in nine cases. J Orthop Trauma. 2002;16:723–9.
37. Marsh DR, Shah S, Elliott J, Kurdy N. The Ilizarov method in nonunion, malunion and infection of fractures. J Bone Joint Surg Br. 1997;79:273–9.
38. Weaver LK. The undersea and hyperbaric medical society, hyperbaric oxygen therapy indications. In: North Palm Beach, F. 13th ed. Best Publishing; 2014.
39. Gill AL, Bell CN. Hyperbaric oxygen: its uses, mechanisms of action and outcomes. QJM. 2004;97:385–95.
40. Kawashima M, Tamura H, Nagayoshi I, Takao K, Yoshida K, Yamaguchi T. Hyperbaric oxygen therapy in orthopedic conditions. Undersea Hyperb Med. 2004;31:155–62.
41. Mader JT, Adams KR, Wallace WR, Calhoun JH. Hyperbaric oxygen as adjunctive therapy for osteomyelitis. Infect Dis Clin N Am. 1990 Sep;4(3):433–40.
42. Fang RC, Galiano RD. Adjunctive therapies in the treatment of osteomyelitis. Semin Plast Surg. 2009;23:141–7.
43. Savvidou OD, Kaspiris A, Bolia IK, Chloros GD, Goumenos SD, Papagelopoulos PJ, Tsiodras S. Effectiveness of hyperbaric oxygen therapy for the management of chronic osteomyelitis: a systematic review of the literature. Orthopedics. 2018;41(4):193–9. https://doi.org/10.3928/01477447-20180628-02.
44. Chen CY, Lin KP, Lu SH, Chen YJ, Lin CF. Adjuvant hyperbaric oxygen therapy in the treatment of hemodialysis patients with chronic osteomyelitis. Ren Fail. 2008;30:233–7.
45. Chen CE, Shih ST, Fu TH, Wang JW, Wang CJ. Hyperbaric oxygen therapy in the treatment of chronic refractory osteomyelitis: a preliminary report. Chang Gung Med J. 2003;26:114–21.
46. Skeik N, Porten BR, Isaacson E, et al. Hyperbaric oxygen treatment outcome for different indications from a single center. Ann Vasc Surg. 2015;29:206–14.

Chapter 12
Hyperbaric Oxygen Therapy and Burns

Ranajit Chatterjee and Lalit Gupta

12.1 Introduction

Thermal burns pose a significant global health challenge, causing substantial suffering and even death. The impact of burn injuries is profound, leading to severe pain, tissue damage, and various complications such as infections and scarring. In India, the burden of burn cases is evident, with an estimated annual incidence of 6–7 million burn injuries in India alone [1]. Numerous factors contribute to the high incidence of burns in India. Illiteracy and lack of education regarding safety practices increase the risk of burn accidents, particularly in domestic settings. Poverty creates unsafe living conditions and limited access to resources, further exacerbating the likelihood of burn injuries. Moreover, low levels of safety consciousness and awareness lead to risky behaviors, compounding the problem. Additionally, the absence of organized burn care facilities in some regions can delay prompt and appropriate treatment, leading to more severe outcomes for burn victims.

Hyperbaric oxygen therapy (HBOT) consists of intermittently administering 100% oxygen at pressures greater than 1 atmosphere in a pressure vessel [2, 3]. It has been used in the management of various medical conditions, including thermal burns. Thermal burns are injuries caused by exposure to heat, resulting in damage to the skin and underlying tissues. The use of HBOT in the treatment of thermal burns aims to increase the supply of oxygen to the burnt area to improve healing, reduce tissue edema, enhance immune function, and improve the microcirculation in the burnt area [3, 4].

R. Chatterjee
Department of Critical Care, Swami Dayanand Hospital, Delhi, India

L. Gupta (✉)
Department of Anaesthesia and Critical Care, Maulana Azad Medical College and Lok Nayak Hospital, New Delhi, India

A. G. D'Almeida, J. Hidalgo (eds.), *Evidence-Based Hyperbaric Medicine*,
https://doi.org/10.1007/978-3-032-06346-5_12

12.2 Pathophysiology

The pathophysiology of thermal burns involves a complex interplay of cellular and molecular events. The initial injury leads to tissue damage, inflammation, and the release of inflammatory mediators. This inflammatory response can result in tissue hypoxia and impaired wound healing. HBOT has been proposed to counteract these effects by providing a high concentration of oxygen to the damaged tissues, promoting angiogenesis, reducing inflammation, and enhancing tissue repair [4].

Studies conducted with humans and animals have shown consistent and significant results in using HBOT to manage thermal burns. These studies have demonstrated the potential of HBOT in preventing skin ischemia, reducing edema, and improving wound healing [4–6].

However, it is important to note that the use of HBOT as an adjunct therapy for thermal burns remains controversial due to limited and conflicting evidence [7, 8]. HBOT has shown promise as a potential adjunct therapy in the treatment of thermal burns. It has been reported to improve wound healing, reduce edema, and enhance tissue repair. However, further research is needed to establish its efficacy and determine the optimal protocols for its use in thermal burn management [8].

12.3 Infection and Thermal Burns

Infection is a common complication of thermal burns and can lead to significant morbidity and mortality [2, 8]. Some key points about infection with thermal burns:

1. *Bacterial Colonization*: Shortly after the burn occurs, bacteria from the surrounding environment and the patient's skin can colonize the wound. This initial colonization is a normal part of the wound healing process. However, if the bacterial load becomes excessive or pathogenic bacteria dominate, it can lead to infection.
2. *Risk Factors*: Several factors can increase the risk of infection in thermal burns, including the size and depth of the burn, delay in medical treatment, presence of foreign materials in the wound, and underlying health conditions that weaken the immune system.
3. *Types of Infections*: Burn wounds can be susceptible to both localized and systemic infections. Localized infections are confined to the wound site, while systemic infections can spread throughout the body, potentially leading to sepsis, a life-threatening condition.
4. *Common Pathogens*: The most common bacteria responsible for burn wound infections are *Staphylococcus aureus*, including methicillin-resistant *Staphylococcus aureus*, and *Pseudomonas aeruginosa*. These bacteria are opportunistic pathogens that can flourish in the warm, moist environment of a burn wound.

The use of HBOT in the management of thermal burns has been shown to reduce the risk of infection and improve outcomes [8]. HBOT works by increasing the supply of oxygen to the damaged tissues, promoting wound healing, and enhancing immune function [9]. It has been reported to reduce the risk of infection by enhancing the bactericidal activity of white blood cells, reducing bacterial growth, and promoting the formation of new blood vessels [3, 9]. In a meta-analysis of the effect of HBOT on thermal burns, those who received HBOT had a significantly lower incidence of wound infections compared to those who did not receive HBOT [10]. Other studies also concluded that HBOT reduced the incidence of sepsis in patients with thermal burns [5, 11].

12.4 Evidence of HBOT on Thermal Burns

Studies conducted with humans and animals have shown consistent and significant results in using HBOT to manage thermal burns. These studies have demonstrated the potential of HBOT in preventing skin ischemia, reducing edema, and improving wound healing. In a case–control study, patients with thermal burns who received HBOT had a significantly shorter hospital stay and a lower incidence of wound infections compared to those who did not receive HBOT [5].

HBOT indeed offers several advantages in the management of second- and third-degree burn injuries, particularly when administered within the first 48–72 hours after the thermal injury occurs. [2, 12, 13]

1. *Mitigation of Ischemia Reperfusion Injury*: HBOT helps increase the oxygen saturation in the body up to 12 times that of breathing air at sea level. This increased oxygen supply can reduce ischemia–reperfusion injury, which occurs when blood flow is restored to damaged tissues after a period of reduced blood flow. The added oxygen helps "bring back to life" the jeopardized tissue, preventing further tissue death and signaling to the body that the damaged area is not a foreign invader.
2. *Promotion of New Tissue Growth*: HBOT continues to promote new tissue growth beyond the initial 72 hours. It aids in the manufacturing of new blood vessels (neoangiogenesis), which is crucial for supplying nutrients and oxygen to the healing tissue. Additionally, HBOT supports the production of fibroblasts responsible for collagen synthesis, a vital component of wound healing.
3. *Reduction of Inflammation*: HBOT reduces inflammation in the body, which can be significant in burns where inflammation may hinder the healing process. By modulating the inflammatory response, HBOT helps create a more favorable environment for healing to take place.
4. *Infection Control*: Oxygen is a potent weapon for white blood cells to kill bacteria. HBOT's ability to provide increased oxygen levels can enhance the immune system's ability to combat infections, which are common complications in severe burns.

It is crucial to note that HBOT can offer significant benefits for burn injuries. However, it is not a standalone treatment and should be used as part of a comprehensive burn care plan. Standard burn treatments, such as wound care, infection control, and surgical interventions, remain essential components of burn management.

12.5 Effects of HBOT on Immunological Markers

HBOT has been reported to enhance immune function by increasing the production of white blood cells and enhancing their bactericidal activity. It has also been shown to reduce the production of inflammatory cytokines, which can contribute to tissue damage and impaired wound healing [14–16].

In a study of patients with thermal burns, HBOT was found to increase the production of interleukin-8, a cytokine involved in the recruitment of white blood cells to the site of injury [14]. This increase in interleukin-8 production was associated with improved wound healing and reduced incidence of wound infections.

Here are some of the effects of HBOT on immunological markers:

1. *Increased Oxygen Levels*: HBOT significantly increases the supply of oxygen to the body, including tissues and cells involved in the immune response. Higher oxygen levels can enhance the functioning of immune cells, such as neutrophils, macrophages, and lymphocytes.
2. *Enhanced Neutrophil Function:* Neutrophils are crucial immune cells responsible for defending the body against bacterial infections. HBOT has been shown to increase the oxidative burst activity of neutrophils, making them more effective in killing bacteria.
3. *Improved Microbial Killing*: The higher oxygen levels during HBOT create an oxidative environment that is toxic to certain bacteria, including anaerobic pathogens. This can directly enhance the body's ability to combat bacterial infections.
4. *Modulation of Cytokines*: HBOT has been observed to influence the production and release of cytokines, which are signaling molecules involved in immune responses. It can reduce the production of pro-inflammatory cytokines, leading to an anti-inflammatory effect.
5. *Stimulation of Growth Factors*: HBOT can induce the release of growth factors, such as vascular endothelial growth factor, which plays a key role in wound healing and tissue repair. This can support the regeneration of damaged tissues, including those affected by infections.
6. *Anti-Edema Effect*: HBOT can help reduce tissue edema (swelling) in certain conditions, which may be beneficial in cases of inflammatory responses or infections.
7. *Immune Cell Recruitment*: HBOT has been shown to enhance the recruitment of immune cells to wound sites, aiding in tissue repair and infection control.

8. *Antibacterial Properties*: HBOT itself has direct bactericidal effects, contributing to the control of bacterial infections.

12.6 Effects of HBOT on Bacteriology of Tissue Culture in Areas of Deep Dermal Burns

HBOT has been shown to reduce bacterial growth in tissue cultures from areas of deep dermal burns. In a study of patients with thermal burns, tissue cultures from areas treated with HBOT had significantly lower bacterial counts compared to those from areas not treated with HBOT. HBOT has also been reported to enhance the bactericidal activity of white blood cells, reducing bacterial growth and promoting the formation of new blood vessels. These effects can contribute to the reduction of bacterial infections in patients with thermal burns [8, 17].

HBOT has shown promise as a potential adjunct therapy in the treatment of thermal burns. It has been reported to reduce the risk of infection, improve wound healing, and enhance immune function. However, further research is needed to establish its efficacy and determine the optimal protocols for its use in thermal burn management [17–19].

1. Bactericidal Action: HBOT can exert direct bactericidal effects on various pathogenic bacteria. The high concentration of oxygen delivered during HBOT creates an oxidative environment that is toxic to certain types of bacteria. This can help in reducing the bacterial load in the burn wound.
2. Enhanced Immune Response: HBOT has been shown to enhance the function of white blood cells, particularly neutrophils, which play a crucial role in the body's defense against bacterial infections. Improved immune response can help combat and control bacterial growth in the burn wound.
3. Anaerobic Bacteria Suppression: Deep dermal burns, which often involve tissue necrosis and reduced blood flow, can create an environment favorable for the growth of anaerobic bacteria (bacteria that thrive in the absence of oxygen). HBOT, by providing high levels of oxygen, creates an aerobic environment that can suppress the growth of anaerobic bacteria.
4. Reduction of Biofilm Formation: Bacterial biofilms are communities of bacteria that adhere to the wound surface and can protect bacteria from the body's immune response and antimicrobial treatments. HBOT has been shown to disrupt and reduce biofilm formation, enhancing the effectiveness of other antimicrobial treatments.
5. Promotion of Wound Healing: HBOT promotes wound healing by increasing oxygen supply to the tissues, which aids in tissue repair and regeneration. A well-oxygenated wound environment is less conducive to bacterial growth, as many bacteria thrive in low-oxygen conditions.

6. Control of Opportunistic Infections: Burn wounds are vulnerable to opportunistic infections due to compromised skin barriers. HBOT can help control these infections and prevent their spread to deeper tissues.
7. Reduction of Inflammation: HBOT can reduce excessive inflammation in the burn wound. Inflammation is a response to infection, but when it becomes prolonged and severe, it can hinder the healing process and exacerbate tissue damage. By controlling inflammation, HBOT contributes to a more favorable environment for wound healing and infection control.

12.7 Procedure of Giving Hyperbaric Therapy in Burns

HBOT is a specialized treatment that involves breathing pure oxygen in a pressurized chamber [8, 19, 20]. The procedure for giving HBOT in burns typically involves the following steps:

1. *Assessment*: The patient is assessed to determine the extent and severity of the burn injury. This assessment includes a physical examination, laboratory tests, and imaging studies.
2. *Preparation*: The patient is prepared for the HBOT procedure, which involves changing into a hospital gown and removing any metal objects.
3. *Chamber entry*: The patient is placed in a hyperbaric chamber, which is a sealed chamber that can be pressurized to increase the concentration of oxygen. The patient breathes pure oxygen through a mask or hood while inside the chamber.
4. *Compression Phase*: The chamber is gradually pressurized with 100% pure oxygen. The chamber is pressurized to the prescribed level, which is typically 2.0–2.5 atmospheres absolute (ATA). The patient may experience a sensation of pressure in their ears, similar to what is felt during changes in altitude (like during a flight). The medical team will instruct the patient on techniques, such as swallowing or yawning, to equalize the pressure in their ears. The duration of the treatment session varies depending on the patient's condition and the severity of the burn injury.
5. *Treatment Phase*: Once the desired pressure is achieved, the patient breathes in pure oxygen for the prescribed duration, typically between 60 and 120 minutes per session. During this time, the patient may rest or engage in light activities, such as reading or listening to music.
6. *Decompression Phase*: After completing the treatment session, the pressure inside the chamber is gradually reduced back to normal atmospheric pressure. The patient may again experience ear-popping sensations during this phase.
7. *Post-Treatment Care*: After the session, the patient is monitored for a short period to ensure that they are stable and have no adverse reactions. The patient is monitored for any adverse effects of the treatment, such as ear pain or dizziness. The patient may require multiple sessions of HBOT to achieve the desired therapeutic effect.

8. *Session Frequency*: The number of HBOT sessions and the overall treatment duration will depend on the severity of the burn injury, the patient's response to the therapy, and the medical team's treatment plan.

12.8 Discussion

The use of HBOT in the treatment of thermal burns remains controversial due to limited and conflicting evidence. However, studies have shown that HBOT can reduce the risk of infection, improve wound healing, and enhance immune function in patients with thermal burns [2, 6, 8]. One of the potential benefits of HBOT in the treatment of thermal burns is its ability to increase the supply of oxygen to the damaged tissues, promoting wound healing and reducing tissue edema. HBOT has also been reported to enhance immune function by increasing the production of white blood cells and enhancing their bactericidal activity.

Despite these potential benefits, the use of HBOT in the treatment of thermal burns requires careful consideration of the risks and benefits. HBOT can cause adverse effects such as ear pain, sinus pain, and lung damage [4, 21–26]. Some of the side effects and considerations associated with HBOT in burn patients are as follows:

1. *Barotrauma to the Ears*: Barotrauma, which refers to injuries caused by changes in pressure, is common in the ears, particularly in burns affecting the head and neck. This can lead to ear-related complications. To mitigate this risk, routine ear, nose, and throat evaluations are recommended, and early myringotomy (a surgical incision of the eardrum) may be performed to relieve pressure and prevent further damage.
2. *Hypotension and Fluid Management*: In larger burn injuries, adequate fluid and electrolyte resuscitation during the first 24 hours can be challenging. Some patients have experienced hypotension (low blood pressure) shortly after exiting the hyperbaric chamber. This might be due to hypovolemia (low blood volume) that was masked during HBOT. Careful assessment of volume status by using dynamic parameters and volume replacement is crucial before, during, and after hyperbaric treatment. To address this, some units have increased fluid intake during ascent to compensate for any masked hypovolemia.
3. *Experience and Expertise*: Burn patients with severe injuries are among the most challenging cases in medicine. Units planning to offer HBOT to burn patients should be well-versed in the management of critical care patients in the hyperbaric setting and familiar with the specific issues faced by burn patients. The hyperbaric team must have experience in managing central lines, ventilators, and all aspects of critical care within the hyperbaric chamber.
4. *Effect of 100% oxygen*: During HBOT, patients breathe 100% oxygen under increased atmospheric pressure. Under certain circumstances, the increased

oxygen levels can lead to an excessive buildup of oxygen free radicals in the central nervous system, which can trigger seizures.

5. *Eye surgeries*: Recent history of eye surgery or history of glaucoma may be a contraindication to HBOT as expansion or contraction of gas in the eye, if any, due to high pressure can damage the eye.
6. *Severe Reactive Airways Disease*: Conditions such as severe asthma or chronic obstructive pulmonary disease with reactive airways disease may be exacerbated by HBOT.
7. *Untreated Pneumothorax*: A pneumothorax (collapsed lung) that is not yet treated should be considered a contraindication, as the increased pressure in the chamber could worsen the condition, and in cases, pulmonary edema is also reported due to a sudden change in intrathoracic pressure.
8. *Cost*: It is also a costly and time-consuming treatment that requires specialized equipment and trained personnel.

12.9 Conclusion

HBOT has shown promise as a potential adjunct therapy in the treatment of thermal burns. It has been reported to reduce the risk of infection, improve wound healing, and enhance immune function. However, further research is needed to establish its efficacy and determine the optimal protocols for its use in thermal burn management. Patient safety and appropriate wound management remain top priorities in the treatment of thermal burns.

Its incorporation into routine practice requires more extensive research, a well-equipped and expertly staffed hyperbaric facility, and careful consideration of patient safety and individual medical conditions. Until further evidence and experience are available, HBOT should be considered on a case-by-case basis, with the goal of optimizing burn care and patient outcomes. While HBOT holds promise, it should be used cautiously and administered by experienced health care providers trained in hyperbaric medicine and burn care.

References

1. Gupta JL, Makhija LK, Bajaj SP. National programme for prevention of burn injuries. Indian J Plast Surg. 2010;43(Suppl):S6–S10.
2. Villanueva E, Bennett MH, Wasiak J, Lehm JP. Hyperbaric oxygen therapy for thermal burns. Cochrane Database Syst Rev. 2004;2004(3):CD004727.
3. HBOT and burn treatment: How it works and why it's effective [Internet]. Nationalhyperbaric.com. Available from: https://www.nationalhyperbaric.com/hbot-treatments-and-conditions/burn-treatment
4. Edwards M, Cooper JS. Hyperbaric treatment of thermal burns. Treasure Island: StatPearls Publishing; 2023.

5. Oley MH, Oley MC, Aling DMR, Kalangi JA, Islam AA, Hatta M, et al. Effects of hyperbaric oxygen therapy on the healing of thermal burns and its relationship with ICAM-1: a case-control study. Ann Med Surg. 2021;61:104–9.
6. Alyafi T, Al-Marzouki A-HH, Al Hassani AN. Therapeutic outcome of burn patients treated with hyperbaric oxygen. Cureus. 2021;13(10):e18671.
7. Grover I, Neuman T. Hyperbaric oxygen therapy. In: Encyclopedia of respiratory medicine. Elsevier; 2006. p. 292–6.
8. Memar MY, Yekani M, Alizadeh N, Baghi HB. Hyperbaric oxygen therapy: antimicrobial mechanisms and clinical application for infections. Biomed Pharmacother. 2019;109:440–7.
9. Hyperbaric oxygen therapy [Internet]. Hopkinsmedicine.org. 2022. Available from: https://www.hopkinsmedicine.org/health/treatment-tests-and-therapies/hyperbaric-oxygen-therapy
10. Huang C, Zhong Y, Yue C, et al. The effect of hyperbaric oxygen therapy on the clinical outcomes of necrotizing soft tissue infections: a systematic review and meta-analysis. World J Emerg Surg. 2023;18:23.
11. Camporesi EM, Bosco G. Mechanisms of action of hyperbaric oxygen therapy. Undersea Hyperb Med. 2014;41(3):247–52.
12. Thom SR, Mendiguren H, Nebolon M, Campbell D, Kilpatrick L. Temporary inhibition of human neutrophil B2 intgrin function by hyperbaric oxygen. Clin Res. 1994;42:130A.
13. Hyperbaric oxygen therapy for treating second- and third-degree burns [Internet]. Woundsource.com. Available from: https://www.woundsource.com/blog/hyperbaric-oxygen-therapy-treatment-second-and-third-degree-burns.
14. de Wolde SD, Hulskes RH, de Jonge SW, Hollmann MW, van Hulst RA, Weenink RP, Kox M. The effect of hyperbaric oxygen therapy on markers of oxidative stress and the immune response in healthy volunteers. Front Physiol. 2022;13:826163.
15. Benkő R, Miklós Z, Ágoston VA, Ihonvien K, Répás C, Csépányi-Kömi R, Kerék M, Béres NJ, Horváth EM. Hyperbaric oxygen therapy dampens inflammatory cytokine production and does not worsen the cardiac function and oxidative state of diabetic rats. Antioxidants. 2019;8(12):607.
16. Vezzani G, Socias S, Bianco A, Paoli A, Caberti L, Cantadori L. Inflammatory mediators and other biomarkers in co-intoxicated patients after hyperbaric oxygen therapy (HBO2). Acta Med Mediter. 2016:32.
17. Gill AL, Bell CNA. Hyperbaric oxygen: its uses, mechanisms of action and outcomes. QJM. 2004;97(7):385–95.
18. Ortega MA, Fraile-Martinez O, García-Montero C, Callejón-Peláez E, Sáez MA, Álvarez-Mon MA, García-Honduvilla N, Monserrat J, Álvarez-Mon M, Bujan J, Canals ML. A general overview on the hyperbaric oxygen therapy: applications, mechanisms and translational opportunities. Medicina (Kaunas). 2021;57(9):864.
19. Choudhury R. Hypoxia and hyperbaric oxygen therapy: a review. Int J Gen Med. 2018;11:431–42.
20. Hyperbaric Oxygen Therapy. Mayoclinic.org. 2022. Available from: https://www.mayoclinic.org/tests-procedures/hyperbaric-oxygen-therapy/about/pac-20394380.
21. Smolle C, Lindenmann J, Kamolz L, Smolle-Juettner F-M. The history and development of hyperbaric oxygenation (HBO) in thermal burn injury. Medicina. 2021;57(1):49.
22. Weaver LK, Churchill S. Pulmonary edema associated with hyperbaric oxygen therapy. Chest. 2001;120:1407–9. https://doi.org/10.1378/chest.120.4.1407.
23. Domachevsky L, Rachmany L, Barak Y, Rubovitch V, Abramovich A, Pick CG. Hyperbaric oxygen-induced seizures cause a transient decrement in cognitive function. Neuroscience. 2013;247:328–34. https://doi.org/10.1016/j.neuroscience.2013.05.052.
24. McMonnies CW. Hyperbaric oxygen therapy and the possibility of ocular complications or contraindications. Clin Exp Optom. 2015;98(2):122–5.

25. For Tissue Damage, Including Wound Care. Hyperbaric Oxygen Therapy (HBOT). Hca.wa.gov. Available from: https://www.hca.wa.gov/assets/program/021513_hbot_final_report[1].pdf
26. Heyboer M 3rd, Sharma D, Santiago W, McCulloch N. Hyperbaric oxygen therapy: side effects defined and quantified. Adv Wound Care (New Rochelle). 2017;6(6):210–24.

Chapter 13
Hyperbaric Oxygen Therapy for Hearing Loss

Ranajit Chatterjee and Lalit Gupta

13.1 Introduction

Idiopathic sudden sensorineural hearing loss (ISSNHL) is defined by a sudden and unexplained decrease of hearing sensitivity in at least three consecutive audiometric frequencies, resulting in a 30 dB or more hearing loss in 72 hours or fewer [1]. The source of this illness is unknown; however, it can result in permanent hearing loss, causing substantial morbidity.

ISSNHL is now treated with corticosteroids, vasodilators, immunosuppressants, and antiviral medicines. Corticosteroids are the most extensively used; however, they are not without controversy and restrictions [2]. The standard practice standards for the treatment of ISSNHL have not been uniformly defined, leading to a variety of corticosteroid regimens with varying kinds, doses, and delivery methods.

Oral corticosteroids are typically provided in a tapering regimen lasting 10–14 days. However, the success rate of this method is not totally good, with only around 61% of patients recovering [3]. Intratympanic corticosteroid injections have been used to administer medicine directly into the inner ear when systemic steroids have not been successful. Nonetheless, problems such as tympanic membrane perforations, myringitis, and otitis media have been reported.

When combined with steroid medication, hyperbaric oxygen therapy (HBOT) has emerged as a possible supplementary treatment for ISSNHL [4]. This therapy includes inhaling pure oxygen in a pressurized chamber, which allows a much higher oxygen concentration to dissolve in the circulation and reach tissues throughout the body. According to research, when HBOT is used with traditional therapy

---

R. Chatterjee
Department of Critical Care, Swami Dayanand Hospital, Delhi, India

L. Gupta (✉)
Department of Anaesthesia and Critical Care, Maulana Azad Medical College and Lok Nayak Hospital, New Delhi, India

A. G. D'Almeida, J. Hidalgo (eds.), *Evidence-Based Hyperbaric Medicine*,
https://doi.org/10.1007/978-3-032-06346-5_13

techniques such as corticosteroids, the results for ISSNHL are significantly improved [2–4].

13.2 Anatomy and Physiology of Hearing and the Role of HBOT

The inner ear is responsible for maintaining hearing function and includes a vital structure called the cochlea, which has a high demand for oxygen. If the cochlea experiences hypoxia (low oxygen levels), it can lead to progressive degenerative changes, fibrosis, neuron loss, endolymphatic hydrops (excessive fluid accumulation), and ultimately hearing loss. Unlike other organs with direct blood supply, the cochlea relies on oxygen diffusion through the perilymph and cortilymph for oxygen delivery [4, 5].

To supply oxygen to the inner ear, the labyrinthine artery (internal auditory artery) plays a crucial role. This artery branches off from either the anterior inferior cerebellar artery (in 85% of cases) or the basilar artery (in 15% of cases) [4]. It accompanies the vestibulocochlear nerve through the internal acoustic meatus into the inner ear. Studies using animal models have shown that occlusion (blockage) of the labyrinthine artery leads to progressive degenerative changes, fibrosis, new bone formation, and hearing loss [5, 6].

13.3 Indications

HBOT has shown promise in treating sudden sensorineural hearing loss (SSNHL) . This therapy involves administering pure oxygen in a pressurized chamber, which can increase the oxygen tension in the perilymph and potentially restore hearing in a significant number of patients. The efficacy of HBOT may depend on various factors, including the degree of patency (openness) of the labyrinthine artery and the ability to increase oxygen tension in the perilymph [5].

Numerous prospective randomized controlled trials have demonstrated the benefits of HBOT over placebo for hearing loss treatment [4–6]. The best results are achieved when patients receive HBOT within 14 days of symptom onset and when it is combined with steroids (either systemically or intratympanic, delivered directly into the middle ear). Steroids are typically given at an initial dose of 1 mg/kg/day and tapered over 2–3 weeks, unless there are contraindications [7].

Patients with moderate to severe hearing loss, indicated by a loss of more than 40 dB, are considered good candidates for HBOT. The American Academy of Otolaryngology recommends considering HBOT as a treatment option up to 3 months after symptom onset and advises against the routine use of antivirals, thrombolytics, vasodilators, vasoactive substances, or antioxidants for this condition [8].

Even if patients have not responded to an initial course of steroids, they can still benefit from a combination of intratympanic steroids and HBOT, even up to 10 weeks after symptom onset [7, 8]. To evaluate patients, an otolaryngologist and audiologist should perform an audiogram, brain MRI (to rule out any retro cochlear pathology), and a full autoimmune and vasculitis evaluation, along with an auditory brainstem response test.

During the course of HBOT (usually consisting of 20 treatments), follow-up audiograms should be conducted, and additional audiograms should be done 6 months after completing the therapy. Patients should be educated about the natural history of the condition, the benefits and risks of interventions, and the limitations of existing evidence regarding treatment efficacy. They should also be counseled on the possibility of incomplete recovery of hearing and be made aware of the potential benefits of using amplification, hearing-assistive technology, and other supportive measures.

13.4 Procedure of Giving Hyperbaric Therapy for Hearing Loss

HBOT for SSNHL involves administering pure oxygen in a pressurized chamber to increase the oxygen levels in the bloodstream and tissues, including the inner ear. The increased oxygen concentration is believed to improve the oxygen supply to the cochlea, potentially promoting healing and restoring hearing function [4, 5, 9, 10]. Here is how HBOT is typically given for SSNHL:

1. Pretreatment Evaluation: Before starting HBOT, a thorough evaluation of the patient's medical history and audiological assessment is conducted. This evaluation helps determine if the patient meets the criteria for HBOT and if there are any contraindications.
2. Treatment Schedule: HBOT is typically administered as a series of sessions, referred to as "dives." Each dive involves the patient entering a hyperbaric chamber where the air pressure is increased to higher than atmospheric pressure.
3. Pressurization: The patient is placed inside the hyperbaric chamber, which can be a monoplace chamber (designed for one person) or a multiplace chamber (designed to accommodate multiple patients). The chamber is then pressurized with 100% pure oxygen to the prescribed treatment pressure.
4. Treatment Duration: Each HBOT session usually lasts around 60–90 minutes, depending on the specific protocol and the patient's response. During the session, the patient breathes in pure oxygen through a mask or a hood.
5. Treatment Frequency: The number of HBOT sessions and the treatment schedule may vary based on the severity of the hearing loss and the physician's recommendations. Generally, patients undergo one or more dives per day, with treatments typically conducted on weekdays (Monday to Friday) for several weeks.

6. Concomitant Steroid Therapy: In many cases, HBOT is combined with systemic (oral or intravenous) or intratympanic corticosteroid therapy to enhance the chances of recovery. The use of steroids is often initiated alongside or prior to starting HBOT.
7. Monitoring: During HBOT, patients are closely monitored by health care professionals to ensure their safety and comfort. Vital signs and symptoms are regularly assessed.
8. Post-Treatment Evaluation: After completing the prescribed number of HBOT sessions, the patient's hearing is reevaluated to determine the treatment's effectiveness. Follow-up audiograms may be performed at specific intervals to monitor the patient's progress.

It is important to note that the exact protocol and treatment plan for HBOT in SSNHL may vary based on individual patient characteristics, the severity of hearing loss, and the health care provider's expertise. HBOT for SSNHL is considered a specialized treatment, and it should be administered under the supervision of qualified health care professionals in a certified hyperbaric facility.

13.5 Mechanism of Action of HBOT in Healing Sensory Neural Hearing Loss

The mechanism of action of HBOT in healing SSNHL is not fully understood, and research in this area is ongoing. However, several proposed mechanisms have been suggested based on the known physiological effects of hyperbaric oxygen. Here are some potential ways HBOT may contribute to healing SSNHL:

1. Improved Oxygenation: HBOT involves exposing the body to 100% pure oxygen at increased atmospheric pressure. This leads to a significant increase in the amount of dissolved oxygen in the bloodstream, which can enhance oxygen delivery to tissues with compromised blood flow, including the cochlea. Improved oxygenation may aid in cellular repair and support the survival of sensory hair cells and neurons in the inner ear.
2. Reduction of Hypoxia: In cases of SSNHL, the inner ear may experience hypoxia (low oxygen levels) due to reduced blood flow or microvascular damage. HBOT may help counteract this hypoxic state by providing an abundant supply of oxygen, which could mitigate the progression of degenerative changes and preserve cellular function.
3. Anti-Inflammatory Effects: Hyperbaric oxygen has been shown to reduce inflammation by modulating immune responses and decreasing the production of pro-inflammatory cytokines. In SSNHL, inflammation may play a role in causing or exacerbating damage to the inner ear. HBOT's anti-inflammatory effects may help minimize inflammation-associated tissue damage and promote healing.

4. Angiogenesis: HBOT has been reported to promote the formation of new blood vessels, a process known as angiogenesis. By stimulating angiogenesis, HBOT could potentially improve blood flow to the cochlea, supporting the delivery of essential nutrients and oxygen to promote healing.
5. Neuroprotection: Studies suggest that HBOT may have neuroprotective effects, protecting neurons and nerve cells from damage caused by oxidative stress and other harmful factors. In SSNHL, these neuroprotective properties could help prevent further damage to the auditory nerve and support neural recovery.
6. Enhanced Tissue Repair: HBOT has been associated with increased collagen synthesis, improved wound healing, and enhanced tissue repair. These effects may aid in the restoration of damaged structures within the cochlea and contribute to functional recovery.

It is important to note that while there is promising evidence supporting the use of HBOT for SSNHL, the exact mechanisms of its action are complex and multifactorial. Moreover, the response to HBOT may vary among individuals, and not all patients with SSNHL may experience significant improvement through this therapy. As research continues, a deeper understanding of HBOT's effects on SSNHL will likely emerge, further elucidating its potential as a therapeutic option for this condition.

13.6 Contraindications for HBOT

While HBOT is generally considered safe, there are specific contraindications that need to be taken into account before administering the treatment [11–17]. These contraindications include the following:

1. Confinement Anxiety: Some individuals may experience severe anxiety or claustrophobia when placed in a pressurized chamber, making HBOT unsuitable for them.
2. Severe Congestive Heart Failure: Patients with severe congestive heart failure may not be suitable candidates for HBOT, as the increased pressure in the chamber can put extra strain on the heart.
3. Severe Reactive Airways Disease: Conditions such as severe asthma or chronic obstructive pulmonary disease with reactive airways disease may be exacerbated by HBOT.
4. Untreated Pneumothorax: A pneumothorax (collapsed lung) that is not yet treated should be considered a contraindication, as the increased pressure in the chamber could worsen the condition, and in cases, pulmonary edema is also reported due to a sudden change in intrathoracic pressure.
5. Concomitant Doxorubicin or Bleomycin Therapy: The use of certain chemotherapeutic drugs, such as doxorubicin or bleomycin, alongside HBOT may interfere with their efficacy or lead to adverse effects. Concurrent doxorubicin

use and HBOT can increase the risk of doxorubicin-mediated cardiotoxicity. Therefore, doxorubicin should be stopped at least 24 hours before HBOT.
6. Disulfiram, by blocking superoxide dismutase, can increase the risk of oxygen toxicity (seizures and pulmonary toxicity) and should not be used concurrently with HBOT.
7. Recent history of eye surgery or history of glaucoma may be a contraindication to HBOT as expansion or contraction of gas in the eye, if any, due to high pressure can damage the eye.
8. During HBOT, patients breathe 100% oxygen under increased atmospheric pressure. Under certain circumstances, the increased oxygen levels can lead to an excessive build-up of oxygen free radicals in the central nervous system, which can trigger seizures. So, pre-existing seizure disorder is a contraindication for HBOT.

In addition to the contraindications for HBOT, there are specific contraindications related to systemic corticosteroid use, which is often used in combination with HBOT for certain conditions [14, 18–20]. These include the following:

1. Psychiatric Illness: Patients with certain psychiatric illnesses, such as severe depression or psychosis, may not be suitable candidates for systemic corticosteroids due to potential exacerbation of their mental health condition.
2. Diabetes: Corticosteroids can affect blood glucose levels and may not be recommended for patients with uncontrolled diabetes.
3. Peptic Ulcer Disease: Systemic corticosteroids can exacerbate peptic ulcers and should be used with caution in individuals with this condition.
4. Breastfeeding: Systemic corticosteroids can be excreted in breast milk and may not be suitable for breastfeeding mothers.
5. Liver Disease: Corticosteroids are metabolized in the liver, and patients with severe liver disease may have impaired drug metabolism, making systemic corticosteroids contraindicated or requiring dosage adjustments.

In cases where systemic corticosteroids are contraindicated, intra-tympanic steroids (administered directly into the middle ear) may be a preferable alternative. It is essential for health care providers to carefully assess each patient's medical history and individual circumstances before recommending HBOT or corticosteroid treatment, ensuring that the benefits outweigh the risks for the specific condition being treated.

13.7 Conclusion

HBOT has emerged as a promising and innovative approach in the management of hearing loss, particularly in cases of SSNHL. The evidence from numerous perspectives randomized controlled trials demonstrates that HBOT can significantly improve outcomes in patients with SSNHL when used in combination with conventional treatments, such as systemic or intratympanic corticosteroids.

The optimal timing and frequency of HBOT, as well as its efficacy in specific subgroups of patients, remain areas of ongoing investigation. However, encouraging results have been observed, particularly when treatment is initiated within the first 2 weeks of symptom onset. Patients with moderate to severe hearing loss have shown the most significant benefit, and combining HBOT with steroids seems to yield more favorable outcomes. Despite the promising findings, it is essential to acknowledge that not all patients respond equally to HBOT, and individual variability exists in treatment outcomes.

As our understanding of its mechanisms of action and patient selection criteria continues to evolve, HBOT may become a more established and standardized treatment option, offering renewed hope for individuals with hearing loss and contributing to the advancement of audiological care.

References

1. Kuhn M, Heman-Ackah SE, Shaikh JA, Roehm PC. Sudden sensorineural hearing loss: a review of diagnosis, treatment, and prognosis. Trends Amplif. 2011;15(3):91–105.
2. Plontke SK, Meisner C, Agrawal S, Cayé-Thomasen P, Galbraith K, Mikulec AA, Parnes L, Premakumar Y, Reiber J, Schilder AG, Liebau A. Intratympanic corticosteroids for sudden sensorineural hearing loss. Cochrane Database Syst Rev. 2022;7(7):CD008080.
3. Leung MA, Flaherty A, Zhang JA, Hara J, Barber W, Burgess L. Sudden sensorineural hearing loss: primary care update. Hawaii J Med Public Health. 2016;75(6):172–4.
4. Bayoumy AB, de Ru JA. The use of hyperbaric oxygen therapy in acute hearing loss: a narrative review. Eur Arch Otorhinolaryngol. 2019;276(7):1859–80.
5. Murphy-Lavoie HM, Mutluoglu M. Hyperbaric Treatment of Sensorineural Hearing Loss. StatPearls Publishing; Treasure Island (FL): USA, 2023.
6. Belal A Jr. Pathology of vascular sensorineural hearing impairment. Laryngoscope. 1980;90(11 Pt 1):1831–9.
7. Hu A, Parnes LS. Intratympanic steroids for inner ear disorders: a review. Audiol Neurootol. 2009;14(6):373–82.
8. Chandrasekhar SS, Tsai Do BS, Schwartz SR, Bontempo LJ, Faucett EA, Finestone SA, et al. Clinical practice guideline: Sudden hearing loss (update). Otolaryngol Head Neck Surg. 2019:161(S1).
9. Ortega MA, Fraile-Martinez O, García-Montero C, Callejón-Peláez E, Sáez MA, Álvarez-Mon MA, García-Honduvilla N, Monserrat J, Álvarez-Mon M, Bujan J, Canals ML. A general overview on the hyperbaric oxygen therapy: applications, mechanisms and translational opportunities. Medicina (Kaunas). 2021;57(9):864.
10. Germonpre P, Levie P, Dehalleux C, Caers D. ENT indications for hyperbaric oxygen therapy. B-ENT [Internet]. 2016;Suppl 26(1):87–106. Available from: http://b-ent.be/Content/files/sayilar/21/2016-12-S26-1-087-Germonpre.pdf
11. Baude J, Cooper JS. Hyperbaric contraindicated chemotherapeutic agents. Treasure Island: StatPearls Publishing; 2020.
12. Camporesi EM. Side effects of hyperbaric oxygen therapy. Undersea Hyperb. Med. 2014;41:253–7.
13. Heyboer M, Sharma D, Santiago W, McCulloch N. Hyperbaric oxygen therapy: side effects defined and quantified. Adv. Wound Care. 2017;6:210–24.

14. Cooper JS, Phuyal P, Shah N. Oxygen toxicity. Treasure Island: StatPearls Publishing; 2021.
15. Weaver LK, Churchill S. Pulmonary edema associated with hyperbaric oxygen therapy. Chest. 2001;120:1407–9. https://doi.org/10.1378/chest.120.4.1407.
16. Domachevsky L, Rachmany L, Barak Y, Rubovitch V, Abramovich A, Pick CG. Hyperbaric oxygen-induced seizures cause a transient decrement in cognitive function. Neuroscience. 2013;247:328–34. https://doi.org/10.1016/j.neuroscience.2013.05.052.
17. McMonnies CW. Hyperbaric oxygen therapy and the possibility of ocular complications or contraindications. Clin Exp Optom. 2015;98(2):122–5.
18. Gawdi R, Cooper JS. Hyperbaric contraindications. Treasure Island: StatPearls Publishing; 2023.
19. Marshall GT Thirlby RC, Bredfeldt JE, Hampson NB. Treatment of gastrointestinal radiation injury with hyperbaric oxygen. Undersea Hyperb Med. 2007;34(1):35–42.
20. Kazi SE, Hoque S. Acute psychosis following corticosteroid administration. Cureus. 2021;13(9):e18093.

Chapter 14
Hyperbaric Oxygen Therapy in Diabetes Mellitus

Safaa Hilal

14.1 Introduction

Hyperbaric oxygen therapy (HBOT) is a medical treatment that involves breathing pure oxygen in a pressurized chamber [1]. HBOT works by increasing the concentration of oxygen in the body, which helps reduce inflammation, promote tissue repair, and stimulate the growth of new blood vessels. It is typically administered in a specialized chamber where the air pressure is higher than normal atmospheric pressure. This allows the lungs to gather more oxygen than would be possible by breathing pure oxygen at normal air pressure [2, 3]. The introduction of HBOT as part of a treatment regimen involves integrating it with other medical interventions to address specific health issues. For example, HBOT may be used in conjunction with antibiotics to treat certain infections, or it may be combined with surgery and wound care for non-healing wounds. The goal of incorporating HBOT into treatment is to enhance the overall effectiveness of the treatment plan and improve patient outcomes [4, 5]. HBOT has emerged as a potential adjunctive treatment for diabetic complications due to its ability to improve tissue oxygenation, enhance wound healing, and mitigate inflammation. This chapter aims to explore the role of HBOT in the management of diabetes mellitus (DM), focusing on its mechanisms of action, clinical applications, and evidence-based outcomes [11, 12].

S. Hilal (✉)
Department of Anaesthesiology, ICU and Pain Management Menoufia University, Shibin Al Kawm, Menoufia, Egypt

A. G. D'Almeida, J. Hidalgo (eds.), *Evidence-Based Hyperbaric Medicine*,
https://doi.org/10.1007/978-3-032-06346-5_14

14.2 Mechanism of Action

HBOT involves breathing pure oxygen in a pressurized chamber. In the context of DM , HBOT is believed to work through several mechanisms:

1. *Increased Oxygen Delivery:* HBOT raises the level of oxygen in the bloodstream, which can improve oxygen delivery to tissues that may have reduced blood flow due to diabetes-related vascular complications [6].
2. *Angiogenesis:* HBOT may stimulate the formation of new blood vessels (angiogenesis) in areas with poor circulation, helping to improve blood flow and tissue oxygenation.
3. *Reduced Inflammation:* Chronic inflammation is common in diabetes and can contribute to tissue damage. HBOT has anti-inflammatory effects, which may help reduce inflammation in diabetic tissues.
4. *Improved Wound Healing:* One of the primary applications of HBOT in diabetes is in the treatment of diabetic foot ulcers (DFUs). By promoting angiogenesis, reducing inflammation, and enhancing tissue oxygenation, HBOT can accelerate wound healing and reduce the risk of infection [7, 8].
5. *Antimicrobial Activity:* HBOT can enhance the body's ability to fight certain infections, including those that may complicate DFUs.
6. *Preservation of Ischemic Tissues:* In diabetic patients with peripheral arterial disease, HBOT can help preserve ischemic tissues by providing them with much-needed oxygen.

Overall, HBOT offers a multi-faceted approach to managing complications of DM, particularly in promoting wound healing and tissue repair [9, 10].

14.3 Indications

DM presents a significant health care challenge globally, with its complications affecting multiple organ systems. HBOT in DM has been explored in various studies, but the evidence base is still evolving. Here are some key points regarding the use of HBOT in DM:

1. *Reducing Complications:* Some studies suggest that HBOT may help reduce the risk of amputations in diabetic patients with foot ulcers by promoting wound healing and preventing infection.
2. *Neuropathy:* There is limited evidence suggesting that HBOT may have beneficial effects on diabetic neuropathy, such as improving sensory perception and nerve conduction. However, more research is needed to establish its efficacy in this area.
3. *Microvascular Complications:* HBOT has been proposed as a potential therapy to address microvascular complications associated with diabetes, such as diabetic

retinopathy and nephropathy. However, the evidence supporting its effectiveness in these areas is still inconclusive [13, 14].

14.4 Evidence-Based Practice

Clinicians should adhere to evidence-based guidelines and protocols for the use of HBOT in diabetic patients, staying updated with the latest research findings and recommendations [15].

14.5 Implementation

Here is how HBOT is typically implemented in patients with DM:

1. *Assessment:* Patients undergo a thorough evaluation by health care professionals to determine if HBOT is appropriate for them. This includes assessing the severity of their diabetes, any existing complications, and the specific condition being treated (e.g., DFUs).
2. *Preparation:* Patients are educated about the procedure and its potential benefits and risks. They may need to undergo some tests to ensure that they can safely tolerate HBOT, such as blood tests to assess oxygen levels and lung function.
3. *Treatment Sessions:* Patients are placed inside a hyperbaric chamber, which is pressurized to levels higher than atmospheric pressure. They breathe pure oxygen during the treatment sessions, which typically last from 60 to 120 minutes. The number of sessions needed varies depending on the individual's condition and response to treatment.
4. *Monitoring:* Patients are closely monitored during HBOT sessions to ensure their safety. Vital signs such as heart rate, blood pressure, and oxygen saturation are routinely checked to assess the progress of the wound.
5. *Post-Treatment Care:* After completing HBOT sessions, patients may continue with follow-up appointments to monitor their progress. Additional treatments or adjustments to their diabetes management plan may be recommended.
6. *Multidisciplinary Approach:* Wound care, infection management, vascular interventions, and diabetes control measures such as blood sugar monitoring and medication management.
7. *Research and Continuous Improvement:* Health care professionals stay updated on the latest research and guidelines related to HBOT in diabetes management.

It is important to note that while HBOT shows promise in improving outcomes for diabetic patients, it may not be suitable for everyone, and its efficacy can vary depending on individual factors. Therefore, the decision to undergo HBOT should be made in consultation with health care providers who can assess the potential benefits and risks based on each patient's unique circumstances [4, 16].

14.6 Complications and Side Effects

HBOT carries some risks when used in individuals with DM. These risks primarily stem from potential complications related to the effects of increased oxygen levels in the body and the potential for worsening certain diabetic conditions. Some risks include the following:

1. *Worsening Retinopathy:* A complication affecting the eyes, due to increased oxygen levels, potentially leading to abnormal blood vessel growth in the retina [17].
2. *Neuropathy Complications:* Diabetic neuropathy, which affects the nerves, can be worsened by HBOT due to the potential for increased oxidative stress on the nerves [18].
3. *Hypoglycemia:* HBOT can increase oxygen delivery to tissues, which may lead to increased glucose metabolism.
4. *Delayed Wound Healing:* While HBOT is often used to promote wound healing, in some cases, particularly in individuals with poorly controlled diabetes, it may not have the desired effect and could potentially delay wound healing [19].
5. *Barotrauma:* There is a risk of barotrauma, such as ear or sinus barotrauma, as a result of the pressure changes experienced during HBOT sessions.
6. *Infection:* There is a risk of infection, particularly in individuals with DFUs, as HBOT chambers provide a warm, moist environment that can promote bacterial growth [20].

14.7 Patient Management

Hyperbaric oxygen (HBO) rapidly improves tissue-specific insulin sensitivity and mitochondrial capacity in humans with type 2 diabetes, one single treatment of HBO with 100% O_2 achieved the following outcomes: (1) rapid improvement in insulin sensitivity in skeletal muscle, liver, and WAT; (2) marked improvement in mitochondrial functionality in all these tissues; (3) parallel stimulation of both ROS and antioxidative defense in skeletal muscle and WAT; (4) improved myocellular insulin signaling; and (5) no relevant effects on systemic inflammation [21, 22].

The therapeutic effect of HBOT in patients with severe to profound idiopathic sudden sensorineural hearing loss. There were no differences in hearing improvement between the HBOT and control group (SSNHL) patients with severe to profound SSNHL. However, the hearing recovery of the DM patients in the HBOT group was better than that of those in the control group. These findings imply that HBOT can be considered as one of the treatment methods for patients with severe to profound SSNHL and DM [23, 24].

The effect of HBOT on hematological indices and biochemical parameters in patients with diabetic foot [25]. In diabetic wounds, when inflammation is severe, cytokine levels are found to be high. Oxidative stress is increased during inflammation. CRP release from hepatocytes is also increased by pro-inflammatory cytokines [26]. As mentioned earlier HBOT suppresses inflammation, and it has been shown that HBOT decreases blood CRP levels in diabetic rats [27]. It has also been reported that a reduction in serum CRP and ESR values was reported in patients with diabetic foot wounds who received 120 minutes of HBOT for 20 days at a pressure of 2.5 ATA [28]. Adjuvant HBOT improved hematological indices in diabetic wound patients and had a beneficial effect on biochemical parameters, particularly glucose and CRP levels [29].

14.8 Potency of HBOT on Oral Candidiasis on DM

Hyperglycemia plays a crucial role in influencing the emergence of DM complications. Oral candidiasis can be prevented by maintaining oral hygiene and controlling blood sugar levels through proper medication [6]. However, since impaired immune response also plays an important role in pathogenic mechanisms that contribute to DM complications, a novel strategic therapy that affects those two mechanisms of action should be considered developed [30, 31]. HBOT showed promising results as an approach to overcoming oral complications in DM. This study aimed to determine the potency of HBOT on the blood glucose level, the amount of lymphocytes, and the expression of antibody anti-Candida in oral candidiasis DM [32]. It has been shown that hyperbaric oxygen has fungicidal effects against various fungi and yeasts. While it is not considered a standalone treatment, HBOT may complement conventional antifungal therapies. By creating an environment less favorable for Candida growth, HBOT can potentially enhance the efficacy of antifungal medications. Furthermore, there is evidence suggesting that HBOT, when combined with amphotericin B, can inhibit the growth of *Candida albicans*. This underscores the potential for synergistic effects between HBOT and antifungal agents in addressing fungal infections [33, 34].

An increase in the number of lymphocytes will be followed by an increase in antibodies that function to protect the body from foreign bodies, bacteria, and fungi. Lymphocytes release cytokines that can enhance the cellular immune response and modulate the antifungal activity of polymorphonuclear leukocytes and macrophages. Based on research conducted by Forsyth and Matthew, it is demonstrated that the proliferation of *Candida albicans* can be impeded by lymphocytes. This inhibition occurs through direct interactions with *Candida albicans* hyphae, involving intricate molecular mechanisms [35, 36].

Notably, IL-12-activated CD8þ lymphocytes play a role in directly hindering fungal growth, IL-12-activated NK cells release IFN-γ directly, and the SD11b/CD18 molecule serves as the primary structure in the attachment of lymphocytes to the fungal hypha. Lymphocytes serve as the host's primary defense against fungal infections of the mucosal surfaces and epidermis. An increase in the number of lymphocytes may represent the first step in producing an antifungal effect against *Candida albicans* [37, 38].

Administration of HBOT 2.4 ATA 3 for 30 minutes with 5-minute intervals inhaling ordinary air and performed for 5 consecutive days had a great effect on increasing the number of lymphocytes in diabetic rats, so that they could suppress the growth of *Candida albicans* fungi and accelerate the healing of oral candidiasis. In concordance with Dhingra et al., HBOT could inhibit fungal growth on the fifth day of therapy [39]. Further research on optimizing the duration of the therapy and combination with antifungal agents might reveal the potency of HBOT in oral candidiasis DM [40].

In diabetes, a longer duration of inflammation is observed. The consequence is longer osteoclast activity and bone resorption, resulting in a longer period of periodontal destruction. Other potential influences of diabetes on periodontal disease are as follows:

- Increased production of free oxygen radicals;
- Gingival epithelial barrier modifications;
- Shifts in the dental plaque microbiome.

A postulated mechanism linking periodontitis and diabetes is the influence of peri-pathogens and inflammatory mediators released locally in periodontal tissues. Then, due to their presence in the bloodstream, a systemic inflammatory response is triggered. In consequence, insulin signaling and insulin resistance are impaired. Additionally, increased levels of HbA1c contribute to a higher risk of diabetic complications [41, 42].

In a randomized controlled trial, a reduction in HbA1c levels after periodontal treatment was observed—a reduction of approximately 3–4 mmol/mol (about 0.3–0.4%) over a period of 3–4 months after periodontal treatment. The reduced plaque may likely be responsible for the reduction in the inflammatory process in the periodontal tissues, which reduces systemic inflammation and the activation of the immune system [43, 44].

14.9 HBOT—Medical Applications

The mechanism of action allows the flushing out of toxic gases, stimulates fibroblast proliferation and neovascularization, increases bacterial killing by a free radical mechanism, and suppresses inflammation by inhibiting leukocyte adhesion to the endothelium. Increased blood oxygen content allows recovery from hypoxia and circulatory disorders, enhances wound healing and the regeneration of damaged tissues, and improves fibrous scar remodeling. The aforementioned mechanisms help in the treatment of refractory conditions such as osteoarthritis, radiation necrosis, or diabetic foot. Increasing the amount of dissolved oxygen in tissue with a deficit of it creates a favorable environment for wound reconstruction and healing [45, 46].

14.10 Application of HBOT in DFUs

HBOT could effectively increase the complete healing rate of DFU and reduce the amputation rate, but it would increase the incidence of adverse reactions, while it had no significant effect on mortality [47]. Effect of hyperbaric oxygen treatment on Diabetic foot ulcers. In a meta-analysis studying the effects after hyperbaric oxygen treatment, cellular and biochemical changes in the tissues of diabetic wounds support wound healing, which further leads to an increase in growth factors and fibronectin to hasten cellular proliferation, migration, and the production of extracellular matrix molecules. Additionally, a variation in the methodology used to measure ulcer size and the length of the evaluation could be a factor in the results being non-significant. To use the usefulness of hyperbaric oxygen treatment in reducing ulcer size in patients with DFUs, more studies or robust randomized controlled trials with a high sample size are needed [48, 49].

The examined data showed that hyperbaric oxygen treatment revealed significantly higher healed ulcers, higher adverse events, lower mortality, and higher ulcer area reduction compared to standard treatment in patients with DFUs. However, hyperbaric oxygen treatment and standard treatment had no significant difference in amputation and healing time in patients with DFUs. Yet, attention should be paid to its values since most of the selected examinations had a low sample size (11 out of 17 examinations were ≥100), and some of the comparisons had a low number of selected studies [50–52].

14.11 Future Directions

There is growing interest in exploring the potential of HBOT in managing other diabetic complications, such as diabetic retinopathy (affecting the eyes) and diabetic neuropathy (nerve damage). Research in these areas is ongoing, and while some studies have shown promising results, more evidence is needed to establish the effectiveness of HBOT in these contexts [53, 54].

As technology and understanding of HBOT mechanisms advance, future developments may include more personalized treatment approaches tailored to individual patient characteristics and wound types. This could involve optimizing treatment parameters such as pressure levels, duration of sessions, and frequency of treatments to maximize therapeutic benefits while minimizing potential risks [55, 56].

Overall, while HBOT holds promise in the management of diabetic complications, including foot ulcers, retinopathy, and neuropathy, further research and clinical trials are necessary to fully elucidate its potential benefits, optimize treatment protocols, and expand its applications in diabetic care [7].

14.12 Conclusions

HBOT presents a multifaceted approach in managing complications arising from DM. By harnessing mechanisms such as increased oxygen delivery, angiogenesis, inflammation reduction, and antimicrobial activity, HBOT offers a promising adjunctive therapy to traditional treatment modalities. Clinical evidence suggests its efficacy in promoting wound healing, mitigating infection risks and potentially addressing diabetic neuropathy and microvascular complications. However, the implementation of HBOT requires careful patient selection, monitoring, and consideration of potential complications such as worsened retinopathy and neuropathy. Despite ongoing research and promising results in various diabetic complications, further studies are needed to establish its efficacy, optimize treatment protocols, and explore its potential in managing other diabetic complications. As technology advances, personalized HBOT approaches tailored to individual patient needs may enhance therapeutic outcomes and broaden its applications in diabetic care. Overall, while HBOT holds great promise, continued research and clinical trials are essential to unlock its full potential in improving outcomes for individuals living with DM.

References

1. Feldmeier J, Carl U, Hartmann K, Sminia P. Hyperbaric oxygen: does it promote growth or recurrence of malignancy? Undersea Hyperb Med. 2003;30(1):1–18. PMID: 12916472
2. Camporesi EM, Bosco G. Mechanisms of action of hyperbaric oxygen therapy. Undersea Hyperb Med. 2014;41(3):247–52. PMID: 25109086
3. Löndahl M. Hyperbaric oxygen therapy as an adjunctive treatment for diabetic foot ulcers. Med Clin North Am. 2013;97(5):957–80. https://doi.org/10.1016/j.mcna.2013.03.011.
4. Kranke P, Bennett M, Roeckl-Wiedmann I, Debus S. Hyperbaric oxygen therapy for chronic wounds. Cochrane Database Syst Rev. 2004;2:CD004123. https://doi.org/10.1002/14651858.CD004123.pub2.
5. Zhang Q, Chang Q, Cox RA, et al. Hyperbaric oxygen attenuates apoptosis and decreases inflammation in an ischemic wound model. J Invest Dermatol. 2008;128(8):2102–12. https://doi.org/10.1038/jid.2008.33.
6. Thom SR. Hyperbaric oxygen: its mechanisms and efficacy. Plast Reconstr Surg. 2011;127(Suppl 1):131S–41S. https://doi.org/10.1097/PRS.0b013e3181fbe2bf.
7. Hunt TK, Pai MP. The effect of varying ambient oxygen tensions on wound metabolism and collagen synthesis. Surg Gynecol Obstet. 1972;135(4):561–7.
8. Abidia A, Laden G, Kuhan G, et al. The role of hyperbaric oxygen therapy in ischaemic diabetic lower extremity ulcers: a double-blind randomized controlled trial. Eur J Vasc Endovasc Surg. 2003;25(6):513–8. https://doi.org/10.1053/ejvs.2002.1904.
9. Cianci P, Petrone G, Drago L, et al. Hyperbaric oxygen therapy in diabetic foot treatment. Acta Chir Belg. 2016;116(4):223–7. https://doi.org/10.1080/00015458.2016.1193305.
10. Londahl M. Hyperbaric oxygen therapy as an adjunctive treatment for diabetic foot ulcers. Int J Low Extrem Wounds. 2016;15(3):220–8. https://doi.org/10.1177/1534734616662896.
11. Diabetic Foot Ulcers: Driver VR, et al. The costs of diabetic foot: the economic case for the limb salvage team. J Vasc Surg. 2010;52(3 Suppl):17S–22S. https://doi.org/10.1016/j.jvs.2010.06.003. Löndahl M. Hyperbaric oxygen therapy as adjunctive treatment of

diabetic foot ulcers. Med Clin North Am. 2013;97(5):957–980. https://doi.org/10.1016/j.mcna.2013.03.010
12. Delayed Wound Healing: Londahl M, Katzman P, Nilsson A, Hammarlund C. Hyperbaric oxygen therapy facilitates healing of chronic foot ulcers in patients with diabetes. Diabetes Care. 2010;33(5):998–1003. https://doi.org/10.2337/dc09-1749. Abidia A, et al. The role of hyperbaric oxygen therapy in ischaemic diabetic lower extremity ulcers: a double-blind randomized-controlled trial. Eur J Vasc Endovasc Surg. 2003;25(6):513–518. https://doi.org/10.1053/ejvs.2002.1905
13. Radiation-Induced Tissue Damage: Bennett MH, Feldmeier J, Hampson NB, Smee R, Milross C. Hyperbaric oxygen therapy for late radiation tissue injury. Cochrane Database Syst Rev. 2016;4(4):CD005005. https://doi.org/10.1002/14651858.CD005005.pub4. Al-Waili NS, Butler GJ. Effects of hyperbaric oxygen on inflammatory response to wound and trauma: possible mechanism of action. Sci World J. 2006;6:425–441. https://doi.org/10.1100/tsw.2006.109
14. Diabetic Retinopathy: Palojärvi A, Vähätupa M, Kuusela T. Hyperbaric oxygen therapy in retinopathy. Diabetes. 1967;16(6):431–433. https://doi.org/10.2337/diab.16.6.431. Ljubimov AV, et al. Molecular mirages in diabetic retinopathy. Eye (Lond). 2018;32(5):897–905. https://doi.org/10.1038/s41433-017-0002-4
15. Abidia A, Laden G, Kuhan G, et al. The role of hyperbaric oxygen therapy in ischaemic diabetic lower extremity ulcers: a double-blind randomized-controlled trial. Eur J Vasc Endovasc Surg. 2003;25(6):513–8. https://doi.org/10.1053/ejvs.2002.1891.
16. Zamboni WA, Wong HP, Stephenson LL, Pfeifer MA. Evaluation of hyperbaric oxygen for diabetic wounds: a prospective study. Undersea Hyperb Med. 1997;24(3):175–9.
17. Thom SR. Hyperbaric oxygen: its mechanisms and efficacy. Plast Reconstr Surg. 2009;123(5S):110S–7S. https://doi.org/10.1097/PRS.0b013e3181a2c877.
18. Feldmeier JJ. Hyperbaric oxygen therapy and delayed radiation injuries (soft tissue and bony necrosis): 2012 update. Undersea & hyperbaric medicine: journal of the Undersea and Hyperbaric Medical Society, Inc. 2017;44(3):257–62. [PMID: 28641541]
19. Kranke P, Bennett MH, Martyn-St James M, Schnabel A, Debus SE. Hyperbaric oxygen therapy for chronic wounds. Cochrane Database Syst Rev. 2015;2015(6):CD004123. https://doi.org/10.1002/14651858.CD004123.pub4.
20. Mathieu D, Marroni A, Kot J. Tenth European Consensus Conference on Hyperbaric Medicine: recommendations for accepted and non-accepted clinical indications and practice of hyperbaric oxygen treatment. Diving Hyperb Med. 2010;40(4):240–51. [PMID: 21560691]
21. Theresia Sarabhai et al/Published: 30 September 2022.
22. Deafness NIo, Disorders OC. NIDCD Fact Sheet: Sudden Deafness (US Department of Health and Human Services, 2018).
23. Alexander TH, Harris JP. Incidence of sudden sensorineural hearing loss. Otol Neurotol. 2013;34(9):1586–9.
24. Mattox DE, Simmons FB. Natural history of sudden sensorineural hearing loss. Ann Otol Rhinol Laryngol. 1977;86(4):463–80.
25. Byl FM Jr. Sudden hearing loss: eight years' experience and suggested prognostic table. Laryngoscope. 1984;94(5):647–61.
26. Liu R, Li L, Yang M, et al. Systematic review of the effectiveness of hyperbaric oxygenation therapy in the management of chronic diabetic foot ulcers. Mayo Clin Proc. 2013;88:166–75.
27. Sharma R, Sharma SK, Mudgal SK, et al. Efficacy of hyperbaric oxygen therapy for diabetic foot ulcer, a systematic review, and meta-analysis of controlled clinical trials. Sci Rep. 2021;11:2189.
28. Gunes AE, Aktas S. Effect of hyperbaric oxygen therapy on complete blood count. Undersea Hyperb Med. 2017;44:357–64.
29. Adil GF, Jasim NA, Narjis AHA. Hematological changes among divers. Med J Basrah Uni. 2006;24:60–5.

30. Sinan M, Ertan NZ, Mirasoglu B, et al. Acute and long-term effects of hyperbaric oxygen therapy on hemorheological parame-ters in patients with various disorders. Clin Hemorheol Microcirc. 2016;62:79–88.
31. Mulawarmanti D, Parisihni K, Widyastuti W. The impact of hyperbaric oxygen therapy on serum C-reactive protein levels, osteoprotegerin expression, and osteoclast numbers in induced-periodontitis diabetic rats. Eur J Dent. 2020;14:404–9.
32. Chen C, Wu R, Hsu M, et al. Adjunctive hyperbaric oxygen therapy for healing of chronic diabetic foot ulcers: a randomized controlled trial. J Wound Ostomy Continence Nurs. 2017;44:536–45.
33. Chang JS, Chang E, Lee Y, et al. Hyperbaric oxygen exposure atten-uates circulating stress biomarkers: a pilot interventional study. Int J Environ Res Public Health. 2020;17:7853.
34. Cruz-Villanueva SR, Ramirez-Nava JC, Moreno-Luna JA, et al. Effect of Hyperbaric Oxygen Therapy (HBOT) on insulin resis-tance associated with abdominal obesity in Wistar rats with dietary sucrose-induced metabolic syndrome. J Nutr Sci Vitaminol (Tokyo). 2021;67:292–300.
35. Woo J, Min JH, Lee YH, Roh HT. Effects of hyperbaric oxygen therapy on inflammation, oxidative/antioxidant balance, and muscle damage after acute exercise in normobaric, normoxic and hypobaric, hypoxic environments: a pilot study. Int J Environ Res Public Health. 2020;17(20):7377.
36. Korpinar S, Uzun H. The effect of hyperbaric oxygen at different pressures on oxidative stress and antioxidant status in rats. Medicina (B Aires) 2019;55(02):1–8 22; Li FQ, Ma CF, Shi LN, et al. Diagnostic value of immunoglobulin G antibodies against Candida enolase and fructose bisphosphate aldolase for candidemia. BMC Infect Dis. 2013;13:253.
37. Samaranayake YH, Samaranayake LP. Experimental oral candidiasis in animal models. Clin Microbiol Rev. 2001;14(02):398–429.
38. Laihad FM, Sudiana IK, Guritno MS. Literature review: hyperbaric oxygen therapy on mucormycosis infection in oral cavity. Folia Medica Indonesiana. 2017;53(02):163–8.
39. Andriani D, Setyaningtyas D, Nafi'ah. Efek ekstrak acanthus ilicifolius terhadap ekspresi antibodi anticandida albicans pada tikus wistar terimunosupresi oral kandidiasis. Denta Jurnal Kedokteran Gigi. 2017;11(01):35–41.
40. Segal E, Menhusen MJ, Shawn S. Hyperbaric oxygen in the treatment of invasive fungal infections: a single-center experience. Isr Med Assoc J. 2007;9(05):355–7.
41. Forsyth CB, Mathews HL. Lymphocyte adhesion to Candida albi-cans. Infect Immun. 2002;70(02):517–27.
42. Dhingra S, Buckey JC, Cramer RA. Hyperbaric oxygen reduces Aspergillus fumigatus proliferation in vitro and influences in vivo disease outcomes. Antimicrob Agents Chemother. 2018;62(03):17–8.
43. WHO. Available online: https://www.who.int/health-topics/oral-health#tab=tab_1. Accessed on 2 Jan 2023
44. IDF Diabetes Atlas. Available online: https://diabetesatlas.org/atlas/ninth-edition;2019. Accessed on 2 Jan 2023
45. Shinomiya N. Molecular mechanisms of hyperbaric oxygen therapy. In: Shinomiya N, Asai Y, editors. Hyperbaric oxygenation therapy, vol. 1. Singapore: Springe; 2020. p. 3–20.
46. Resanović I, Zarić B, Radovanović J, Sudar-Milovanović E, Gluvić Z, Jevremović D, Isenović ER. Hyperbaric oxygen therapy and vascular complications in diabetes mellitus. Angiology. 2020;71:876–85.
47. Rekomendacje Grupy Roboczej Polskiego Towarzystwa Stomatologicznego i Narodowego Programu Ochrony Antybiotyków w Zakresie Stosowania Antybiotyków w Stomatologii. Available online: https://stomatologia-zalecenia-25_01-net.pdf. (antybiotyki.edu.pl). Accessed on 20 Apr 2023
48. Eley B, Soory M, Manson JD. Periodontics, vol. 15. 6th ed. Churchill Livingstone: Livingstone; 2010. p. 233.
49. Papapanou PN, Sanz M, Buduneli N, Dietrich T, Feres M, Fine DH, Flemmig TF, Garcia R, Giannobile WV, Graziani F, et al. Periodontitis: consensus report of workgroup 2 of the 2017

world workshop on the classification of periodontal and Peri—implant diseases and conditions. J Periodontol. 2018;89(Suppl. S1):S173–82.
50. Received: 7 December 2023 Accepted: 15 Dec 2023. https://doi.org/10.1111/iwj.14621
51. Int Wound J. 2024;21:e14621. https://doi.org/10.1111/iwj.14621.
52. Imam MS, Mohamed EA, Abdelrahim. First published: 05 Oct. Citations: 2; 2023. https://doi.org/10.1111/iwj.14427.
53. Bennett MH, Feldmeier J, Hampson NB, Smee R, Milross C. Hyperbaric oxygen therapy for late radiation tissue injury. Cochrane Database Syst Rev. 2016;4:CD005005.
54. Kalani M, Jörneskog G. Nader's commentary on hyperbaric oxygen therapy. Springer; 2012.
55. Goldman RJ. Hyperbaric oxygen therapy for wound healing and limb salvage: a systematic review. PM & R: The Journal of Injury, Function, and Rehabilitation. 2009;1(5):471–89.
56. Löndahl M, Katzman P, Nilsson A, Hammarlund C, Eneroth M. Hyperbaric oxygen therapy facilitates healing of chronic foot ulcers in patients with diabetes. Diabetes Care. 2011;34(5):1115–20.

Chapter 15
Diabetic and Ischemic Wound

Tamanna Bajracharya, Prastab Parajuli, and Asmita Giri

15.1 Introduction

Ischemic and diabetic wounds are predominant chronic wounds that are encountered in clinical practice. A chronic wound is a full-thickness skin defect that fails to heal after 3 months of standard care [1]. These commonly arise from a vascular (arterial insufficiency and venous stasis), pressure, or diabetic ulcer, but can be sometimes due to infections, traumas, burns, surgical complications, and immune diseases. Nonhealing, chronic wounds pose a substantial negative impact on both the quality of life of patients and health care systems. The presence of co-morbidities, such as diabetes or peripheral artery disease, and increased age have a major contribution to the impairment of the healing process of an ulcer, thus resulting in chronic wounds [1, 2].

15.2 Clinical Features

15.2.1 Arterial Insufficiency Ulcers

- Patients present with signs and symptoms of arterial insufficiency, such as claudication and/or rest pain, depending on the severity.
- Typically located in the most distal part of the toes where there is the least blood flow, or in areas with the potential for pressure such as foot web spaces and over phalangeal heads.

T. Bajracharya (✉) · P. Parajuli · A. Giri
Critical Care Medicine, BnB HospitalGwarko, Lalitpur, Bagmati Province, Nepal

A. G. D'Almeida, J. Hidalgo (eds.), *Evidence-Based Hyperbaric Medicine*,
https://doi.org/10.1007/978-3-032-06346-5_15

- Have sharply demarcated "punched out" margins and are associated with minimal exudate [3].
- The bed of the ulcers is usually pale, non-granulating, and necrotic attributing to inadequate blood flow.
- The surrounding skin may be dusky erythematous, cool to touch, hairless, thin, and brittle, with a shiny texture.
- There may be thickening or loss of toenails.
- Gangrene of the extremities may also occur.
- Dorsalis pedis and posterior tibial artery pulsation may be diminished or even absent. The ankle-brachial index may be low [4].

15.2.2 Venous Ulcers

- Typically located between mid-calf and the ankle, with the medial and lateral malleolus being the most common sites [3].
- Ulceration may be discrete or circumferential with an irregular, gently sloping edge with an ulcer bed often covered with a fibrinous layer mixed with granulation tissue [3].
- The patients generally describe a dull ache and swelling that improve with elevation.
- The skin surrounding the ulcer is eczematous, presenting with scaling, weeping, and crusting, and is intensely pruritic.
- The limb is usually edematous, firm, and warm with reddish-brown hyperpigmentation (Fig. 15.1).

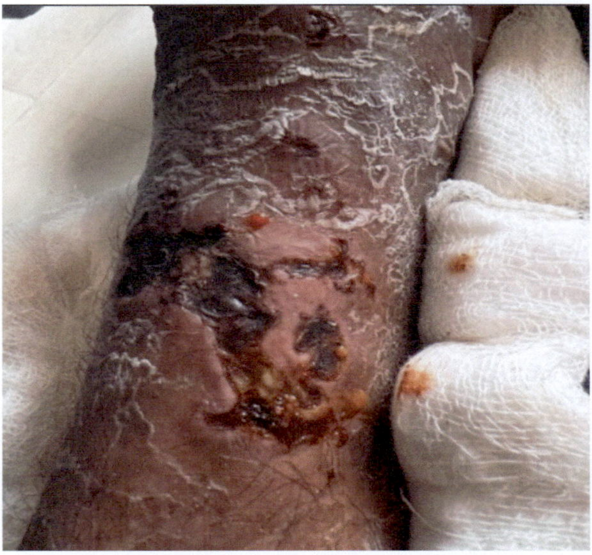

Fig. 15.1 Venous ulcer. (Courtesy: Dr. Parash Shrestha)

15.2.3 Pressure Ulcers

- Pressure ulcers usually develop in the skin and soft tissue overlying bony prominences, common areas being sacrum, ischial tuberosity, calcaneum, medial and lateral metatarsal heads, and fibula heads.
- These can present as intact skin or as an open ulcer.
- Stages of pressure ulcers have been given by the National Pressure Ulcer Advisory Panel staging system.
  Stage 1: Non-blanchable erythema of intact skin.
  Stage 2: Partial-thickness skin loss with exposed dermis.
  Stage 3: Full-thickness skin loss, in which fat is visible in the ulcer. Fascia, muscle, tendon, ligament, cartilage, and/or bone are not exposed.
  Stage 4: Full-thickness skin and tissue loss. Full-thickness skin and tissue loss with exposed or directly palpable fascia, muscle, tendon, ligament, cartilage, or bone in the ulcer.
  Unstageable Pressure Injury: in which the extent of tissue damage within the ulcer cannot be confirmed because it is obscured by slough or eschar (Fig. 15.2).

15.2.4 Diabetic Ulcers

- Usually not painful.
- Mixed neuropathic and vascular disease.
- Located in pressure sites, planter surface, heels, and bony prominences.

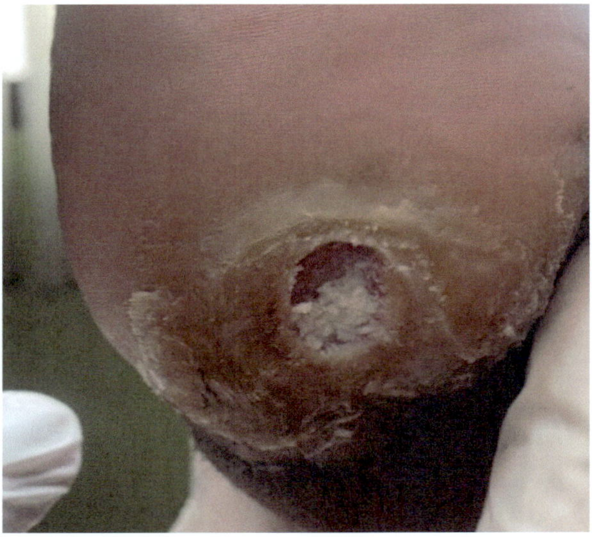

Fig. 15.2 Pressure ulcer. (Courtesy: Dr. Parash Shrestha)

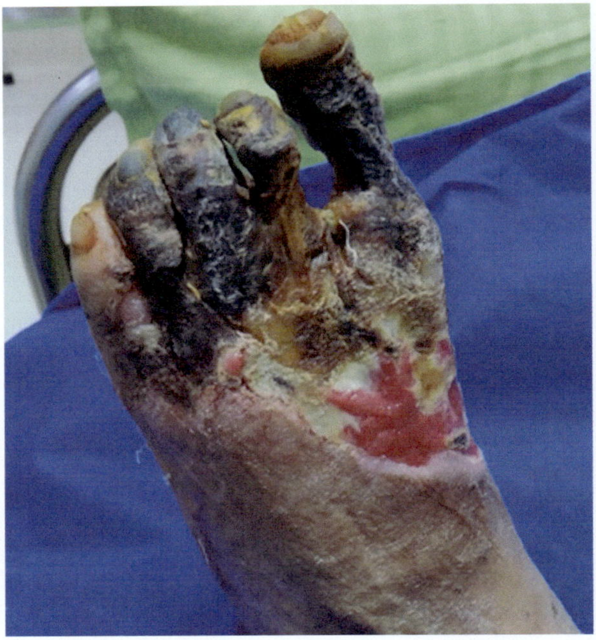

Fig. 15.3 Diabetic ulcer. (Courtesy: Dr. Parash Shrestha)

- Have a thin undermined border with a black-gray or yellow base.
- Surrounding skin is usually pale and has a reticular pattern.
- Callus or bullae around the wound.
- Sometimes Charcot's, hammertoe deformity present.
- Pulses usually present and unreliable ABI index.
- Wagner classification can be used to grade diabetic foot ulcer:
  Grade 0—intact skin.
  Grade 1—superficial ulcer of the skin or subcutaneous tissue.
  Grade 2—ulcers extend into tendon, bone, or capsule.
  Grade 3—deep ulcer with osteomyelitis, or abscess.
  Grade 4—partial foot gangrene.
  Grade 5—whole foot gangrene (Fig. 15.3).

15.3 Etiology

Based on the causative etiologies, the Wound Healing Society classifies chronic wounds into four categories: pressure ulcers, venous ulcers, arterial insufficiency ulcers, and diabetic ulcers [5].

15.3.1 Pressure Ulcers

Pressure ulcers, as their name implies, are areas of tissue necrosis caused by unrelieved pressure to soft tissue compressed between a bony prominence and an external surface for a prolonged period of time. Pressure injuries affect 6–18% of hospitalized patients [6, 7]. The average hospital length of stay for patients diagnosed with pressure ulcers is three times that of patients who do not develop pressure ulcers [8]. The etiologic factors involved in their development are biomechanical forces (confined pressure, shearing forces, and friction), moisture, and local ischemia. Pressure ulcers particularly affect comorbid and elderly patients, especially those who are chronically ill, bed- or wheelchair-bound, and patients in the intensive care unit. Ischemia-reperfusion injury, inadequate lymphatic drainage, cellular deformation, excess cellular apoptosis, and extracellular matrix breakdown are the major factors during pressure injury, which cause a chronic inflammatory state and dysregulated healing [9].

15.3.2 Venous Ulcers

A venous ulcer occurs most commonly on the lower extremities. It accounts for 70–80% of leg ulcers presenting for evaluation [10]. The overall prevalence of this condition is 2% rising to 5% in those over 65 years of age [11]. Venous ulcers are more common in women and older persons. The primary risk factors are older age, obesity, previous leg injuries, deep venous thrombosis, post-thrombotic syndrome, varicose veins, and phlebitis [12].

These ulcers affect the venous microvasculature and the macrovascular system. The macrovasculature involves abnormalities with hemodynamics. In the lower extremities, blood flows from the superficial perforating veins to the deep veins, with valves in each system to ensure unidirectional blood flow. When the calf muscles contract, the blood flow from the deep veins into the inferior vena cava. Any defect, such as venous dilation, incompetent valves, and venous reflux, results in venous insufficiency. Several demographics, genetic, and environmental factors could trigger such conditions. This chronic insufficiency and stasis lead to venous hypertension and venous stasis. The glycocalyx and endothelium present in microvasculature are affected by changes in shear stress and activation of leukocytes and adhesion molecules. The microvascular system is composed of a network of capillaries, post-capillary venules, interstitium, and lymphatic vessels that respond to overexpressed inflammatory pathways and upregulation of cytokines, chemokines, matrix metalloproteinases, iron-free radicals, and activated oxygen and nitrogen [13].

15.3.3 Arterial Ulcers

Arterial ischemic ulcers compose about 5–20% of all nonhealing lower extremity ulcers [14]. Many diseases and disorders can cause peripheral arterial ulcers, including Raynaud's disease, arteriosclerosis obliterans, Buerger's disease, arterial emboli or thrombi, and obliterative or cutaneous vasculopathy. Arterial ulcers are often associated with a history of atherosclerosis, hypertension, hyperlipidemia, diabetes, smoking, prolonged bedridden patients due to illness or disability, and elderly patients [14]. These ulcers are usually located on the leg or foot area but can occur in any pressure point area in the presence of reduced blood perfusion. They are caused by inadequate tissue blood perfusion of the lower extremities, resulting in tissue hypoxia and tissue damage [3]. They are often painful, and the pain associated with the ischemic ulcer has been described as a combination of nociceptive and neuropathic pain [15]. The three macrovascular mechanisms involved in the pathogenesis of arterial ulcers are extramural strangulation, mural thickening or accretion, and intramural restriction of blood flow, which occurs with considerable overlapping [16].

15.3.4 Diabetic Ulcers

Statistics indicate that 15–25% of persons with diabetes mellitus will get a diabetic foot ulcer (DFU) [17] with an annual incidence of 2–4% [18]. The global prevalence of diabetic foot was 6.3% (95%CI: 5.4–7.3%) with the rate being highest in North America [19]. The increasing incidence of diabetes and increased longevity of diabetic patients are linked with rising burdens due to DF s [20]. Worsening of DFUs leads to lengthy hospital stays and surgical interventions such as debridement and even amputation. Diabetic foot was found to be more common in males compared to females, and more prevalent in type 2 than in type 1 diabetic patients.

The risk factors of DFU can be personal or foot-specific factors. The patients with advanced age, lower BMI, long-standing diabetes, uncontrolled diabetes, diabetic retinopathy, nephropathy, hypertension, history of smoking, cardiovascular disease, black Hispanic race, people from low-income and low literacy rate backgrounds, and people with poor nutritional status were more likely to develop diabetic foot. Joint mobility limitation and toe and foot deformities are at a high risk of developing foot ulcers [19, 21, 22]. Diabetic wounds are associated with an increased risk of death [23]. The underlying etiology of DFU is classified into three types: purely neuropathic (35%), purely ischemic (15%), and mixed neuroischemic (50%) [24]. Factors related to diabetes that contribute to the pathogenesis of DFUs include neuropathic, vascular, and immune system components, all of which are related with the hyperglycemic state [22].

15.3.5 Neuropathy

The hyperglycemic conditions increased the production of some enzymes, such as aldose reductase and sorbitol dehydrogenase. These enzymes convert glucose into sorbitol and fructose. As these sugar products accumulate, the synthesis of nerve cell myoinositol is decreased, affecting nerve conduction. Hyperglycemia produces free reactive oxygen species (ROS) which damage the blood supply and metabolism and structure of the peripheral nerve [25].

Sensory neuropathy leads to loss of proprioception, pain, and temperature sensation, which predisposes to unrecognized minor trauma and contributes to abnormal gait. Pre-ulcerative lesions or minor wounds remain unnoticed and are repeatedly re-traumatized, resulting in ulcer formation. Motor neuropathy precipitates muscle wasting, flexor-extensor imbalance, foot deformities (equinus deformity, clawed toes, hammertoes (toes in permanent flexion), and Charcot's deformity (flattening of the medial longitudinal arches)), abnormal gait, and consequently abnormal pressure distribution that predisposes new pressure points to ulceration. Autonomic neuropathy results in reduced sweating that causes dry, fragile skin prone to spontaneous cracking, reduced sympathetic nerve-induced vasoconstriction, and microvascular dysregulation of the skin that contributes to local edema and ultimately impaired healing [26].

There are three stages in the evolution of diabetic ulcers. Sensory, motor, and autonomic neuropathy leads to the development of a callus, which is the first stage of the formation of a diabetic ulcer. Repetitive trauma to the callus leads to subcutaneous hemorrhage, and finally, its erosion leads to the formation of an ulcer [27].

15.3.6 Vasculopathy

Diabetes is strongly associated with the development and acceleration of peripheral arterial disease. The peripheral arterial disease causes narrowing or blockage of blood vessels in the extremities, usually the lower extremities, that results in decreased perfusion leading to ischemic ulcer [28]. Diabetes also affects the microvascular beds by altering the basement membrane structure, the integrity of the capillary wall, the regulatory function of the endothelium, and the tendency for microvascular thrombosis. These micro and macrovascular changes result in tissue ischemia and impaired wound healing.

15.3.7 Immunopathy

Diabetic patient poses ineffective inflammatory response, impaired angiogenesis, neuropathy, barrier disruption, and subsequent polymicrobial infection, which strongly favor impaired wound healing [25].

15.4 Molecular Pathophysiology of Diabetic and Ischemic Wounds

Naturally, wound repair proceeds through various phases that involve an inflammatory response and cellular migration, proliferation, matrix deposition, and tissue remodeling. Wound healing begins immediately following injury. There is the activation of the hemostasis mechanism, where a platelet plug is formed to prevent blood loss and provides a preliminary fibrin matrix for cell migration. Platelets also secrete growth factors and cytokines. It is then followed by the recruitment of inflammatory and other cells such as neutrophils, monocytes, and macrophages. Neutrophils release ROS and protease that prevent bacterial contamination and cleanse the wound of cellular debris. Blood monocytes arrive at the wound site and differentiate into macrophages, which not only remove bacteria and nonviable tissue by phagocytosis but also release various growth factors and cytokine-recruiting fibroblast, endothelial cells, and keratinocytes. Once the inflammation phase starts to diminish, and immune cells undergo apoptosis, the proliferation phase sets in. In the proliferative phase, keratinocytes begin to close the wound gap, new blood vessels develop through angiogenesis, and fibroblasts take the place of the original fibrin clot with granulation tissue. Finally, the deposited matrix is remodeled further by fibroblasts, blood vessels regress, and myofibroblasts cause overall wound contraction [29]. Despite such innate healing properties of wounds, multiple aspects of an individual attenuate the healing process. Although all types of chronic wounds appear to have nothing in common pathophysiology, closer examination of their similarities can lead to the conclusion that all chronic wounds are caused by a combination of causes rather than a single deficiency. Each component of pathogenesis is deleterious, but, in aggregate, they collectively overwhelm the healing response in many patients [30]. Some common features shared by each of these wounds include prolonged or excessive inflammation, persistent infections, formation of drug-resistant microbial films, and the inability of dermal and or epidermal cells to respond to reparative stimuli. However, the underlying pathologies differ among various types of chronic wounds, making it challenging to treat [31].

15.4.1 The Role of Inflammatory Response

Interruption or dysregulation of one or more phases of the normal wound-healing process leads to nonhealing (chronic) wounds. Inflammation is prolonged in chronic wounds, and it is believed that these wounds might be trapped in a chronic inflammatory state that fails to progress [32]. Chronic wound tissue and fluid analysis indicate a misbalanced environment between inflammatory and anti-inflammatory signals [33, 34]. The increased proinflammatory cellular infiltrates are composed largely of neutrophils and macrophages. As a result, the deregulation of several key proinflammatory cytokines, such as IL-1β and tumor necrosis factor-α (TNFα), prolongs the inflammatory phase and delays healing. An increase in IL-1β and TNFα leads to elevated metalloproteinases that excessively degrade the local Extracellular matrix and thus impair cell migration [34]. Recent studies have implicated the inflammasome, a multiprotein complex of the innate immune system responsible for the activation and release of IL-1β in the development of chronic wounds [35].

15.4.2 The Role of Bacteria

Contamination of wounds with microbial is inevitable. All chronic wounds show significant bacteria count [36]. The host immune response to bacteria is inflammation, chiefly an influx of polymorphonuclear leukocytes that release proteases and oxidants, which degrade cytokines and the extracellular matrix. In chronic wounds, there is an excess of protease level, which leads to proteolytic destruction of the extracellular matrix and prevents the wound from moving forward into the proliferative phase, and also amplify the inflammatory cycle, which leads to a delay in wound healing [37].

15.4.3 The Role of Angiogenesis and Vasculogenesis

Both angiogenesis (sprouting of capillaries from existing blood vessels) and vasculogenesis (mobilization of bone marrow-derived endothelial progenitors) are essential components of tissue repair as they support cells at the wound site with nutrition and oxygen [38]. Inadequate local angiogenesis is considered to be a contributing factor to impaired healing. Proteins with antiangiogenic properties, such as myeloperoxidase, exhibit high expression levels in chronic wounds of diabetic patients, whereas angiogenic stimulators, such as extracellular superoxide dismutase, are generally decreased. Such an antiangiogenic environment leads to elevated cell death, demonstrated by Annexin A5, which is exclusively found in chronic wound exudates [39]. Deprivation of proangiogenic factors, such as members of the vascular endothelial growth factor family in vascular leg ulcers and chemokine (C-X-C motif) ligand 9 expression in pressure ulcer, prevents normal angiogenesis [40–43].

15.4.4 The Role of the Senescent Cell Population

Chronic wounds are characterized by a senescent cell population of keratinocytes, endothelial cells, fibroblasts, and macrophages, which demonstrate impaired proliferative and secretory capacities, and are made unresponsive to typical wound-healing signals. Fibroblasts in particular from venous and pressure ulcers have a diminished ability to proliferate [44]. The senescent cells in chronic wounds are attributed to oxidative stress that leads to DNA damage-related cell cycle arrest or to abnormal metabolic changes in diabetic patients.

15.4.5 The Role of Ischemia-Reperfusion Injury

Cyclic ischemia-reperfusion injury remains a novel concept as it relates to chronic ulcers [45]. Ischemia-reperfusion injury is characterized by a sequence of biochemical and cellular events that cause extensive cellular damage through pathways that lead to leukocyte and complement activation, oxidative stress, and microvasculature dysfunction [46].

During the ischemic event, there is a lack of oxygen and essential nutrient supply, which impairs cellular metabolism. At a cellular level, there is the reduction of ATP production through impairment of mitochondrial oxidative phosphorylation, which results in loss of the transmembrane potential and an influx of various ionic species, leading to cell swelling and activation of enzymes responsible for cell membrane disruption. In addition, ischemia induces the expression of endothelial adhesion molecules and cytokines that prime the tissue for further insult by creating a proinflammatory state. Upon reperfusion, leukocytes become activated, and the inflammatory cascade ensues, causing deleterious cellular reactions and tissue damage. The sudden influx of oxygen causes the overproduction of ROS, a process termed oxidative stress, which causes cytotoxic injury to surrounding tissues [47]. Impaired vasorelaxation due to a decrease in nitrous oxide expression during reperfusion also contributes significantly to microvascular dysfunction [48].

15.5 Management of Diabetic and Ischemic Wounds

Management begins with a detailed history and assessment of the wound status. Chronic relevant illnesses such as diabetes, deep vein thrombosis, and hypertension should be looked for and optimized, as this might impact wound healing as in diabetes. The lifestyle of the patient, including smoking/alcohol use and mobility, should be evaluated. The nutritional status of the patient should also be assessed, as this is significant for wound healing.

The plan should be made for optimization of chronic illnesses, lifestyle modification, and building up the nutritional status of the patient along with the treatment of the ulcer. Treatment should be individualized and should have a multi-disciplinary approach.

The leg should be evaluated for ulcer size, site, appearance, wound base, and extension. Peripheral pulses should be assessed. This examination helps in differentiating different ulcer types and helps in forming a treatment plan for the patient.

Signs of neuropathy should be looked for during the assessment of the patient. The ulcer should be concomitantly evaluated for signs of local and systemic infection, as this is also the cause of wound healing failure. Neuropathy can mask the presence of deep infections or abscesses. Hence, clinical suspicion must remain high when insensate patients complain of pain or flu-like symptoms. Once diagnosed, infection-complicating chronic wounds must be treated aggressively. This includes thorough debridement, surgical drainage of abscesses, debridement of infected bone, and bone and tissue culture-guided antimicrobial therapy [31].

Blood investigations along with radiological evaluation of the involved limb and ulcer should be done. Angiography with revascularization might be necessary at times and should be planned during the evaluation of the patient, especially in suspected arterial ulcers, with the goal of improving the blood flow to the wound site and augmenting healing.

Debridement has long been recognized as a critical component of wound care. Sharp debridement removes nonviable tissue and slough along with bacterial biofilms that prolong the inflammatory response in the chronic wound. Thorough debridement converts the chronic wound from one that is excessively inflamed to more of an acute profile that can jump-start the wound toward a healing trajectory [49]. Ulcerectomy involving complete excision of ulcers down to healthy bleeding tissue also results in the healing of DFUs [49]. Maintenance debridement with enzymes (collagenase) is frequently used to gently remove slough or to enzymatically debride thick crusts (especially in neuroischemic wounds). Simple hydrogels or hydrocolloid dressings can provide for slow autolytic debridement of slough and dried crusts, especially in ischemic patients or those who cannot undergo surgical debridement [31].

Most wounds have excessive pressure as their proximate cause; it is important that the high pressures must be ameliorated before healing can take place. This is the concept of off-loading of pressure, which sometimes involves surgical off-loading too.

15.6 Basic Treatment

Basic treatment options for different wound types can be summarized as follows [16]:

Venous: Leg elevation, compression therapy, aspirin, pentoxifylline (Trental), surgical management/debridement.

Arterial: Revascularization, antiplatelet medications, management of risk factors.

Neuropathic: Off-loading of pressure, surgical offloading/ surgical internal decompression/ debridement, topical growth factors; tissue-engineered skin.

Pressure: Off-loading of pressure; debridement, reduction of excessive moisture, shear, and friction; adequate nutrition.

Many wound protocols and randomized controlled trials have observed that wound area reduction by 53% at a 4-week interval of basic treatment, had chances of complete recovery at 12 weeks, as compared to wound failure to do so in 4-week intervals. Advanced treatment options can be planned in such cases [50, 51, 52].

15.7 Advanced Treatment

15.7.1 Hyperbaric Oxygen Therapy

The proposed mechanisms for hyperbaric oxygen therapy (HBOT) to have a therapeutic role in chronic wounds include increased oxygen transport capacity of plasma (independent of red blood corpuscle number and function), improved function of the leukocyte oxygen-dependent peroxidase system, reduced tissue edema due to the osmotic effect of oxygen, stimulation of progenitor stem cell mobilization and angiogenesis, and improved fibroblast function [28]. If there is a superimposed infection, HBOT also inhibits bacterial growth (particularly anaerobes), generates free radicals that destroy bacterial cellular structures, and improves the oxygen-dependent transport of antibiotics.

In 2015, a Cochrane review concluded that HBOT increased the rate of ulcer healing in DFUs at 6 weeks but not at longer-term follow-up, with no significant difference in the risk of major amputation [53].

There may be a role for the use of HBOT to accelerate ulcer healing in diabetic patients with nonhealing neuropathic ulcers and low-grade ischemia who have failed to respond to conventional wound care. However, HBOT does not prevent major limb amputation and should not be used as an alternative to revascularization in patients with CLTI. On this background, the Global Vascular Guidelines on CLTI Management strongly recommend that physicians do not offer HBOT to patients with severe, uncorrected ischemia (i.e., Wlfi ischemia grade 2/3; level of evidence—B) [28].

15.7.2 Split-Thickness Skin Grafts

The benefit of *split-thickness skin graft* (STSG) to aid the apposition of the chronic wound edges and subsequent closure of the wound has been shown. Anderson et al. in their review suggested that an at-risk patient population such as those with peripheral vascular disease (PVD), end stage renal disease (ESRD), and current smokers may require additional treatment with STSG to promote chronic wound healing. Dermal substitutes in conjunction with STSG and negative pressure wound therapy in conjunction with STSG can be an option that is being studied. STSG is becoming an option as long as the vascular supply is intact [53].

15.7.3 Biologic and Regenerative Medicine Approaches

Biologic and regenerative medical treatments (including gene therapy and cellular therapy) have been developed to improve wound healing and prevent or limit the extent of amputation. These treatments are aimed at promoting therapeutic angiogenesis which is defined as the new growth of blood vessels from pre-existing vasculature in response to growth factor stimulation [53].

Stem cell therapy is another type of regenerative therapy that involves the differentiation of stem cells into vascular cells and the induction of angiogenic growth factor expression. Stem cell-based therapies offer tremendous potential for skin regeneration following injury and disease. Mesenchymal stem cells can assist with the regeneration of damaged vascular tissue in differentiated or undifferentiated states. Experimental studies have shown early re-epithelization and a significant increase in angiogenesis in groups receiving stem cell therapy [54].

15.7.4 MicroRNA

Research regarding microRNA (miRNA) function in the regulation of wound healing and developing improved miRNA modulation techniques in the skin are being studied [16].

The role of the *C282Y mutation* along with *integrin receptor activation/inhibition* is another treatment option being evaluated for chronic wound healing [16].

15.8 Conclusion

Diabetic and ischemic wounds are common chronic wounds with multifactorial etiology and are associated with significant morbidity. They are challenging to treat regardless of the underlying etiology. However, a multidisciplinary approach with an understanding of etiopathology can help understand the nature of the wound, which will ultimately guide for successful treatment. Treating the underlying medical condition, consistent offloading, and creating an optimal wound-healing environment are all key to wound healing, and patient education regarding optimization of chronic disease conditions, limb care, and nutritional buildup is necessary for avoiding recurrence. More research is needed regarding the validity and usefulness of several advanced treatment options being evaluated to use regularly in the future, which, if successful, might help a number of patients with these wounds.

References

1. Vuerich R, Groppa E, Vodret S, Ring NAR, Stocco C, Bossi F, et al. Ischemic wound revascularization by the stromal vascular fraction relies on host-donor hybrid vessels. NPJ Regener Med. 2023;8(1):8.
2. Rodrigues M, Kosaric N, Bonham CA, Gurtner GC. Wound healing: a cellular perspective. Physiol Rev. 2019;99(1):665–706.
3. Grey JE, Enoch S, Harding KG. ABC of wound healing: venous and arterial leg ulcers. BMJ. 2006;332(7537):347–50.
4. Yadav M, Haseen MA, Rizvi SAA, Yadav M. Role of ankle brachial pressure index (ABI) in screening patients with risk factors for developing peripheral vascular disease. Indian J Vasc Endovasc Surg. 2022;9(2):139–44.
5. The Wound Healing Society. Chronic wound care guidelines. http://woundheal.org/documents/final_pocket_guide_treatment.aspx. 2006. Accessed March 2023.
6. Li Z, Lin F, Thalib L, Chaboyer W. Global prevalence and incidence of pressure injuries in hospitalised adult patients: a systematic review and meta-analysis. Int J Nurs Stud. 2020;105:103546.
7. Tubaishat A, Papanikolaou P, Anthony D, Habiballah L. Pressure ulcers prevalence in the acute care setting: a systematic review, 2000-2015. Clin Nurs Res. 2018;27(6):643–59.
8. Mervis JS, Phillips TJ. Pressure ulcers: pathophysiology, epidemiology, risk factors, and presentation. J Am Acad Dermatol. 2019;81(4):881–90.
9. Niemiec SM, Louiselle AE, Liechty KW, Zgheib C. Role of microRNAs in pressure ulcer immune response, pathogenesis, and treatment. Int J Mol Sci. 2020;22(1):64.
10. O'Donnell TF, Passman MA, Marston WA, Ennis WJ, Dalsing M, Kistner RL, et al. Management of venous leg ulcers: clinical practice guidelines of the Society for Vascular Surgery® and the American Venous Forum. J Vasc Surg. 2014;60(2):3S–59S.
11. Eberhardt RT, Raffetto JD. Chronic venous insufficiency. Circulation. 2014;130(4):333–46.
12. Nelson EA, Adderley U. Venous leg ulcers. BMJ Clin Evid. 2016;2016.
13. Raffetto JD, Ligi D, Maniscalco R, Khalil RA, Mannello F. Why venous leg ulcers have difficulty healing: overview on pathophysiology, clinical consequences, and treatment. J Clin Med. 2020;10(1):29.
14. Mayrovitz HN, Wong S, Mancuso C. Venous, arterial, and neuropathic leg ulcers with emphasis on the geriatric population. Cureus. 2023;15(4).
15. Kogure T, Sumitani M, Abe H, Hozumi J, Inoue R, Mietani K, et al. Ischemic ulcer pain is both nociceptive and neuropathic pain based on a discriminant function analysis using the McGill Pain Questionnaire. J Pain Palliat Care Pharmacother. 2017;31(2):98–104.
16. Agale SV. Chronic leg ulcers: epidemiology, aetiopathogenesis, and management. Ulcers. 2013;2013:1.
17. Yazdanpanah L, Shahbazian H, Nazari I, Arti HR, Ahmadi F, Mohammadianinejad SE, et al. Incidence and risk factors of diabetic foot ulcer: a population-based diabetic foot cohort (ADFC study)—two-year follow-up study. Int J Endocrinol. 2018;2018:1.
18. Crawford F, McCowan C, Dimitrov BD, Woodburn J, Wylie G, Booth E, et al. The risk of foot ulceration in people with diabetes screened in community settings: findings from a cohort study. QJM. 2011;104(5):403–10.
19. Zhang P, Lu J, Jing Y, Tang S, Zhu D, Bi Y. Global epidemiology of diabetic foot ulceration: a systematic review and meta-analysis. Ann Med. 2017;49(2):106–16.
20. Lipsky BA, Berendt AR, Cornia PB, Pile JC, Peters EJ, Armstrong DG, et al. 2012 Infectious Diseases Society of America clinical practice guideline for the diagnosis and treatment of diabetic foot infections. Clin Infect Dis. 2012;54(12):e132–e73.
21. McDermott K, Fang M, Boulton AJ, Selvin E, Hicks CW. Etiology, epidemiology, and disparities in the burden of diabetic foot ulcers. Diabetes Care. 2023;46(1):209–21.
22. Clayton W Jr, Elasy TA. A review of the pathophysiology, classification, and treatment of foot ulcers in diabetic patients. Clin Diabetes. 2009;27(2):52–8.

23. Walsh J, Hoffstad O, Sullivan M, Margolis D. Association of diabetic foot ulcer and death in a population-based cohort from the United Kingdom. Diabet Med. 2016;33(11):1493–8.
24. Sidawy AP, Perler BA. Rutherford's vascular surgery and endovascular therapy, E-Book. Elsevier Health Sciences; 2018.
25. Burgess JL, Wyant WA, Abdo Abujamra B, Kirsner RS, Jozic I. Diabetic wound-healing science. Medicina. 2021;57(10):1072.
26. Hicks CW, Selvin E. Epidemiology of peripheral neuropathy and lower extremity disease in diabetes. Curr Diab Rep. 2019;19:1–8.
27. Oliver TI, Mutluoglu M. Diabetic foot ulcer. 2019.
28. Conte MS, Bradbury AW, Kolh P, White JV, Dick F, Fitridge R, et al. Global vascular guidelines on the management of chronic limb-threatening ischemia. Eur J Vasc Endovasc Surg. 2019;58(1):S1–S109. e33. https://doi.org/10.1016/j.ejvs.2019.05.006.
29. Wilkinson HN, Hardman MJ. Wound healing: cellular mechanisms and pathological outcomes. Open Biol. 2020;10(9):200223.
30. Mustoe TA, O'shaughnessy K, Kloeters O. Chronic wound pathogenesis and current treatment strategies: a unifying hypothesis. Plast Reconstr Surg. 2006;117(7S):35S–41S.
31. FrykbergRobert G. Challenges in the treatment of chronic wounds. Adv Wound Care. 2015;4:560.
32. Eming SA, Hammerschmidt M, Krieg T, Roers A. Interrelation of immunity and tissue repair or regeneration. In: Seminars in cell & developmental biology. Elsevier; 2009. p. 517–27.
33. Eming SA, Koch M, Krieger A, Brachvogel B, Kreft S, Bruckner-Tuderman L, et al. Differential proteomic analysis distinguishes tissue repair biomarker signatures in wound exudates obtained from normal healing and chronic wounds. J Proteome Res. 2010;9(9):4758–66.
34. Beidler SK, Douillet CD, Berndt DF, Keagy BA, Rich PB, Marston WA. Inflammatory cytokine levels in chronic venous insufficiency ulcer tissue before and after compression therapy. J Vasc Surg. 2009;49(4):1013–20.
35. Stojadinovic O, Minkiewicz J, Sawaya A, Bourne JW, Torzilli P, de Rivero Vaccari JP, et al. Deep tissue injury in development of pressure ulcers: a decrease of inflammasome activation and changes in human skin morphology in response to aging and mechanical load. PLoS One. 2013;8(8):e69223.
36. Bowler PG. Wound pathophysiology, infection and therapeutic options. Ann Med. 2002;34(6):419–27.
37. McCarty SM, Percival SL. Proteases and delayed wound healing. Adv Wound Care. 2013;2(8):438–47.
38. Eming SA, Brachvogel B, Odorisio T, Koch M. Regulation of angiogenesis: wound healing as a model. Prog Histochem Cytochem. 2007;42(3):115–70.
39. Krisp C, Jacobsen F, McKay MJ, Molloy MP, Steinstraesser L, Wolters DA. Proteome analysis reveals antiangiogenic environments in chronic wounds of diabetes mellitus type 2 patients. Proteomics. 2013;13(17):2670–81.
40. Leu A, Leu H-J, Franzeck U, Bollinger A. Microvascular changes in chronic venous insufficiency—a review. Cardiovasc Surg. 1995;3(3):237–45.
41. Hoffmann DC, Willenborg S, Koch M, Zwolanek D, Müller S, Becker A-KA, et al. Proteolytic processing regulates placental growth factor activities. J Biol Chem. 2013;288(25):17976–89.
42. Edsberg LE, Wyffels JT, Brogan MS, Fries KM. Analysis of the proteomic profile of chronic pressure ulcers. Wound Repair Regen. 2012;20(3):378–401.
43. Romagnani P, Lasagni L, Annunziato F, Serio M, Romagnani S. CXC chemokines: the regulatory link between inflammation and angiogenesis. Trends Immunol. 2004;25(4):201–9.
44. Stanley A, Osler T. Senescence and the healing rates of venous ulcers. J Vasc Surg. 2001;33(6):1206–11.
45. Hu MS, Borrelli MR, Lorenz HP, Longaker MT, Wan DC. Mesenchymal stromal cells and cutaneous wound healing: a comprehensive review of the background, role, and therapeutic potential. Stem Cells Int. 2018;2018:6901983. https://doi.org/10.1155/2018/6901983.

46. Eltzschig HK, Collard CD. Vascular ischaemia and reperfusion injury. Br Med Bull. 2004;70(1):71–86.
47. Toledo-Pereyra LH, Lopez-Neblina F, Toledo AH. Reactive oxygen species and molecular biology of ischemia/reperfusion. Ann Transplant. 2004;9(1):81–3.
48. Seal JB, Gewertz BL. Vascular dysfunction in ischemia-reperfusion injury. Ann Vasc Surg. 2005;19(4):572–84.
49. Piaggesi A, Schipani E, Campi F, Romanelli M, Baccetti F, Arvia C, et al. Conservative surgical approach versus non-surgical management for diabetic neuropathic foot ulcers: a randomized trial. Diabet Med. 1998;15(5):412–7.
50. Association AD. Consensus development conference on diabetic foot wound care: 7-8 April 1999, Boston, Massachusetts American Diabetes Association Diabetes care. 1999;22(8):1354–60.
51. Sheehan P, Jones P, Caselli A, Giurini JM, Veves A. Percent change in wound area of diabetic foot ulcers over a 4-week period is a robust predictor of complete healing in a 12-week prospective trial. Diabetes Care. 2003;26(6):1879–82.
52. Veves A, Sheehan P, Pham HT. A randomized, controlled trial of Promogran (a collagen/oxidized regenerated cellulose dressing) vs standard treatment in the management of diabetic foot ulcers. Arch Surg. 2002;137(7):822–7.
53. Edwards D, Black AT, Spielfogel WD. A multidisciplinary approach to managing ischemic wounds and current treatment options. Curr Treat Options Cardiovasc Med. 2021;23(7):51.
54. Qin HL, Zhu XH, Zhang B, Zhou L, Wang WY. Clinical evaluation of human umbilical cord mesenchymal stem cell transplantation after angioplasty for diabetic foot. Exp Clin Endocrinol Diabetes. 2016;124(8):497–503.

Chapter 16
Hyperbaric Oxygen Therapy for Diabetic Foot Ulcers

Vitória Duarte, Catarina Ivo, David Veríssimo, and Mafalda Marcelino

16.1 Case Presentation

A 72-year-old male presented with a left foot ulcer, marked by healing and recurrence over a 6-month period. His past history included heavy tobacco use for more than 40 years and a recently diagnosed onset of type 2 diabetes. The initial examination noted a heavily exudative ulcer on the dorsum of his left foot. The patient was in exquisite pain, particularly upon elevation of his lower extremity, which was cool to the touch. The wound edges were irregular, and there was obvious depth to the ulcer. The patient was afebrile.

During the patient's subsequent hospitalization, magnetic resonance imaging and X-rays did not reveal bone marrow edema, osteolysis, or deep abscess. Cultures revealed multiple bacterial organisms, and the patient was prescribed IV antibiotics, including vancomycin and piperacillin/tazobactam.

Question—What should be the next step in the management of this patient?
Answer—Vascular evaluation

Assessment of the adequacy of the circulation is an important component of the evaluation of all ulcers, particularly those in patients with diabetes. Symptoms of claudication or extremity pain at rest, and physical findings of absent pulses, cool temperature, or pallor on elevation should raise suspicion about the presence of peripheral artery disease.

A vascular evaluation of the patient revealed multi-segmental occlusions of multiple arteries of the lower extremity, both proximal and distal to the popliteal artery. A vascular surgeon performed subsequent revascularization. The patient's pain

V. Duarte (✉) · C. Ivo · D. Veríssimo · M. Marcelino
Department of Endocrinology, Hospital das Forças Armadas, Lisbon, Portugal
e-mail: vita_pires@hotmail.com; mcatarinaivo@gmail.com; d.verissimo87@gmail.com; marcelino.mafalda@gmail.com

A. G. D'Almeida, J. Hidalgo (eds.), *Evidence-Based Hyperbaric Medicine*,
https://doi.org/10.1007/978-3-032-06346-5_16

level decreased significantly after the endovascular intervention, and the ulcer responded to initial management that focused solely on regular cleaning.

16.2 Principles of Management

1. **Prevention—**Patients with diabetes are at risk of lower-limb amputation because of the high incidence of chronic wounds and diabetic foot ulcers. The lifetime incidence of foot ulcers in diabetic patients is around 25%. After successful healing, the recurrence rate is 65% within 3 years [1]. Therefore, the prevention of foot ulcers is paramount to reduce the risks to the patient.

Diabetic foot ulcers have a multifactorial etiology, in which neuropathy, ischemia, and infection all play a part [2]. First, peripheral neuropathy leads to loss of protective sensation and foot deformity. Thus, plantar pressures are redistributed, and some foot areas sustain chronic high pressure, which ultimately results in ulceration. This is aggravated by autonomic neuropathy, which is responsible for callus formation and dry skin, susceptible to cracking. The latter creates gates of entry for bacteria, leading to potential deep-tissue infection. Second, wound healing may also be impaired in cases with concomitant lower extremity ischemia due to peripheral arterial disease. Finally, diabetic patients are susceptible to infection, mainly due to impaired immune response.

2. **Diagnosis—**The first step in managing diabetic foot ulcers is assessing, grading, and classifying the ulcer. Foot ulcers may be classified in terms of severity, in order to facilitate a logical approach to treatment and aid in the prediction of outcome [3]. The most commonly used classification system is the Wagner system. Grade I ulcers are superficial, involving the full skin thickness but no underlying tissues. Grade II ulcers are deeper, penetrating down to ligaments and muscles, but not involving bone or abscess formation. Grade III ulcers are deep ulcers with cellulitis or abscess formation, often complicated with osteomyelitis. Grade IV ulcers have localized gangrene, and grade V ulcers have extensive gangrene involving the entire foot (Table 16.1).

3. **Treatment—**Diabetic ulcers require complex multimodal treatment including glycemic control, local wound care, revascularization, treatment of infections, and off-loading. According to the IDF Clinical Practice Recommendations on the Diabetic Foot, treatment should occur in a stepwise approach. The first and most urgent step is to treat any infection that is present. Infections can be graded according to the severity to determine what class of antibiotic to use and whether to treat the patient in an outpatient or inpatient setting.

The mainstay of therapy for diabetic foot ulcers is offloading of pressure. The preferred treatment for a neuropathic plantar ulcer is a knee-high offloading device.

Table 16.1 Wagner classification for diabetic foot ulcers originally described by Wagner FW, 1979

Grade	Description
0	No open wound, but high risk due to deformities or callus
1	Superficial ulcer involving only the skin surface
2	Deep ulcer extending into tendon, bone, or joint capsule
3	Deep ulcer with abscess, osteomyelitis, or joint sepsis
4	Localized gangrene of the forefoot or toes
5	Extensive gangrene involving the entire foot

Other options include bed rest, crutches, or felted foam in combination with appropriate footwear.

If present, arterial insufficiency needs to be managed. In patients with either an ankle pressure <50 mmHg or an ankle-brachial index <0.5, consider vascular imaging and revascularization. As a team, diabetologists, podiatrists, and vascular surgeons significantly improve clinical outcomes.

The basics of wound care must consist of regular debridement of fibrous or nonviable tissue and creating a moist environment.

Nonetheless, despite optimal treatment, most ulcers in diabetic patients with concomitant limb ischemic are refractory to wound healing. Major amputation rates have been reported at 5–23% 2 years after revascularization. This has prompted the search for effective alternative or additive treatment options.

16.3 Evidence Contour

For diabetic foot ulcers that fail to demonstrate improvement (>50% wound area reduction) after a minimum of 4 weeks of standard wound therapy, we may consider adjunctive wound therapy options. These include negative pressure therapy, platelet-derived growth factor, and hyperbaric oxygen therapy (HBOT), among others.

1. **Negative pressure wound therapy (NPWT)** involves the application of airtight occlusive dressings and local subatmospheric pressure to a wound in order to accelerate wound healing. There is low-certainty evidence to suggest that NPWT may be helpful in postoperative diabetic foot ulcers compared with

dressings [4]. However, the recommendations for NPWT and the superiority over other modalities in the management of nonsurgical diabetic foot ulcers remain without consensus.

2. **Growth factors**—Tissue growth factors promote cellular proliferation and angiogenesis and thereby improve ulcer healing. However, further trials investigating the effect of growth factors in diabetic foot ulcers are needed before firm conclusions can be drawn [5]. The safety profiles of the growth factors are also unclear.
3. HBOT has been suggested as a valuable addition to conventional treatment for a variety of indications, including necrotizing soft tissue infections and chronic wounds in patients with diabetes. HBOT for diabetic ulcers involves intermittent administration of 100% oxygen, usually in daily sessions of 90 minutes each, at pressures of 1.5–3.0 atmospheres absolute in an airtight cabin. By increasing the blood oxygen content, HBOT creates a favorable gradient for the diffusion of oxygen into the tissues. In hypoxic tissues, the enhanced oxygen supply has multiple effects that may benefit wound healing. By increasing the expression of vascular endothelial growth factor and fibroblast growth factor, HBOT may enhance angiogenesis and fibroblast proliferation. In addition, the resulting hyperoxia may cause vasoconstriction, thereby decreasing tissue edema. By reducing the expression of pro-inflammatory cytokines, HBOT reduces inflammation, while simultaneously enhancing the bacterial killing activity of leukocytes.

Previous clinical trials and systematic reviews on the effectiveness of HBOT as an adjunct to standard wound care have provided conflicting evidence [6]. In order to assess the benefit of adjunctive HBOT, a systematic literature search was conducted (Table 16.2). Only randomized controlled trials (RCTs) were included in the benefit assessment. The selection of the studies was based on their relevance and sample size [7–11]. The results of the individual studies are organized by outcomes and discussed below.

Table 16.2 Baseline wound characteristics and HBOT regimens

	Faglia, 1996	Duzgun, 2008	Londahl, 2010	Fedorko, 2015	Santema, 2018
N	68	100	94	103	120
Wagner grade					
Grade 2	13%	18%	26%	45%	51%
Grade 3	25%	37%	56%	50%	30%
Grade 4	62%	45%	18%	5%	19%
Wound duration	?	>4 weeks	>3 months	>4 weeks	>4 weeks
Vascular status	Ischemic	?	Ischemic	Ischemic	Ischemic
HBOT sessions	38	30–45	40	30	30–40
HBOT duration (min)	90	90	85	90	90

Table 16.3 Outcomes of the individual RCTs. I—intervention group (HBOT); C—control group

	Faglia, 1996	Duzgun, 2008	Londahl, 2010	Fedorko, 2015	Santema, 2018
Wound healing	I = 51% C = 49%	I = 66% C = 0%	I = 51% C = 27%	I = 20% C = 22%	I = 55% C = 48%
Major amputations	I = 9% C = 33%	I = 0% C = 34%	I = 6% C = 2%	I = 22,5% C = 24,1%	I = 12% C = 22%
Minor amputations	I = 58% C = 35%	I = 8% C = 48%	I = 8% C = 9%	I = 28,6% C = 24,1%	I = 25% C = 26,6%
HBOT benefit	Amputation ($P = 0.016$)	Wound healing and amputation ($p < 0.05$)	Wound healing ($P = 0.03$)	**No benefit**	**No benefit**

In all studies, HBOT was provided in the intervention group as an additional measure to standard wound care; the control group received the respective standard wound care. Standard therapy in all RCTs entailed wound care, including dressing changes, local debridement, revascularization, off-loading, and infection control with appropriate antibiotic therapy.

Regarding wound healing, the study by *Duzgun* et al. is often quoted as the justification for HBOT utility in treating diabetic wounds. However, these results should be interpreted with caution because it is difficult to explain a zero healing rate in a random cohort of 50 control group patients. The two most recent studies (*Fedorko* et al. and *Santema* et al.) show no benefit of adjunctive HBOT compared with standard wound care (Table 16.3).

Concerning the risk of amputation, a difference can be observed across ulcer grades. The majority of patients in the *Fedorko (2015)* and *Santema (2018)* RCTs presented Wagner grade 2 ulcers, where HBOT did not offer an additional advantage in reducing the risk for amputation. However, previous studies have focused on more severe ulcers (grade 4). That can explain the benefit of HBOT in patients included in the *Faglia* et al. and *Duzgun* et al. RCTs.

Although it is not possible to determine which patients will universally fail to benefit from HBOT, it is feasible, however, to model the outcome of some patients. Hyperbaric oxygen treatment is unlikely to be effective in patients with unfavorable $TcPO_2$ values [12]. This also holds true for very old patients, with a history of smoking and chronic kidney disease. Renal failure patients with two or more lesions and a Wagner score of 3 or higher are unlikely to improve following HBOT [13, 14]. Unfortunately, these are also the very patients who are least likely to benefit from any other type of intervention. Furthermore, wounds exhibiting impaired growth factor production, low chemotactic responsiveness, or normal levels of tissue oxygenation are not appropriate for HBO therapy.

HBOT can generally be considered a safe treatment modality, which is reflected by the low frequency of adverse events in the trials included in this review [15]. Reported side effects include barotraumatic otitis, inability to equalize middle ear pressure, hypoglycemia, dizziness, oxygen-induced seizure (one case), and worsening of cataract (one case).

16.4 Conclusion

HBOT is a safe and well-tolerated adjunctive therapy to heal lower-extremity lesions. The available evidence on the effectiveness of HBOT for the treatment of diabetic foot ulcers is not solid. Although there is some indication of a beneficial effect on wound healing, it is currently unknown which patients are likely to benefit from HBOT and which patients are not. Before referral for HBOT, a patient should have failed to improve on conventional treatment. Also, a vascular consultation should be offered prior to HBOT. Potential candidates for HBOT usually have Wagner III, IV, and V lesions. The latest findings suggest that cigarette smoking, old age, and reduced peripheral perfusion are associated with a reduced response to HBOT.

References

1. Ibrahim A, Jude E, Langton K, Harkless L, Gawish H, et al. IDF clinical practice recommendations on the diabetic foot. International Diabetes Federation; 2017.
2. Del Core M, Ahn J, Lewis R, Raspovic K, Lalli T, Wukich D. The evaluation and treatment of diabetic foot ulcers and diabetic foot infections. Foot Ankle Orthop. 2018:1–11.
3. Schaper N, van Netten J, Apelqvist J, Bus S, Hinchlife R, Lipsky B. IWGDF Guidelines on the prevention and management of diabetic foot disease. International Working Group on the Diabetic Foot (IWGDF); 2019.
4. Maranna H, Lal P, Mishra A, Bains L, Sawant G, Bhatia R, Kumar P, Beg M. Negative pressure wound therapy in grade 1 and 2 diabetic foot ulcers: a randomized controlled study. Diabetes Metab Syndr Clin Res Rev. 2021;15:365–71.
5. Martí-Carvajal AJ, Gluud C, Nicola S, Simancas-Racines D, Reveiz L, Oliva P, Cedeño-Taborda J. Growth factors for treating diabetic foot ulcers. Cochrane Database Syst Rev. 2015;(10)
6. O'Reilly D, Pasricha A, Campbell K, Burke N, Assasi N, Bowen JM, et al. Hyperbaric oxygen therapy for diabetic ulcers: systematic review and meta-analysis. Int J Technol Assess Health Care. 2013;29:269–81.
7. Faglia E, Favales F, Aldeghi A, Calia P, Quarantiello A, Oriani G, et al. Adjunctive systemic hyperbaric oxygen therapy in treatment of severe prevalent ischemic diabetic foot ulcer. A randomized study. Diabetes Care. 1996;19:1338e43.
8. Duzgun AP, Satir HZ, Ozozan O, Saylam B, Kulah B, Coskun F. Effect of hyperbaric oxygen therapy on healing of diabetic foot ulcers. J Foot Ankle Surg. 2008;47:515–9.
9. Londahl M, Katzman P, Nilsson A, Hammarlund C. Hyperbaric oxygen therapy facilitates healing of chronic foot ulcers in patients with diabetes. Diabetes Care. 2010;33:998–1003.
10. Fedorko L, Bowen JM, Jones W, et al. Hyperbaric oxygen therapy does not reduce indications for amputation in patients with diabetes with nonhealing ulcers of the lower limb: a prospective, double-blind, randomized controlled clinical trial. Diabetes Care. 2016;39:392–9.
11. Santema K, Stoekenbroek R, Koelemay M, Reekers J, van Dortmont L, Oomen A, et al. Hyperbaric oxygen therapy in the treatment of ischemic lower extremity ulcers in patients with diabetes: results of the DAMO2CLES multicenter randomized clinical trial. Diabetes Care. 2018;41:112–9.
12. Margolis DJ, Gupta J, Hoffstad O, Papdopoulos M, Glick HA, Thom SR, et al. Lack of effectiveness of hyperbaric oxygen therapy for the treatment of diabetic foot ulcer and the prevention of amputation: a cohort study. Diabetes Care. 2013;36:1961–6.

13. Tiaka EK, Papanas N, Manolakis A, Maltezos E. The role of hyperbaric oxygen in the treatment of diabetic foot ulcers. Angiology. 2012;63(4):302–14.
14. Fife CE, Buyukcakir C, Otto G, Sheffield P, Love T, Warriner R 3rd. Factors influencing the outcome of lower-extremity diabetic ulcers treated with hyperbaric oxygen therapy. Wound Repair Regen. 2007;15(3):322–31.
15. Stoekenbroek RM, Santema TB, Legemate DA, Ubbink DT, van den Brink A, Koelemay MJ. Hyperbaric oxygen for the treatment of diabetic foot ulcers: a systematic review. Eur J Vasc Endovasc Surg. 2014;47:647–55.

Chapter 17
Compromised Grafts and Flaps

Sudipta Mukherjee, Pralay Shankar Ghosh, and Santanu Bagchi

17.1 Introduction

Reconstructive surgery with flaps and grafts is an evolving modality in the current era. With the rapid advancement of onco-surgery, tissue gaps are filled with grafts or flaps. With the advancement of microvascular surgeries, free tissue transfer is becoming more and more common. Vascular insufficiency is the most common post-operative complication in this subgroup. It can be both arterial (more common) or venous, eventually leading to compromised blood flow to the transferred tissue. Immediate surgical intervention is the primary modality, along with other corrective measures, to restore blood flow. But it is not always a feasible option. In case of a compromised graft, an increase in oxygen tension in the tissue can improve graft survival. Hyperbaric oxygen therapy (HBOT) can play an important role in this regard. It can improve graft viability, leading to a reduction in regrafting or repeat flap procedures [1].

17.2 Flaps and Grafts

Tissue grafts and flaps are used for reconstruction of anatomical gaps created by tissue loss [2]. This tissue loss can happen due to trauma or due to surgical debridement or debulking of pathological tissue in case of malignancy, chronic disease, burn, and soft tissue infection. It can be approached in two ways. In the "reconstructive ladder" approach, it starts with a simple wound closure technique (e.g., secondary intention and primary closure) to an advanced one (e.g., free flap). In the

S. Mukherjee (✉) · P. S. Ghosh · S. Bagchi
Department of Critical Care Medicine, Tata Medical Center, Kolkata, West Bengal, India

A. G. D'Almeida, J. Hidalgo (eds.), *Evidence-Based Hyperbaric Medicine*,
https://doi.org/10.1007/978-3-032-06346-5_17

"reconstructive elevator" approach, a complex surgical option has been chosen from the beginning with individualization as per the patient's and wound characteristics [3].

Flap and graft are different in terms of their vascular supply. Grafts lack their blood supply and depend on the recipient bed for initial nutrition, vascularization, and survival (Graft take). It can have a single type of tissue (simple graft) or multiple tissue types of different sizes (composite graft). The normal physiological course of "graft take" is important to identify graft compromise early. The initial pale color (due to lack of vascularity) of the graft passes through a bluish congestive phase to a pink blush. Graft compromise mostly happens within the first 48 hours, leading to dusky appearance, followed by superficial skin changes (epidermolysis) and necrosis.

Flaps have their own inherent blood supply while transferring from donor to recipient tissue. There are different kinds of flaps (e.g., rotational flap, random pattern flap, pedicled flaps, etc.), but "free tissue transfer" needs special mention. Free tissue transfer undergoes microvascular anastomosis at the donor bed; it has its unique challenges in terms of complications such as arterial insufficiency, venous congestion, ischemia–reperfusion (IR) injury, and so on. All these need immediate surgical intervention as an initial step, along with other conservative management. Rotational flaps have their own blood supply, and undue tension or torsion needs to be avoided on the vascular pedicle to prevent vascular compromise.

17.3 Mechanism of Graft/Flap Failure

Hypoxia is the most common physiological factor of flap / graft compromise. Normally, the oxygen tension in the grafted tissue varies from 5 to 20 mm Hg. Reconstruction failure can occur due to multiple reasons, such as poor perfusion of flap bed, irradiated flap bed, large flap (compared to the vascular supply), or IR injury. This may lead to an undue chain of events such as surgical intervention (local wound care, vacuum-assisted closure, debridement, or revascularization), loss of tissue, morbidity, and psychological stress to the patient and family along with time and financial implications. Sometimes, the plasmatic imbibition of oxygen from the recipient bed is inadequate compared to the metabolic demand of the graft, leading to compromised graft survival.

17.4 Hyperbaric Oxygen as Therapeutic Options

Hyperbaric oxygen (HBO) does not have any prophylactic role in healthy uncompromised flap or graft [4]. So, routine usage is not recommended presently. Preventive measures are mostly related to the evaluation of the compromised wound bed and its preparation. But, in a significant no of cases, this is difficult to identify a “compromised recipient site,” and even on identification, definitive therapeutic options are lacking. Along with surgical interventions, HBOT of the wound bed can be considered to improve oxygen tension in the tissue. In a meta-analysis of eight studies, HBOT has been shown to augment healing in acute complicated wounds [5]. In the same way, HBOT has shown some role as salvage therapy with improved survival and outcome of skin grafts and flaps.

17.5 Physiological Rationale

HBOT is usually given at a pressure of 2–2.5 atmosphere absolute (ATA), and it can increase dissolved oxygen content in the blood by ten-fold. Total oxygen-carrying capacity has been shown to increase by 7% in an animal model without the contribution of hemoglobin. In a conventional scenario, this dissolved oxygen is clinically insignificant, but, during HBOT, due to high partial pressure of oxygen in arterial blood (PaO_2), plasmatic imbibition of oxygen leads to increased oxygen tension at different tissues, including the graft. This increase in tissue oxygenation had been demonstrated by Sheffield by measuring transcutaneous oxygenation [6]. After the initiation of wound healing, further continuation of oxygen supply requires restoration of vascular supply by capillary formation.

This increased oxygenation at the tissue level will cause an increase in vascular endothelial growth factor (VEGF) production [7]—more at the ischemic tissue. VEGF induces nitric oxide synthetase expression on newly formed endothelial cells and increases nitric oxide production, leading to neovascularization—an increase in capillary formation both in numbers and in surface area. This leads to an increase in flap circulation, improved collagen synthesis, increased fibroblast function, and its proliferation, leading to better healing [8].

IR injury is another significant concern for flap surgery once the circulation is restored after an initial ischemic insult. Restoration of blood flow after initial compromise produces a “second blow” to the tissue [9]. The tissue damage is due to increased production of reactive free oxygen radicals, neutrophilic infiltration and adhesion, and eventually vasoconstriction. The role of HBOT in the prevention of free radical injury is apparently contradictory. But there is clinical evidence suggesting that HBOT can significantly mitigate IR injury. There is activation of the antioxidant system along with suppression of lipid peroxidation. It also inhibits neutrophil activation and adhesion via neutrophil beta 2 integrin CD18 surface receptors present on endothelium via an NO-dependent pathway [10, 11]. HBOT also increases VEGF production along with suppression of the extracellular matrix plasminogen system [12]. All these can cause selective vasoconstriction of the arterio-venous shunt at the distal flap, leading to improved perfusion [13] and a decrease in tissue edema.

HBOT can also decrease infectious complications of the wound and surgical site. High oxygen has bacteriostatic and sometimes bactericidal effects on anaerobic organisms, leading to a lesser chance of bacterial overgrowth in these susceptible tissues. High oxygen content also neutralizes bacterial exotoxins, leading to less tissue damage [14].

17.6 Animal Study

The role of HBOT has been evaluated on compromised grafts in different animal models. Compromised grafts include a poor recipient bed; as a result, graft healing and survival are at risk. HBO with 2 ATA was very effective in terms of wound healing in compromised circulation, without significant impact on well-vascularized wounds [15]. It showed an improved epithelialization rate in burn injury. It also showed a positive impact on redo partial thickness skin grafting [16]. Besides, there is histological evidence of improved graft survival with HBOT for chondrocutaneous grafts. Taking 1.5 cm as the "vascularity safe" upper limit of graft, most of the benefit of HBOT is with larger size grafts. Histopathological benefit is also observed in skin flap. Microvascular vessel thrombosis, neutrophilic infiltration, damage to intima, edema, and eventually necrosis are less with HBOT [17].

Not only in random pattern flaps but also in pedicle flaps with direct source artery for its vascular supply, HBOT has shown significant benefit by decreasing flap necrosis [18]. The benefit is more if HBOT had been started early (i.e., immediately after surgery) rather than delayed by 24 hours. In an experimental model with secondary ischemia with free tissue transfer, HBOT has been shown to have significant benefit in terms of flap survival compared to no intervention or 100% oxygen administration. Tolerance of normothermic microvascular flap to prolong secondary ischemia has also increased significantly with HBOT [19]. HBOT has shown its benefit mainly for arterial compromise leading to tissue hypoxemia; it does not have much role in the case of venous congestion leading to graft edema and necrosis (in that case, "Leech therapy" is an option) [20].

HBOT had been compared with different pharmacological interventions, too. When compared with allopurinol and superoxide dismutase for axial pattern ischemic skin flap survival, superoxide dismutase showed promising results and needs further evaluation in a properly designed model [21]. It has been used in combination with free radical scavengers/inhibitors, too. HBOT in combination with superoxide dismutase, catalase, and alpha-tocopherol acetate has shown significant improvement in random-pattern skin flap survival. But there was not much benefit in adding inhibitors like allopurinol with HBOT [22]. HBOT has also been combined with antioxidants like vitamin E and C, and the role of this combination therapy in IR injury caused by free radicals has been evaluated in experimental models. The combination therapy has shown to increase flap viability significantly in animal models. Antioxidant vitamins have also shown positive results even without HBOT [23].

17.7 Clinical Data

There is reasonably good evidence in favor of HBOT for skin grafting. There is a significant increase in graft surface area survival, both for split thickness and full thickness skin grafting—data are stronger for split thickness graft. HBOT is also used as a salvage therapy for larger grafts (>2 cm composite grafts) if there is no recipient vessel present for anastomosis. A significant number (up to 90%) of compromised grafts and flaps have been salvaged with HBOT [24]. HBOT has been shown to have some contribution to the salvage of upper limb crush injuries. These are all small studies [25] or isolated case reports [26]. Mutilated hand and upper limb injuries can be really challenging to salvage. Most of these patients will need initial debridement followed by free flap closure as secondary interventions. Free flaps such as antero-lateral thigh and abdominal groin flap were used. HBOT was initiated early (within 6–7 hours) after reconstructive–revascularization surgeries with significantly good outcomes in terms of limb survival [25]. Similar results were found with the latissimus dorsi flap with forearm tissue gap closure [26] and the superior gluteal artery perforator flap for breast reconstruction [27]. In a small case series of irradiated patients, pharyngostome closure with pectoralis major muscle was evaluated for HBOT with a positive outcome [28]. There are soft positive data after bony resection also. After resection and grafting of mandibular tumor in a small case series, HBOT has been used with apparently good outcome for problematic wound healing [29]. HBOT has been used in combination with antibiotics and free vascularized muscle flap in the treatment of tibial osteomyelitis. A significant number of patients had shown long-term clinical response (e.g., no wound drainage)—especially patients with muscle flap [30]. A similar result was found by Bassetto et al. [31] in their plastic surgery practice, too. There are also contradictory findings. In their small case series of microvascular reconstruction of mandibular osteoradionecrosis, Gal et al. did not find any benefit of HBOT. Preoperative HBOT in this study was found to be more likely to cause post-operative wound infection and surgical complication [32]. In another retrospective study by Nolen et al., post-operative complication after free flap reconstruction of mandibular osteonecrosis were evaluated. Overall complication rate is similar with statistically insignificant increase in post-operative infection rate in the HBO therapy group [33].

In their review, Haltern et al. [34] found HBOT to be reasonably safe in clinical practice. Along with its usage in compromised flaps and grafts, its efficacy has been evaluated in the treatment of other compromised wounds, such as diabetic foot, necrotizing fascitis, and osteoradionecrosis, with reasonable success. The Cochrane review comprising of 229 patients precluded meta-analysis due to heterogeneity of the studies [35], and they could not conclude anything definitive. In the systematic review by Zhou et al. [36], they have included 23 clinical trials comprising 957 patients in the HBOT group compared with 583 patients in the control group. HBOT was offered as a planned intervention within 72 hours of surgery rather than a salvage therapy. They have shown significantly higher flap survival rate compared to the control group. In another retrospective study by Kucur et al. [37], among 260 free flap reconstructive surgeries of the head and neck, flap failure was only 3.5%. Among these, 20 patients with poor wound healing had received HBOT, with only three showing flap loss. HBOT has been used in China for a long time, and they have also published their cumulative experience recently with a positive outcome [36]. Among complicated re-operative surgeries of hypospadias, a meta-analysis by Anand et al. [38] had shown significantly less graft failure and complication rate in the HBOT group. In small studies, this intervention has been shown to be cost-effective also for compromised flaps [39], as it decreases other surgical interventions like debridement besides decreasing morbidity of the patient.

17.8 Timing of HBOT

Timing of HBOT is an important component for clinical success. Early initiation for compromised flaps has shown better outcomes in terms of graft survival and significant delay (>3 days) after flap compromise may lead to poor outcomes in the majority of the cases [40]. In case of suspected intraoperative ischemia and without significant correctable surgical factors, HBOT can be considered during the immediate post-operative period and may need to continue for 3 days. Patient compliance and pre-treatment oxygen concentration have been shown to have a positive impact on clinical outcomes. The present treatment protocol is more associated with "pre-operative" wound bed preparation, especially in cases of a compromised receptor site. Sometimes, HBOT has been used for early healing of the compromised wound bed (e.g., radiated wound bed or diabetic wound) by improving vascularity.

The Tenth European Consensus Conference on Hyperbaric Medicine has made some "accepted" recommendations regarding its usage in compromised flaps and grafts [41]. Compromised skin graft and musculocutaneous flap has a level 2 recommendation; even if there is low quality of real-world evidence, there is a strong agreement among the experts in terms of its utility (Table 17.1).

17.9 Equipment (Francis et al.)

HBOT needs a dedicated pressurized chamber to keep the whole system inside. It can be a mono-place (single patient) or multi-place (multiple patients) chamber. Multi-place chambers are also needed for patients who are on a ventilator or have other accessory equipment along with the patient. Regular inspection and facility checks are mandated in terms of the quality of oxygen and air along with the carbon dioxide exhaustion level. A safety officer is mandatory for each plant, and regular monitoring is needed to prevent sudden unnoticed equipment failure. Another catastrophic complication is fire. There should be a written protocol in terms of its usage from the patients' and medical personnel's perspective. No electronic gadgets or combustible materials are allowed inside, even near the vicinity of the chamber.

Table 17.1 Recommendations for 'accepted' usage of HBO therapy in compromised flaps and grafts (Tenth European Consensus Conference on Hyperbaric Medicine)

Sl no.	Statement	Level of recommendation	Level of evidence
1.	'Suggest' using HBOT in the treatment of compromised skin grafts and flaps	Type 2	Level C
2.	'Recommend' HBOT in all cases of compromised skin grafts and flaps as soon as possible after the diagnosis of compromised grafts/tissues	Type 1	Level B
3.	'Suggest' tissue viability be evaluated by clinical judgement and more objective methods including use of Transcutaneous oximetry (TCOM) or assessment of capillaries by laser Doppler	Type 1	Level B
4.	'Suggest' HBOT at a pressure between 203 and 253 kPa for at least 60 minutes per session (preferably 90–120 min), repeated two or three times in first day, then twice per day or once daily until tissues declared alive or necrotic	Type 2	Level C
5.	'Recommend' HBOT be used both pre- and post-operatively in cases where there is an increased risk for compromised skin grafts and flaps, e.g., irradiated or infected wound bed, immuno-compromised patient	Type 1	Level C

Type 1 = strong recommendation
Type 2 = weak recommendation
Type 3 = Neutral recommendation
Level A = High level of evidence
Level B = Moderate level of evidence
Level c = low level of evidence
Data taken from Mathieu et al. [41]

Special training is required for all medical personnel involved in HBOT. It is advisable to have a 40-hour training capsule for both doctors and HBOT technicians for safe and optimal usage of this medical facility, along with regular training of the safety officer. Acrylic monospace chamber and other sophisticated equipment need special cleaning protocol and technique [42].

17.10 Complications and Contraindications

The main concern of HBOT is related to barotrauma. There can be an increase in close-space air pressure, especially after a local injury, leading to rupture of the covering membrane. This is applicable to the lung and the middle ear. It can cause irritation and rupture of the tympanic membrane—rupture of small vessels leads to damage to different chambers of the ear. An untreated pneumothorax is an absolute contraindication for HBOT. Pulmonary bullae/blebs and emphysematous lung disease are relative contraindications. Other complications are convulsion, pulmonary edema, and hemorrhages. Some drugs can also be considered as relative contraindications like disulfiram (blocks superoxide dismutase that protects against oxygen toxicity of HBOT), cisplatin and sulfamylon (impair wound healing), and bleomycin (interstitial pneumonitis). Other medical conditions that are considered relative contraindications are claustrophobia, sinusitis, seizure disorder, pregnancy, and implanted device (pacemaker and epidural pump) [43]. A rare but dangerous complication is fire followed by an explosion.

17.11 Dosage of HBO

As per the Undersea and Hyperbaric Medical Society, the standard dosage of HBO therapy is 2–2.5 ATA for 1.5–2 hours two times a day [44]. An oxygen break of 10 minutes is to be considered to avoid oxygen seizure. Close clinical monitoring is needed in terms of flap / graft vascularity, stability, and viability. Additional adjuncts such as transcutaneous oximetry (TCOM) and Doppler study can be done for objective monitoring. TCOM value <40 mmHg is suggestive of a compromised flap and warrants continuation of treatment. HBOT can be tapered off once a day after the stability of the flap.

17.12 Conclusion

HBOT can be a good therapeutic option as salvage therapy for compromised grafts and flaps. There are not many randomized controlled trials, and it would be difficult to conduct for such interventions. We need more structured data to conclude regarding this modality. This facility is also not available in most of the tertiary care hospitals. Each state or city should have one or two referral centers for HBOT. It can develop as a good salvage therapeutic option in the coming days.

References

1. Gould LJ, May T. The science of hyperbaric oxygen for flaps and grafts. Surg Technol Int 2016;28:65–72. PMID: 27042776.
2. Francis A, Baynosa CR. Hyperbaric oxygen therapy for the compromised graft or flap. Adv Wound Care. 2017;6(1):23–32.
3. Gottlieb LJ, Krieger LM. From the reconstructive ladder to the reconstructive elevator. Plast Reconstr Surg. 1994;93:1503–4.
4. Vishwanath SCG. Hyperbaric oxygen therapy in free flap surgery: is it meaningful? MJAFI. 2011;67:253–6.
5. Dauwe PB, Pulikkottil BJ, Lavery L, Stuzin JM, Rohrich RJ. Does hyperbaric oxygen therapy work in facilitating acute wound healing: a systematic review. Plast Reconstr Surg. 2014;133(2):208e–15e. https://doi.org/10.1097/01.prs.0000436849.79161.a4. PMID: 24469192.

6. Sheffield PJ. Tissue oxygen measurements with respect to soft tissue wound healing with normobaric and hyperbaric oxygen. HBO Rev. 1985;6:18–46.
7. Sheikh AY, Gibson JJ, Rollins MD, Hopf HW, Hussain Z, Hunt TK. Effect of hyperoxia on vascular endothelial growth factor levels in a wound model. Arch Surg. 2000;135:1293–7.
8. Kleban S, Baynosa RC. The effect of hyperbaric oxygen on compromised grafts and flaps. Undersea Hyperb Med. 2020 Fourth Quarter;47(4):635–48. https://doi.org/10.22462/10.12.2020.13. PMID: 33227840.
9. Francis A, Baynosa R. Ischaemia-reperfusion injury and hyperbaric oxygen pathways: a review of cellular mechanisms. Diving Hyperb Med. 2017;47(2):110–7. https://doi.org/10.28920/dhm47.2.110-117. PMID: 28641323; PMCID: PMC6147229.
10. Godman CA, Joshi R, Giardina C, Perdrizet G, Hightower LE. Hyperbaric oxygen treatment induces antioxidant gene expression. Ann N Y Acad Sci. 2010;1197:178–83.
11. Baynosa RC, Naig AL, Murphy PS, et al. The effect of hyperbaric oxygen on nitric oxide synthase activity and expression in ischemia-reperfusion injury. J Surg Res. 2013;183:355–61.
12. Francis A, Kleban SR, Stephenson LL, Murphy PS, Letourneau PR, Fang XH, Wang WZ, Baynosa RC. Hyperbaric oxygen inhibits reperfusion-induced neutrophil polarization and adhesion via plasmin-mediated VEGF release. Plast Reconstr Surg Glob Open. 2017;5(9):e1497. https://doi.org/10.1097/GOX.0000000000001497. PMID: 29062662; PMCID: PMC5640368.
13. Zamboni WA, Roth AC, Russell RC, Graham B, Suchy H, Kucan JO. Morphologic analysis of the microcirculation during reperfusion of ischemic skeletal muscle and the effect of hyperbaric oxygen. Plast Reconstr Surg. 1993;91:1110–23.
14. Phillips JC. Understanding hyperbaric oxygen therapy and its use in the treatment of compromised skin grafts and flaps. Plast Surg Nurs. 2005 25(2):72–80; quiz 81–2. [PubMed: 15983497].
15. Kivisaari J, Niinikoski J. Effects of hyperbaric oxygen and prolonged hypoxia on the healing of open wounds. Acta Chir Scand. 1975;141:14–9.
16. Korn HN, Wheeler ES, Miller TA. Effect of hyperbaric oxygen on second degree burn wound healing. Arch Surg. 1977;122:732–7.
17. Ağir H, Mersa B, Aktaş S, Olgaç V. Siçan karin deri flebi modelinde, iskemi-reperfüzyon hasarindan hemen sonra ve iki saat sonra uygulanan hiperbarik oksijen tedavisinin histolojik etkileri [Histologic effects of hyperbaric oxygen therapy administered immediately after or two hours after ischemia-reperfusion injury: a rat abdominal skin flap model]. Kulak Burun Bogaz Ihtis Derg. 2003;10(1):18–24. Turkish. PMID: 12529573.
18. Champion WM, McSherry CK, Goulian D. Effect of hyperbaric oxygen on survival of pedicled skin flaps. J Surg Res. 1967;7:583–6.
19. Stevens DM, Weiss DD, Koller WA, Bianchi DA. Survival of normothermic microvascular flaps after prolonged secondary ischemia: effects of hyperbaric oxygen. Otolaryngol Head Neck Surg. 1996;115(4):360–4. https://doi.org/10.1016/S0194-5998(96)70051-7. PMID: 8861891.
20. Lozano DD, Stephenson LL, Zamboni WA. Effect of hyperbaric oxygen and medicinal leeching on survival of axial skin flaps subjected to total venous occlusion. Plast Reconstr Surg. 1999;104:1029–32.
21. Prada FS, Arrunategui G, Alves MC, Ferreira MC, Zumiotti AV. Effect of allopurinol, superoxide-dismutase, and hyperbaric oxygen on flap survival. Microsurgery. 2002;22(8):352–60. https://doi.org/10.1002/micr.10073. PMID: 12497572.
22. Stewart RJ, Moore T, Bennett B, Easton M, Newton GW, Yamaguchi KT. Effect of free-radical scavengers and hyperbaric oxygen on random-pattern skin flaps. Arch Surg. 1994;129(9):982–7; discussion 987–8. https://doi.org/10.1001/archsurg.1994.01420330096017. PMID: 8080381.
23. Tomur A, Etlik O, Gundogan NU. Hyperbaric oxygenation and antioxidant vitamin combination reduces ischemia-reperfusion injury in a rat epigastric Island skin-flap model. J Basic Clin Physiol Pharmacol. 2005;16(4):275–85. https://doi.org/10.1515/jbcpp.2005.16.4.275. PMID: 16438393.

24. Bowersox JC, Strauss MB, Hart GB. Clinical experience with hyperbaric oxygen therapy in salvage of ischemic skin flaps and grafts. J Hyperbaric Med. 1986;1:141–9.
25. Chiang IH, Tzeng YS, Chang SC. Is hyperbaric oxygen therapy indispensable for saving mutilated hand injuries? Int Wound J. 2017;14(6):929–36. doi: https://doi.org/10.1111/iwj.12730. Epub 2017 Mar 1. PMID: 28251838; PMCID: PMC7950024.
26. Serra MP, Longhi P. Salvage of upper limb following a severe crushing trauma: immediate reconstruction with a free flap and subsequent hyperbaric oxygen therapy. Case Rep Med. 2009;2009:568142. https://doi.org/10.1155/2009/568142. Epub 2009 May 27. PMID: 19718265; PMCID: PMC2729425.
27. Park SK, Schank KJ, Engwall-Gill A, Clarkson JHW. Superior gluteal artery perforator flap salvaged via hyperbaric oxygen therapy. BMJ Case Rep. 2022;15(3):e248411. https://doi.org/10.1136/bcr-2021-248411. PMID: 35351757; PMCID: PMC8966518.
28. Cordova A, Corradino B, Pirrello R, Di Lorenzo S, Dispenza C, Moschella F. Surgical treatment of pharyngostomes in irradiated patients. Our experience with musculocutaneous pectoralis major flap and hyperbaric oxygen therapy. Acta Otolaryngol. 2005;125(7):759–64. https://doi.org/10.1080/00016480510027556. PMID: 16012039.
29. Steckeler S, Bötel U, Warninghoff V. Die hyperbare Sauerstofftherapie—Ein adjuvantes Therapieverfahren bei Problemfällen in der knöchernen Wiederherstellungschirurgie [Hyperbaric oxygen therapy—an adjuvant therapeutic procedure with problem cases in reconstructive bone surgery]. Fortschr Kiefer Gesichtschir. 1994;39:164–7. German. PMID: 8088651.
30. Maynor ML, Moon RE, Camporesi EM, Fawcett TA, Fracica PJ, Norvell HC, Levin LS. Chronic osteomyelitis of the tibia: treatment with hyperbaric oxygen and autogenous microsurgical muscle transplantation. J South Orthop Assoc. 1998;7(1):43–57. PMID: 9570731.
31. Bassetto F, Bosco G, Brambullo T, Kohlscheen E, Tocco Tussardi I, Vindigni V, Tiengo C. Hyperbaric oxygen therapy in Plastic Surgery practice: case series and literature overview. G Chir. 2019;40(4):257–75. PMID: 32011977.
32. Gal TJ, Yueh B, Futran ND. Influence of prior hyperbaric oxygen therapy in complications following microvascular reconstruction for advanced osteoradionecrosis. Arch Otolaryngol Head Neck Surg. 2003;129(1):72–6. https://doi.org/10.1001/archotol.129.1.72. PMID: 12525198.
33. Nolen D, Cannady SB, Wax MK, Scharpf J, Puscas L, Esclamado RM, Fritz M, Freiberger J, Lee WT. Comparison of complications in free flap reconstruction for osteoradionecrosis in patients with or without hyperbaric oxygen therapy. Head Neck. 2014;36(12):1701–4. https://doi.org/10.1002/hed.23520. Epub 2014 Jan 20. PMID: 24123657.
34. Haltern C, Siekmann UP, Rump AF, Rossaint R. Hyperbare Oxygenationstherapie (HBO): eine Standortbestimmung [Hyperbaric oxygen therapy (HBO): current standing]. Anasthesiol Intensivmed Notfallmed Schmerzther. 2000;35(8):487–502. German. https://doi.org/10.1055/s-2000-7079. PMID: 10992960.
35. Eskes A, Vermeulen H, Lucas C, Ubbink DT. Hyperbaric oxygen therapy for treating acute surgical and traumatic wounds. Cochrane Database Syst Rev. 2013;12:CD008059. https://doi.org/10.1002/14651858.CD008059.pub3.
36. Zhou YY, Liu W, Yang YJ, Lu GD. Use of hyperbaric oxygen on flaps and grafts in China: analysis of studies in the past 20 years. Undersea Hyperb Med. 2014;41:209–16. PMID: 24984315.
37. Kucur C, Durmus K, Uysal IO, Old M, Agrawal A, Arshad H, Teknos TN, Ozer E. Management of complications and compromised free flaps following major head and neck surgery. Eur Arch Otorrinolaringol. 2016;273(1):209–13. https://doi.org/10.1007/s00405-014-3489-1. Epub 2015 Jan 10. PMID: 25575841.
38. Anand S, Krishnan N, Bajpai M. Utility and safety of hyperbaric oxygen therapy as a rescue treatment in complicated cases of hypospadias: a systematic review and meta-analysis. J Pediatr Urol. 2022;18(1):39–46. https://doi.org/10.1016/j.jpurol.2021.10.004. Epub 2021 Oct 20. PMID: 34696963.

39. Baynosa RC, Zamboni WA. The effect of hyperbaric oxygen on compromised grafts and flaps. Undersea Hyperb Med. 2012;39:857–65.
40. Waterhouse MA, Zamboni WA, Brown RE, Russell RC. The use of HBO in compromised free tissue transfer and replantation, a clinical review. Undersea Hyperbaric Med. 1993;20(Suppl):64.
41. Mathieu D, Marroni A, Kot J. Tenth European Consensus Conference on Hyperbaric Medicine: recommendations for accepted and non-accepted clinical indications and practice of hyperbaric oxygen treatment. Diving Hyperb Med. 2017;47(1):24–32. https://doi.org/10.28920/dhm47.1.24-32. Erratum in: Diving Hyperb Med. 2017 Jun;47(2):131–132. PMID: 28357821; PMCID: PMC6147240.
42. Pougnet R, Fenet O, Loddé B, Cochard G, Henckes A, Pougnet L. Doctors in a hyperbaric medical unit: what is the hyperbaric exposure? Int Marit Health. 2018;69(4):304–5. [PubMed: 30589071].
43. Liao SC, Mao YC, Yang KJ, Wang KC, Wu LY, Yang CC. Targeting optimal time for hyperbaric oxygen therapy following carbon monoxide poisoning for prevention of delayed neuropsychiatric sequelae: a retrospective study. J Neurol Sci. 2019;396:187–92. [PubMed: 30481656].
44. Knobloch K, Redeker J, Vogt PM. The reconstructive ladder in necrotizing fasciitis of the chest wall. Interact Cardiovasc Thorac Surg. 2010;10(3):484–5. [PubMed: 20185854].

Chapter 18
Recommended Indications: Intracranial Abscess

Flávio Marino

18.1 Case Presentation

A 45-year-old immunocompromised male presents to the emergency department with a 2-week history of progressive headache, fever, and altered mental status. He reports a recent dental infection treated with a 10-day course of amoxicillin/clavulanate. On examination, he presents confused, febrile, and signs of increased intracranial pressure, including papilledema. No motor or sensory deficits noted. A head computed tomography (CT) reveals a hypodense lesion with peripheral enhancement.

Question: What is the most probable diagnosis?
Answer: Intracranial abscess.

The term intracranial abscess includes cerebral abscess, subdural empyema, and epidural empyema, and is a relatively rare condition with an estimated incidence of 0.3–1.3 per 100,000 [1, 2]. An overall mortality is estimated at 10–36% [3].

Further investigations, including microbiological analysis of cerebrospinal fluid and magnetic resonance imaging (MRI), confirm the diagnosis of intracranial abscess. The causative organism is identified as *Streptococcus intermedius*, indicating a likely odontogenic source.

F. Marino (✉)
Department of Intensive Care Medicine, Hospital de Vila Franca de Xira, EPE, Vila Franca de Xira, Lisboa, Portugal

A. G. D'Almeida, J. Hidalgo (eds.), *Evidence-Based Hyperbaric Medicine*,
https://doi.org/10.1007/978-3-032-06346-5_18

18.2 Principles of Management

The standard approach to managing intracranial abscess involves a combination of antibiotic therapy and surgical intervention (aspiration, drainage, or excision). When a surgical approach is not possible, optimized medical therapy is still the cornerstone. Prompt diagnosis and treatment are crucial to prevent complications and minimize neurological damage.

1. *Diagnosis*—Intracranial abscess should be suspected in patients presenting with symptoms such as persistent headache, fever, focal neurological deficits, and signs of increased intracranial pressure.

   History of recent infections such as dental infections, chronic or severe sinusitis, otitis and mastoiditis, recent head trauma, or neurosurgery should be questioned and trigger higher suspicion for intracranial abscess diagnosis.

   High-risk groups include immunocompromised individuals, for example, HIV/AIDS patients. It is important to notice that cerebral toxoplasmosis may be the first opportunistic infection in patients with previously undiagnosed HIV infection. For this reason, HIV testing should be proposed to all patients with brain abscess [4].

   Neuroimaging studies, such as CT or MRI, are crucial for confirming the diagnosis and assessing the size, location, and characteristics of the abscess.

   Contrast-enhanced CT usually reveals a peripheral ring-enhanced lesion, with a central area of hypodensity surrounded by varying levels of hypodensity (edema) [5].

   MRI is preferred due to its ability to identify additional lesions, detect at-risk lesions for complications earlier, and minimize the toxicity associated with gadolinium contrast agents. It has also proven beneficial in differential diagnosis, specifically between tumors [5].
2. *Antibiotic Therapy*—Empirical antibiotic therapy should be initiated promptly after obtaining appropriate cultures. Antibiotic selection should be based on the suspected or confirmed pathogens and local antimicrobial susceptibility patterns. Most commonly isolated microorganisms include *Streptococcus* and *Staphylococcus* species [6].

   Bacterial abscesses are typically seen in immunocompetent individuals, whereas immunocompromised patients can be susceptible to infection from a diverse range of organisms, including fungi [2]. Tailoring antibiotic therapy based on case-by-case, culture, and sensitivity results is fundamental.

   Generally, the duration of antibiotic therapy for intracranial abscesses is typically long term, and intravenous antibiotics may be required for a prolonged period. Monitor response to treatment and adjust antibiotics accordingly.
3. *Surgical Intervention*—Surgical intervention is often necessary to evacuate the abscess and achieve source control. The specific surgical approach depends on factors such as abscess location, size, associated complications, and the neurosurgeon's and institutional expertise.

Options for surgical intervention include stereotactic aspiration, craniotomy with abscess drainage, or a combination of both. Minimally invasive and guided approach revolutionizes surgical management [5, 7].

4. *Monitoring and Follow-Up*—Close monitoring of the patient's clinical status, including neurological examination, vital signs, and laboratory parameters, is essential. Serial neuroimaging studies, such as CT or MRI, are performed to assess the response to treatment, evaluate the resolution of the abscess, and monitor for any complications or recurrence.
5. *Multidisciplinary Approach*—Management of intracranial abscess often requires a multidisciplinary team, including neurosurgeons, infectious disease specialists, intensivists, and radiologists.

18.3 Evidence Contour

Controversial aspects of managing intracranial abscess, considering the available evidence include use of corticosteroids, antiepileptic therapy, and use of hyperbaric oxygen therapy (HBOT) as an adjunctive therapy.

1. *Corticosteroids*—Corticosteroid use is not routinely recommended for all cases of intracranial abscesses, and their use should be determined on a case-by-case basis. Due to its anti-inflammatory effects, they may be considered in certain cases to reduce brain swelling and associated symptoms. Concerns about the potential negative impact on outcomes due to immunosuppressive characteristics make its use controversial [8].
2. *Antiepileptic Therapy* may be considered in cases that the patient develops seizures or is at risk of experiencing seizures due to the location or size of the abscess. The duration of antiepileptic therapy depends on the individual patient's response to treatment and the underlying cause of the seizures. In some cases, antiepileptic medications may be required only for a short period, such as during the acute phase of the abscess, while, in other cases, they may be needed for a more extended period, especially if the abscess has caused structural brain damage or if there is an ongoing risk of recurrent seizures.
3. *HBOT*—Controversies surrounding the use of HBOT as an adjunctive treatment for intracranial abscess have been a topic of debate. Since 1996, the Undersea and Hyperbaric Medical Society has approved HBOT as an adjunctive therapy for intracranial abscess [7]. Proponents of HBOT argue that it can improve outcomes and is well tolerated and safe with appropriate therapeutic protocol application, with few side effects, typically not severe [1, 9].

Mechanisms proposed to enhance outcomes include the high atmospheric pressure promoting increased oxygen tension in perfused and infected tissues, generating lysis of cell barriers and enhancing bactericidal effects of antibiotics in anaerobic and mixed infections, enhancing bacteria-killing action and vasoconstriction which cause a minor blood volume and intracranial pressure, protecting against secondary brain injury, and permitting regeneration of the surrounding tissue [10, 11]. Additionally, HBOT may have immunomodulatory effects, reducing inflammation and promoting the immune response [1, 12].

Patient Selection:
According to the Tenth European Consensus Conference on Hyperbaric Medicine, the decision to use HBOT on intracranial abscess should be considered in patients with [13]:

- Multiple abscesses;
- Abscess in a deep or dominant location;
- Compromised host;
- Contra-indication to surgery;
- Lack of response or further deterioration in spite of standard treatment.

Final decision should be based on careful assessment and should take into account logistical issues, especially in critically ill patients, where the level of care should be secure and maintained in transportation and during treatment in the hyperbaric chamber.

Timing and Protocol:
Timing of HBOT initiation in the management of intracranial abscess is not well established. Early initiation may be beneficial, but optimal timing remains uncertain.

HBOT protocol typically involves delivering oxygen at a pressure of 2.0–2.5 atmospheres absolute for 60–90 minutes per treatment, usually, one or two sessions per day [3, 10]. The total number of sessions is unknown, reaching on average 13.4 sessions, and depending on the patient's recovery, including neurological clinical evaluation and repeated CT [3].

References

1. Ortega MA, Fraile-Martinez O, García-Montero C, et al. A general overview on the hyperbaric oxygen therapy: applications, mechanisms and translational opportunities. Medicina. 2021;57:864.
2. Das JM, Tommeraasen MA, Cooper JS. Hyperbaric evaluation and treatment of intracranial abscess.
3. Mathieu D, editor. Handbook on hyperbaric medicine. Dordrecht: Springer; 2006.
4. Sonneville R, Ruimy R, Benzonana N, Riffaud L, Carsin A, Tadié J-M, Piau C, Revest M, Tattevin P. An update on bacterial brain abscess in immunocompetent patients. Clin Microbiol Infect. 2017;23:614–20.
5. Cantiera M, Tattevin P, Sonneville R. Brain abscess in immunocompetent adult patients. Rev Neurol. 2019;175:469–74.
6. Brouwer MC, Coutinho JM, van de Beek D. Clinical characteristics and outcome of brain abscess: systematic review and meta-analysis. Neurology. 2014;82:806–13.
7. Mandour C, Gazzaz M, El Mostarchid B. Hyperbaric oxygen therapy in the treatment of brain abscess: about a case. Roman Neurosurg. 2018;32:125–8.

8. Simjian T, Muskens IS, Lamba N, et al. Dexamethasone administration and mortality in patients with brain abscess: a systematic review and meta-analysis. World Neurosurg. 2018;115:257–63.
9. Costa DA, Amaro CE, Nunes A, Cardoso JS, Daniel PM, Rosa I, Branco JV. Hyperbaric oxygen therapy as a complementary treatment for radiation proctitis: Useless or useful?—A literature review. 2021;27:17.
10. Serrato Perdomo JD, Gutiérrez A, Chacón L, Donato Á. Absceso cerebral bilateral frontal, medicina hiperbárica, cirugía y terapia antimicrobiana en germen extraño. Reporte de caso y revisión de la literatura. Neurol Neurocir Psiquiatr. 2022;50:109–13.
11. Nakahara K, Yamashita S, Ideo K, et al. Drastic therapy for Listerial brain abscess involving combined hyperbaric oxygen therapy and antimicrobial agents. J Clin Neurol. 2014;10:358.
12. de Wolde SD, Hulskes RH, de Jonge SW, Hollmann MW, van Hulst RA, Weenink RP, Kox M. The effect of hyperbaric oxygen therapy on markers of oxidative stress and the immune response in healthy volunteers. Front Physiol. 2022;13:826163.
13. Mathieu D, Marroni A, Kot J. Tenth European Consensus Conference on Hyperbaric Medicine: recommendations for accepted and non-accepted clinical indications and practice of hyperbaric oxygen treatment. 2017;47:9.

Chapter 19
Hyperbaric Medicine in Critical Care

Bruno Sarmento Banheiro, Lucie Cunha, Adelaide Valente, Marcelo Gordinho, Isa Cordeiro, and Manuel Almeida

19.1 Introduction

Hyperbaric oxygen therapy (HBOT) consists in breathing 100% oxygen intermittently while inside a treatment chamber at a pressure higher than at sea level pressure (i.e., 1 atm abs) [1, 2]. In certain circumstances, HBOT is the primary treatment modality, whereas in others, it is an adjunct to surgical or pharmacologic interventions [1, 3–5].

HBOT is a treatment that can be traced back to the 1600s. Nevertheless, oxygen was first described as a treatment in acute care in 1885 [1].

The first well-known chamber was built and run by a British clergyman named Henshaw. He built a structure called the *domicilium* that was used to treat a multitude of diseases [2]. The chamber was pressurized with air or unpressurized using bellows. The idea of treating patients under increased pressure was continued by the French surgeon Fontaine, who built a pressurized, mobile operating room in 1879. Dr. Orville Cunningham, a professor of anesthesia, ran what was known as the "Steel Ball Hospital." The structure, erected in 1928, was six stories high and 64 feet in diameter. The hospital could reach 3 atmospheres of pressure (atm) but was closed in 1930 because of the lack of scientific evidence indicating that such treatment alleviated disease. It was deconstructed during World War II for scrap. The military continued work with hyperbaric oxygen. The work of Paul Bert, who demonstrated the toxic effects of oxygen (producing generalized seizures), as well as the

B. S. Banheiro (✉) · L. Cunha · A. Valente · M. Gordinho · I. Cordeiro · M. Almeida
Centro Hospitalar Universitário do Algarve—Unidade Hospitalar de Portimão—Serviço de Medicina Intensiva 2, Portimão, Faro, Portugal
e-mail: brunoasbg@hotmail.com; sll_cunha@hotmail.com; adelaideclodevalente@gmail.com; mdsgordinho@gmail.com; isafialhocordeiro94@gmail.com; m_almeida3108@hotmail.com

A. G. D'Almeida, J. Hidalgo (eds.), *Evidence-Based Hyperbaric Medicine*,
https://doi.org/10.1007/978-3-032-06346-5_19

work of J. Lorrain-Smith, who demonstrated pulmonary oxygen toxicity, was used with Navy divers. Exposure times to oxygen at different depths of water (and, hence, different levels of pressure) were quantified and tested based on time to convulsions [6, 7].

19.2 Technic/Fundamentals

HBOT is a therapy based on breathing pure oxygen or a gas mixture (heliox, nitrox) in a closed chamber with increased atmospheric pressure [8].

There are two types of chambers: monoplace, a long plastic tube where one patient is breathing pressurized 100% oxygen, and multiplace (Figs. 19.1 and 19.2), where you can fit two or more people. The difference is that people breathe pure oxygen through a facial mask, a close-fitting hood, or an endotracheal tube [9].

The duration and maximum pressure are normally set to 120 minutes and 3 atm, to prevent the side effects of hyperoxygenation [8].

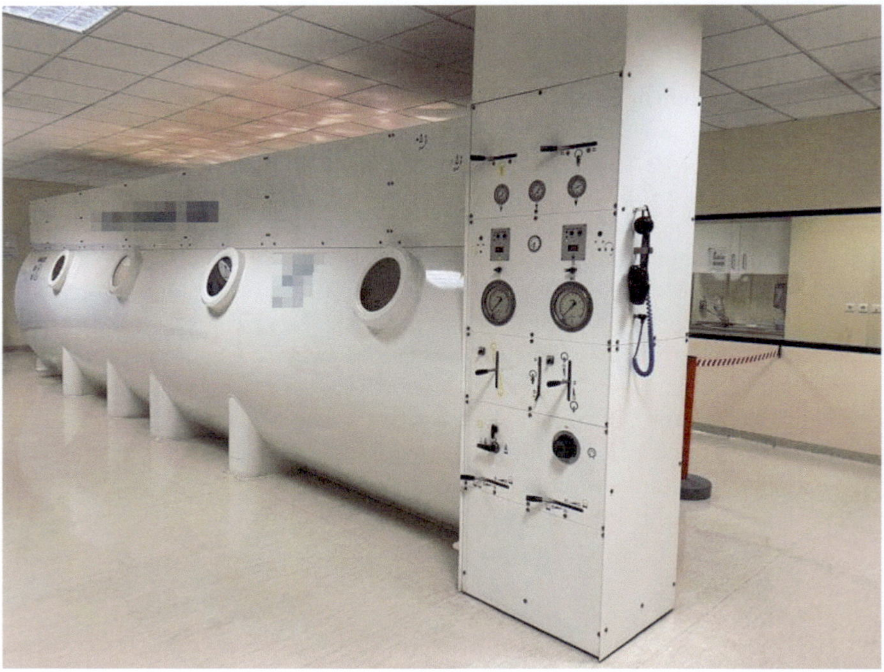

Fig. 19.1 Hyperbaric chamber HAUX-STARMED 2200®

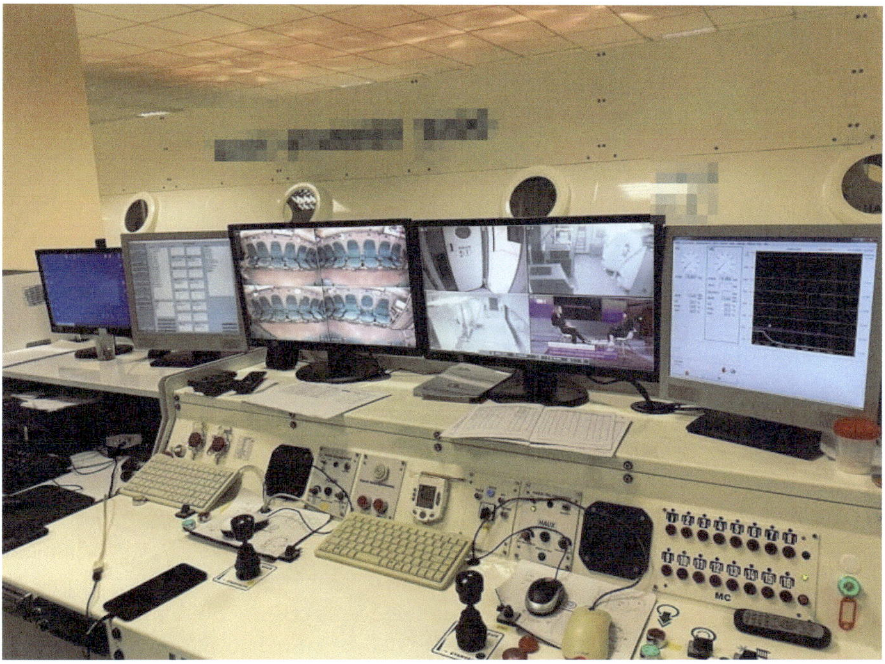

Fig. 19.2 Hyperbaric chamber control room

19.3 Physiology

The understanding of HBOT implies the knowledge of a few basic ideal gas physics laws.

Henry's law determines that the partial pressure of individual gases is caused by multiple impacts of moving molecules against a surface. Therefore, the pressure is directly proportional to the concentration of the gas molecules. Regarding the gases involved in respiratory physiology, such as oxygen, nitrogen, and carbon dioxide, the rate of diffusion of each of these gases is directly proportional to the pressure caused by that gas alone, which is called the partial pressure of that gas [10, 11].

Usually, it is administered 2–3 atm of oxygen through a mask or endotracheal tube, and the surrounding environment is also compressed at the same pressure but with normal air. Most oxygen in the blood is bound to hemoglobin. At normal pressure, about 97% is transported by the hemoglobin, whereas only 3% is dissolved in the plasma. By increasing the pressure and PaO_2 rises above 100 mmHg, the amount

Fig. 19.3 Boyle's law

$$P_1V_1 = P_2V_2$$

P–GASPRESSURE
V–GAS VOLUME
WITH CONSTANT TEMPERATURE

of oxygen present in the blood but not bound to hemoglobin increases significantly. Notably, 3 atm is more than enough to meet resting cellular requirements without any contribution from hemoglobin. The oxygen is in solution, which means that it can reach areas where red blood cells would not be able to go through and can also provide tissue oxygenation in the setting of impaired hemoglobin concentration or function [10, 11].

In carbon monoxide poisoning, besides the ability of oxygenation with the oxygen diluted in the plasma, the high pressure can displace carbon monoxide rapidly from its combination with hemoglobin. With HBOT, the half-life of carbon monoxide decreases from 40–80 to 15–30 minutes [10].

Hyperoxygenation also causes vasoconstriction occurring predominantly at the level of healthy tissues, with attenuation of edema and redistribution of blood volume peripherally in favor of hypoxic tissues, enhancing anti-ischemic and anti-hypoxic effects [12, 13].

HBOT also improves wound healing. By increasing the availability of oxygen in hypoxic lesions, there is increased fibroblast proliferation, angiogenesis, and combat to local infection. There is an increased neutrophil bactericidal activity, limitation of clostridial exotoxin and production of spores, elimination of anaerobes, and inhibition of the growth of several bacterial pathogens. The generation of oxygen free radicals also inhibits bacterial metabolic functions [12, 13].

Boyles's law (Fig. 19.3) also has a major importance in the treatment of some conditions, such as decompression sickness or arterial gas emboli. The volume of the gas is inversely related to its pressure. This means that, by increasing the pressure, the volume of the bubble will decrease [10, 11].

19.4 Clinical Use

Over the last decades, HBOT has been used in numerous diseases, frequently without adequate scientific validation or formal recommendation. This has led to false notions and skepticism in the clinical use of this treatment.

The most recent recommendations for the use of HBOT could be divided as strongly recommended, recommended, and optional [7, 9].

19.5 Therapeutic Uses: Emergent Indications

19.5.1 CO Poisoning

Carbon monoxide binds with a much stronger affinity to hemoglobin than oxygen (240 times). This reduces the capacity of blood to carry oxygen to the tissues. Furthermore, there is an increased affinity of the unoccupied hemoglobin binding sites to the oxygen molecules, reducing the O_2 availability. Concomitantly, the CO can bind to the myoglobin, worsening the tissue hypoxia [5, 9, 13].

HBOT can deliver oxygen dissolved in the plasma, offering a substitute source of tissue oxygenation. It can also accelerate the dissociation of CO from hemoglobin and myoglobin, reducing its half-life from 240–320 to 20 minutes [5].

HBOT should be provided to all patients with confirmed CO poisoning diagnosis presenting with unconsciousness, convulsions, neurologic, cardiac or respiratory impairment, or severe metabolic acidosis [7, 9].

19.5.2 Decompression Illness

Ascension too rapid from divers (or less commonly, a fast ascent to over 5500 m) may cause the partial pressure of nitrogen dissolved in the tissues to exceed the ambient atmospheric pressure, leading to the formation of air bubbles in the blood and tissues. Decompression illness may present with a rash or joint pain or more severe symptoms such as paralysis, confusion, convulsions, and ultimately death [5, 9].

HBOT is the main therapeutic approach. Treatment should be started as soon as possible, with a duration of 2–5 hours or until the symptoms have resolved [5].

19.5.3 Gas Embolism

During numerous procedures, such as the placement of arterial and venous catheters, cardiothoracic surgery, hemodialysis, or mechanical ventilation, air may enter the blood circulation. HBOT, through the increase of the ambient atmospheric pressure, allows an immediate decrease in the volume of the air bubble. Additionally, hyperoxia creates a diffusion gradient to the washout of nitrogen and the entrance of oxygen in the air bubble. As such, HBOT constitutes the first-line treatment and is strongly recommended [5, 7, 9].

19.6 Anaerobic and Mixed Bacterial Soft Tissue Infections

Infections caused by anaerobic bacteria and some mixed infections can result in the loss of local defense mechanisms and tissue destruction due to decreasing tissue oxygen pressures. HBOT increases oxygen transportation (compromised by hemolysis), helping tissue oxygenation, allowing the differentiation of the true extent of the infection and the categorization of the viability of affected tissues. HBOT should be started as soon as possible, always alongside adequate antibiotic treatment and surgical debridement [5, 7, 9, 13].

19.7 Contraindications

The only absolute contraindication for HBOT is an untreated pneumothorax. Placing a patient in a chamber and changing the pressure around them can result in a tension pneumothorax, which can quickly become life-threatening [14].

Concomitant use of doxorubicin was previously thought to be an absolute contraindication because this treatment can increase the doxorubicin cardiotoxicity. Doxorubicin should be stopped at least 24 hours before HBOT. Bleomycin is known to cause interstitial pneumonitis, and a pretreatment evaluation should be performed before HBOT to decide if the treatment is safe. Disulfiram can increase the risk of oxygen toxicity and should not be used concomitantly. Cisplatin can impair wound healing and make the treatment futile [14].

There are several relative contraindications such as obstructive lung disease, asymptomatic pulmonary bleeds, upper respiratory or sinus infection, recent ear or thoracic surgery, upper respiratory infection, allergic rhinitis, history of pneumothorax, epilepsy, optic neuritis, uncontrolled hypertension, uncontrolled heart failure, and claustrophobia [5, 14].

19.8 Side Effects

The HBOT is not free from secondary effects. In general, if pressures do not exceed 300 kPa and the length of treatment is less than 120 minutes, the treatment is safe [5].

The side effects are often mild and reversible but can be severe and life-threatening. The most common fatal complication is fire hazard [15].

Symptomatic reversible barotrauma occurs in 15–20% of treated patients and can include ear damage, sinus damage, ruptured middle ear, or even lung damage. The most common side effect is middle ear barotrauma, followed by sinus barotrauma.

Pulmonary oxygen toxicity can include pulmonary edema, hemorrhage, or respiratory failure. Mild forms of pulmonary toxicity can be present with chest tightness, cough, and reversible falls in pulmonary function that may occur due to repeated treatment [15].

Reversible myopia due to oxygen toxicity on the lens can happen, and it can last for weeks to months. HBOT can also cause fatigue, headache, vomiting, and claustrophobia [15].

Seizures due to central nervous system oxygen toxicity are rare, 1–2%, and usually cause no permanent damage [14, 15].

19.9 Clinical Case

A 53-year-old woman was found at home with reduced consciousness, her pupils were dilated and very sluggish, and her breathing was shallow. According to the neighbors, a structure fire had started around 30 minutes before. The patient was started with an oxygen mask at 6 L/min by emergency medical services personnel and transported to a hospital.

Initial serum carboxyhemoglobin (COHgb) level was 21.9%, and arterial blood gases showed pH 7.33, $PaCO_2$ 32 mmHg, PaO_2 51 mmHg, HCO_3 16 mmol/L, and SaO_2 82%. Additional laboratory tests included normal complete blood count, electrolytes, glucose, and troponin I. Her electrocardiogram showed sinus tachycardia with no ST-T wave changes. Given the elevated COHgb, she was transferred to a facility for HBOT.

Before HBOT, the patient regained consciousness. She had nausea and weakness, but normal vital signs. The patient was prescribed three treatments of 100% oxygen at 2.8 atmospheres for 90 minutes each, recovered uneventfully, and was discharged within 24 hours.

19.10 Future Applications

HBOT can increase blood and tissue oxygenation in an effective way, regardless of hemoglobin transportation. It has unique physical, physiological, and molecular properties that are extremely effective in the management of hypoxemia and hypoxia resulting conditions. As such, the use of HBOT might be extended to a wide range of illnesses and disorders. For example, the potential use of HBOT in the treatment of COVID-19 has been particularly considered, as an effective way to deliver oxygen and mitigate inflammatory reactions. The utility of HBOT to treat inflammatory bowel disease has also been getting attention, as it can have beneficial effects by down-regulating the inflammatory process and improving tissue oxygenation. Its use in the treatment of complications resulting from the injection of cosmetic fillers seems extremely promising [16–18].

References

1. Shultz SM, Hartmann PM. George E Holtzapple (1862–1946) and oxygen therapy for lobar pneumonia: the first reported case (1887) and a review of the contemporary literature to 1899. J Med. 2005;13(4):201–6.
2. Henshaw IN, Simpson A. Compressed air as a therapeutic agent in the treatment of consumption, asthma, chronic bronchitis and other diseases. 1857;5(17):94–6.
3. Chin W, Jacoby L, Simon O, Talati N, Wegrzyn G, Jacoby R, et al. Hyperbaric programs in the United States: locations and capabilities of treating decompression sickness, arterial gas embolisms, and acute carbon monoxide poisoning: survey results. Undersea Hyperb Med. 2016;43(1):29–43.
4. Gill AL, Bell CNA. Hyperbaric oxygen: its uses, mechanisms of action and outcomes. QJMed. 2004;97(7):385–9.
5. Leach RM, Rees PJ, Wilmshurst P. Hyperbaric oxygen therapy. BMJ. 1998;317(7166):1140–3.
6. Kindwall E, Whelan H. Hyperbaric medicine practice. 2nd ed. Flagstaff: Best Publishing Company; 2004. chap 1, 18, 19, 20, 25, 29, 3.
7. Mathieu D, Marroni A, Kot J. Tenth European Consensus Conference on Hyperbaric Medicine: Recommendations for accepted and non-accepted clinical indications and practice of hyperbaric oxygen treatment. Diving Hyperb Med. 2017;47(1):24–32.
8. Albuquerque-e-Sousa JG. Oxigenoterapia hiperbárica (OTHB). Perspectiva histórica, efeitos-fisiológicos e aplicações clínicas. Revista da Sociedade Portuguesa de Medicina Interna. 2007:219–27.
9. Fernandes TDF, et al. Medicina Hiperbárica. Acta Med Port. 2009;22(4):323–34.
10. Hall JE. Guyton and hall textbook of medical physiology. 14th ed. London: W B Saunders; 2021. Chap 40, 41, 45.
11. Neuman TS, Thom SR. Physiology and medicine of hyperbaric oxygen therapy. London: W B Saunders; 2008. Chap 4.
12. Shinomiya N, Asai Y, editors. Hyperbaric oxygenation therapy: molecular mechanisms and clinical applications. 1st ed. Singapore: Springer; 2020. Chap 1.
13. Shah J. Hyperbaric oxygen therapy. J Am Coll Cert Wound Special. 2010;2:9–13.
14. Gawdi R, Jeffrey S. Cooper, hyperbaric contraindications, NBCI, Janeiro; 2021.
15. Leung JK, Lam PK. Hyperbaric oxygen therapy: its use in medical emergencies and its development in Hong Kong. Hong Kong Med J. 2018:191.
16. Paganini M, Bosco G, Perozzo FAG, Kohlscheen E, Sonda R, Bassetto F, et al. The role of hyperbaric oxygen treatment for COVID-19: a review. Adv Exp Med Biol. 2021;1289:27–35.
17. Dulai PS, Gleeson MW, Taylor D, Holubar SD, Buckey JC, Siegel CA. Systematic revier: the safety and efficacy of hyperbaric oxygen therapy for inflammatory bowel disease. Aliment Pharmacol Ther. 2014;39(11):1266–75.
18. Uittenbigaard D, Lansdorp CA, Bauland CG, Boonstra O. Hyperbaric oxygen therapy for dermal ischemia after dermal filler injection with calcium hydroxylapatite: a case report. Undersea Hyperb Med. 2019;46(2):207–10.

Chapter 20
Clinical Evaluation of Patients Proposed for Hyperbaric Oxygen Therapy and Contraindications

Santanu Bagchi, Ahsina Jahan Lopa, and Saurabh Debnath

20.1 Introduction

Hyperbaric oxygen therapy (HBOT) refers to delivering absolutely 100% oxygen at a much higher pressure, usually thrice the ambient atmospheric pressure, within a closed dedicated chamber. The use of this specialized therapeutic modality, contrary to a possible prevalent notion, has been in vogue for a few centuries.

The early description of HBOT, as a treatment modality, has been found way back in 1861 when the first hyperbaric chamber of the United States was established [1]. From the historical perspective, however, the concept of delivering compressed air as a hyperbaric therapy had been found even much earlier, way back in 1662, when Henshaw, a physician from the United Kingdom, utilized it. Subsequent invention of oxygen gas, by renowned British scientist John Priestly in 1775, had an immense impact on the overall science and application of hyperbaric therapy. The use of oxygen in hyperbaric therapy was gaining momentum despite the description of oxygen toxicities, and, in relation to that, the first ever hyperbaric chamber of the world was built at Oshawa, Canada, in 1860. The most well-known chamber from a historical angle was built in Kansas City by Cunningham in 1921 and became operational a few years later. The largest chamber of that period, however, was built in Cleveland, United States, in 1928 [2].

The practical application of the hyperbaric therapy was initially limited to animal models with early description in 1887, where Valenzuela and colleagues selected

S. Bagchi (✉)
Department of Critical Care Medicine,Tata Medical Center, Kokata, West Bengal, India

A. J. Lopa
Department of ICU and Emergency, Brahmanbaria ICU Specialized Hospital, Dhaka, Bangladesh

S. Debnath
AMRI Hospitals, Kolkata, India

A. G. D'Almeida, J. Hidalgo (eds.), *Evidence-Based Hyperbaric Medicine*,
https://doi.org/10.1007/978-3-032-06346-5_20

the rabbit as the animal model to study about the effects of HBOT [3]. The first use of HBOT in decompression sickness was described in 1937 by Behnke and Shaw [4]. Subsequently, there had been reports of HBOT among divers suffering from decompression sickness, particularly during World War II [5]. Over the years, the array of applications of HBOT has grown progressively. Churchill-Davidson, in 1955, used this therapy on cancer patients as an aid to radiation therapy [6]. Another prominent application was reported by Boerema and colleagues around the same period, on cardiac surgery patients with an intention to prolong the circulatory arrest time [7].

20.2 Physiological Aspects of HBOT

Despite the early invention of HBOT, its application in the initial days was quite limited. The primary reason of concern was the oxygen-related toxicities, as initially pointed out by Seguin and Lavoisier in 1789. Subsequently, this concern was also echoed by a few other renowned scientists, like Paul Bert, describing the neurotoxicity, also known as the "Bert effect" [8], and Lorraine Smith, describing the pulmonary toxicities [9]. However, there has been growing interest in the varied applications of HBOT, particularly since the time of World War II, when there was a demonstration of its utility among soldiers with decompression sickness.

Now, the reason or basic principle of HBOT lies in how would a gas (here oxygen) behave within body fluids or tissues, under a dynamic pressure and volume condition, as it had been described by different laws of physics, for example, Henry's law, Boyle's law, or Fick's principle. This application of pure oxygen (or 100% oxygen) at a higher ambient pressure can be at a level between 2 and 3 atmospheres absolute (ATA), within a hyperbaric chamber. When the pressure remains at a level of 2 ATA, there would be an arterial partial pressure of dissolved oxygen (PaO_2) of approximately 1400 mmHg. Similarly, at a higher pressure of 3 ATA, this PaO_2 also increases to approximately 2000 mmHg. Thus, there is a linear relationship between increased ambient pressure and PaO_2, signifying a greater amount of dissolved oxygen in plasma. In this context, the current international standard recommendation from the Undersea and Hyperbaric Medical Society mentions the breathing pressure to be at least 2 ATA or more to be considered a hyperbaric therapy [10]. However, the impact of HBOT is not only limited to increasing dissolved oxygen in plasma and thus ameliorating tissue hypoxia. There happens to be biochemical mechanism of HBOT also, which revolves around the generation of reactive oxygen and nitrogen species. This would activate growth factor receptors and progenitor cells, altering the integrin function as well as altering the synthesis of monocyte chemokine and other mediators of inflammation, such as heat shock proteins, hemoxygenase-1, hypoxia-inducible factor-1, and so on. The earliest application of HBOT, that is, in decompression sickness, utilized the principle of gas bubble physical compression occurring at increased atmospheric pressure [11]. The principle underlying cellular-level mechanism remains the formation of reactive oxygen and nitrogen radicals from pure oxygen therapy and the subsequent impact of these radicals on signal transduction pathways at the cellular level [12].

20.3 Clinical Evaluation

The clinical evaluation of a patient, for proposed HBOT, has some prerequisites. These would include not only patient care evaluation but also other relevant factors such as indication of therapy, any relative or absolute contraindications, the type of chamber available, and so on. Even educating fellow hospital colleagues regarding the general indications is essential for optimal utility of this therapy, and more importantly, detecting an indication of therapy is one of the preliminary steps in patient evaluation. In a somewhat similar fashion, educating the patient about compliance to the hyperbaric chamber protocol, the number of planned therapies, and so on is also essential, as a part of overall assessment.

The current indications of HBOT can be compiled from different resources and guidelines, and it can be summarized in Table 20.1 [13–16].

On the other hand, the contraindications can be absolute or relative. The only absolute contraindication is an untreated pneumothorax. Once pneumothorax has been managed with a chest drain in situ, then with that and keeping the Heimlich valve prior to initiation would be warranted as a prechamber management for starting HBOT on an emergency basis. The relative contraindications can be multiple, for example, congestive cardiac failure (with EF < 35%), uncontrolled hypertension or diabetes mellitus, claustrophobia (particularly in monoplace chambers), congenital spherocytosis with risk for hemolysis, fever with risk of lowering seizure threshold during therapy, chronic sinusitis or recent upper respiratory tract infection (with risk of aggravation and barotrauma), recent ophthalmologic interventions (retinal or cataract related) or optic neuritis due to risk of inadvertent air trapping, recent thoracic surgery with risk of underlying pneumothorax, obstructive airway disorders, seizure history, and so on [17].

Once the requisite history and physical examinations of the patient are over, if urgently indicated, the HBOT should begin soon, with the principle sooner the better. The evaluation of the chamber is also important—the type of chamber available and its suitability for the treatment plan, the limitations of the available chamber from the angle of patient requirement, the capability for mixed gas, the availability of staff, and so on. Some of the monoplace chambers may not allow air breaks during therapy, due to the absence of air hoses, while some may not allow monitoring of the patient's vital parameters during therapy, feasibility of arranging a special ventilator for intubated patients, etc.

In patient assessment, the implications of drug interactions should also not be missed. There are medications that need to be stopped before initiation of HBOT. Recent exposure to Bleomycin (within 1 year) may lead to interstitial pneumonitis and pulmonary fibrosis. Cisplatin may interfere with wound healing, as does Sulfamylon. Doxorubicin has been notorious for causing cardiotoxicities, and

Table 20.1 Indications of HBOT

Carbon monoxide poisoning with or without Cyanide poisoning
Air or gas embolism
Thermal burn injury
Decompression sickness
Acute ischemia due to trauma (e.g., crush injury, compartment syndrome, etc.)
Gas gangrene caused by Clostridial myonecrosis and myositis
Necrotizing soft-tissue infections
Ischemic (and thus compromised) skin grafts and flaps
Delayed injury to both soft tissues and bone, due to radiation
Central retinal artery occlusion
Osteomyelitis (refractory ones)
Anemia due to severe blood loss
Intracranial abscess
Adjunctive therapy to enhance wound healing
Sudden idiopathic sensorineural hearing loss
Diabetic foot (Wagner grade 3 or higher with failed standard therapy)

HBOT should be deferred for at least 3 days after Doxorubicin therapy. Disulfiram may inhibit the protective enzyme against oxygen toxicities, superoxide dismutase. All these or similar medication history must be carefully evaluated prior to initiation of HBOT [18].

From the clinical evaluation point of view, there should be some standardized examinations performed prior to initiation of HBOT [19]. These can be summarized as follows:

1. Patient history and health questionnaire, especially pertaining to indications and contraindications of therapy.
2. General physical examination, keeping in mind the hyperbaric exposure.
3. Pulmonary function tests [including vital capacity (VC), forced vital capacity (FVC), forced expiratory volume in 1 second (FEV1)] in order to ensure that VC/FVC/FEV1 remain within <70% of the normal value of that individual.
4. Baseline resting electrocardiogram in order to exclude patients with acute myocardial ischemia or infarction, bradyarrhythmia, and heart block (particularly grade 3 A-V block).

5. Chest X-ray (preferably both anteroposterior and lateral views) in order to exclude pneumothorax, pleural adhesions, or lung abnormalities.
6. Microscopic external examination of the ear along with observing equalization of pressure, and in case of inadequate clearance of the ear, tymanostomy tubes need to be inserted prior to therapy.
7. Tympanometry in order to assess whether the tympanic membrane is healthy or to carry out further diagnostic assessment if middle ear effusions being present.

20.4 Complications

This highly specialized therapy is not devoid of complications, and there have been many controversies from the innovation of this modality. The concerns primarily revolve around the application of raised barometric pressure and elevated oxygen partial pressure of around 1500–2000 mmHg [19].

20.4.1 Barotraumatic Lesions

This can happen due to either compression or expansion of particularly in a closed space, for example, middle or inner ear cavity, paranasal sinuses, lungs, or even teeth. During the therapy, the pressure equalization problem in the middle ear would manifest as pain or discomfort, being more common among the older population and during the first HBOT session. In extreme situations, rupture of the tympanic membrane might also occur. In contrast to ear, barotrauma in paranasal sinuses would usually manifest as headache or local pain or occasionally nasal bleed even. Sporadic reports of lung barotrauma have been found not only among scuba divers but also among those receiving HBOT [20].

20.4.2 Oxygen Toxicities

The Paul Bert effect affects the central nervous system, and the most dreaded cardinal feature is the occurrence of seizures, usually a generalized one. The possible risk factors would generally include those notorious for lowering the seizure threshold, in general, such as fever, prior epileptic disorder, hypoglycemia, hyperthyroidism, drugs like Penicillin, and so on. There happen to be some specific risk factors too, associated with HBOT and neurological toxicity, and those include drugs like Disulfiram or Acetazolamide (increment in cerebral blood flow) or conditions like hypercarbia, which would again result in cerebral vasodilatation.

Lorraine Smith's effect usually manifests as an occasional substernal burning sensation or dry cough. However, prolonged hyperoxia has a more profound deleterious effect with alveolar flooding and subsequent proliferation of fibroblasts and type 2 pneumocytes. All these would ultimately manifest as pulmonary fibrosis, causing restrictive lung disease and decreased vital capacity. In order to estimate such lung toxicity, a concept called Unit Pulmonary Toxic Dose has been coined [21].

However, this pulmonary toxicity is usually more of a theoretical concern, until and unless HBOT has been used for a prolonged period (daily for a long duration) or in an intense fashion (more than once in a day) or a patient needing ventilation with high oxygen support, in between two HBOT sessions.

20.4.3 Confinement Anxiety

This psychological complication is somewhat an inevitable complication, particularly in a susceptible population. Therapy termination usually does not happen for this complication, though. Proper psychosocial evaluation while taking history with attention to psychotropic drug use is the cornerstone in identifying patients at risk. The multiplace hyperbaric chamber is of great utility in this kind of situation. One should not forget to exclude organic causes also, in case of psychological disturbances.

20.4.4 Ocular Effects

The ocular complications have conflicting evidence. The common complications revolve around myopia and cataract growth. Myopia is usually reversible and has been reported among patients undergoing daily HBOT sessions for a prolonged period [22].

20.5 Conclusion

HBOT is a unique modality that has been in use since the last century, and with time, its applicability is widening gradually. Nevertheless, like any other treatment modality, this therapy also comes with its unique set of complications, albeit less frequently. Therefore, careful patient selection, keeping in mind the indications and contraindications of the therapy, is crucial. The importance of obtaining a thorough medical history, including but not limited to personal, familial, and medication history, along with baseline clinical examinations and some investigations as discussed, cannot be undervalued in any situation. There happens to be an immense promise for the future with this therapy, provided that careful patient selection and evaluation have been done.

References

1. Singh S, Gambert SR. Hyperbaric oxygen therapy: a brief history and review of its benefits and indications for the older adult patient. Ann Longterm Care. 2014;22(7–8):37–42.
2. Edwards ML. Hyperbaric oxygen therapy. Part 1: history and principles. J Vet Emerg Crit Care. 2010;20:284–8.
3. Bean JW. Effects of oxygen at increased pressure. Physiol Rev. 1945;25(1):1–147.
4. Smolle C, Lindenmann J, Kamolz L, Smolle-Juettner F-M. The history and development of hyperbaric oxygenation (HBO) in thermal burn injury. Medicina. 2021;57:49. https://doi.org/10.3390/medicina57010049.
5. Jones MW, Wyatt HA. Hyperbaric, physics. Treasure Island: StatPearls Publishing; 2019.
6. Boerema I. The use of hyperbaric oxygen. Am Heart J. 1965;69:289–92.
7. Boerema I, Meyne NG, Brummelkamp WH, Bouma S, Mensch MH, Kamermans F, Stern Hanf M, van Alderen A. Life without blood. J Cardiovasc Surg. 1960;1:133–47.
8. Dejours P, Dejours S. The effects of barometric pressure according to Paul Bert: the question today. Int JSports Med. 1992;13:S1–5.
9. Hedley-Whyte J. Pulmonary oxygen toxicity: investigation and mentoring. Ulst Med J. 2008;77:39–42.
10. UHMS Position Statement: Low-Pressure Fabric Hyperbaric Chambers Title: Low-Pressure Fabric Hyperbaric Chambers. 2017. Available online: https://www.uhms.org/images/Position-Statements/UHMS_Position_Statement_LP_chambers_revised.pdf
11. Fife CE, Eckert KA, Carter MJ. An update on the appropriate role for hyperbaric oxygen: indications and evidence. Plast Reconstr Surg. 2016;138(3S):107S–116S. https://doi.org/10.1097/PRS.0000000000002714.
12. Thom SR. Hyperbaric oxygen: its mechanisms and efficacy. Plast Reconstr Surg. 2011;12:131S–141S. https://doi.org/10.1097/PRS.0b013e3181fbe2bf.
13. Ortega MA, Fraile-Martinez O, García-Montero C, Callejón-Peláez E, Sáez MA, Álvarez-Mon MA, García-Honduvilla N, Monserrat J, Álvarez-Mon M, Bujan J, et al. A general overview on the hyperbaric oxygen therapy: applications, mechanisms and translational opportunities. Medicina. 2021;57:864. https://doi.org/10.3390/medicina57090864.
14. Centers for Medicare & Medicaid Services. Manual section number 20.29: hyperbaric oxygen therapy. In: Medicare National Coverage Determinations Manual. Version Number 3. US Department of Health and Human Services; 2006.
15. Gesell LB, editor. Hyperbaric oxygen therapy indications. 12th ed. Durham: Undersea and Hyperbaric MedicalSociety; 2008. p. 7–196.
16. Fife CE, Eckert KA, Workman WT. Ethical issues, standards and quality control in practice of hyperbaric medicine. In: Jain KK, editor. Textbook of hyperbaric medicine. 6th ed. New York: Springer; 2016.
17. DuBose KJ, Cooper JS. Hyperbaric Patient Selection. [Updated 2022 Aug 10]. In: StatPearls [Internet]. Treasure Island: StatPearls Publishing; 2023. Available from: https://www.ncbi.nlm.nih.gov/books/NBK499820/
18. Howell RS, Criscitelli T, Woods JS, Gillette BM, Gorenstein S. Hyperbaric oxygen therapy: indications, contraindications, and use at a tertiary care center: 1.3 www.aornjournal.org/content/cme. AORN J. 2018;107(4):442–53.
19. Plafki C, Peters P, Almeling M, Welslau W, Busch R. Complications and side effects of hyperbaric oxygen therapy. Aviat Space Environ Med. 2000;71:119–24.
20. Mueller PHJ, Tetzlaff K, Neubauer B, Mutzbauer TS. Pulmonary barotrauma during hyperbaric oxygen therapy: a case report. Undersea Hyperbaric Med. 1998;25(Suppl):34.
21. Marroni A, Uriani G, Longoni C. Pulmonary eftects. In: Oriani G, Marroni A, Wattel F, editors. Handbook on hyperbaric medicine. New York: Springer; 1996. p. 75–80.
22. Lyne AJ. Ocular effects of hyperbaric oxygen. Trans Ophthalmol Soc U K. 1978;98:66–8.

Chapter 21
The Effect of High Pressures on Human Body Physiology

Ahsina Jahan Lopa, Payel Bose, and Kazi Ismail Hossain

21.1 Introduction

High pressure is a concept not directly tackled by many physicians or physiologists. However, it is a condition that is found in many situations. This application is growing today as the increased interest in deep-sea exploration has opened up an increasing number of people exposing themselves to higher-than-normal atmospheric pressure conditions. Immersion in water results in additional pressure due to the weight of the water exerted via force on the diver. Because water is incompressible, there is an increase of 1 atm of pressure for every 33 feet of seawater (fsw)/10 meters seawater (msw), or 34 feet of freshwater (ffw)/10.3 meters freshwater (mfw). As salt water is denser than fresh water, when a diver is underwater, they are exposed to the weight of the water column above them and the weight of the atmosphere [1].

It should be noted that with the increasing high-pressure applications, the harmful, beneficial, and neutral effects of pressure are of growing interest to medical researchers. High pressure proceeds to affect the human body, a multi-system organism, by altering the body's circulatory, respiratory, and neural functions as well as having direct effects on cells and tissues.

A. J. Lopa (✉)
Department of ICU and Emergency, Brahmanbaria ICU Specialized Hospital, Brahmanberia, Bangladesh

P. Bose
Critical Care Medicine, Medica Superspecialty Hospital, Kolkata, West Bengal, India

K. I. Hossain
Department of ICU, National Institute of Neurosciences and Hospital, Dhaka, Bangladesh

A. G. D'Almeida, J. Hidalgo (eds.), *Evidence-Based Hyperbaric Medicine*,
https://doi.org/10.1007/978-3-032-06346-5_21

21.2 The Impact of High Pressures on the Respiratory System

21.2.1 Changes in Lung Function

The residual volume increases, and the vital capacity decreases. At pressures greater than 100 m of seawater, the vital capacity may decrease by as much as 50%. The increase in residual volume is probably due to closure of small airways and resultant absorption of the air they contain. Considerable difficulty in breathing results from a decreased flow rate. This is due to an increase in airway resistance and the viscous flow properties of air at high density. High airway closure pressures at the end of expiration result in air trapping, and ventilation/perfusion mismatch occurs in the lung. This may result in a fall in arterial PO_2. It has been shown that an inspiratory gas mixture at high density reduces diaphragmatic contractility. This may result in fatigue of the respiratory muscles. The most extreme case of inability to breathe at high pressure is a sudden and dramatic drop in the inspired gas mixture due to closure of a pressure-proof system. This simulates sudden decompression, and in patients with severe obstructive lung disease, it has been observed to cause pneumothorax [2].

21.2.2 Effects on Gas Exchange

Henry's law states that the amount of gas that will dissolve in a liquid at a given temperature is directly proportional to the partial pressure of the gas. In other words, as pressure goes up, so too does the volume of gas dissolved in liquids. Increased pressure, therefore, will lead to over-oxygenation of the blood with further increases causing more radical effects. In a healthy individual breathing air at 101 kPa, oxygen partial pressure in the alveoli is 14 kPa. If the partial pressure of oxygen increases to 20 kPa, such as when breathing oxygen from a cylinder, up to 3% of "extra" oxygen will dissolve in the blood. When breathing pure oxygen at 253 kPa in a hyperbaric chamber, oxygen partial pressure in the alveoli rises to 72 kPa, and 9% of "extra" oxygen is dissolved in blood. Within 30 minutes, this level of oxygen is toxic to the lungs. Ultrastructural changes include damage to the alveolar epithelium and capillary endothelium, with leakage of protein and red blood cells into the alveolar space [3, 4]. Fibrosis and edema further reduce gas exchange and function of the lungs simulated by breathing oxygen at 253 kPa for a period of weeks, which is comparable to that of a patient suffering from acute respiratory distress syndrome.

21.2.3 Pulmonary Barotrauma

Barotrauma is physical damage to body tissues caused by a difference in pressure between a gas space inside, or in contact with the body, and the surroundings. The initial injury is often due to overpressure; the gas in the space is at a higher pressure than the surroundings, and the resultant pressure difference causes the gas to diffuse into the surrounding tissues. On depressurization, the trapped gas will expand and can cause damage to the tissues, either by tearing them directly or by preventing the gas from diffusing out of the tissues, which will cause the gas to reform into bubbles on further decompression [4, 5]. When the transpulmonary pressures are more than 60–70 mmHg, it can lead to rupture of alveoli with their blood vessels, and the alveoli will then be flooded with blood and debris and will collapse. Air leak will occur according to the site of ruptured alveoli, either central to the mediastinum, causing pneumomediastinum or pneumoprecadium, or peripheral, causing surgical emphysema or pneumothorax [6].

21.2.4 Pulmonary Edema

Pulmonary edema is the movement of fluid out of the capillaries of the lung and into the lung's air spaces. This results in impaired gas exchange and may cause respiratory failure. It is caused by changes in Starling forces, damage to the capillary-alveolar membrane, and decreased lymphatic clearance of pulmonary edema. High-pressure pulmonary edema is a type of non-cardiogenic pulmonary edema that occurs as a result of an abrupt rise in pulmonary capillary pressure. This is mainly seen in self-contained underwater breathing apparatus (SCUBA) diving and is a result of the abnormal breathing patterns and stress associated with the equipment and the environment of the dive.

21.2.5 Effects of High Pressures on the Airways

A narrowing of the lower airways is the most likely of the many effects of high pressures to be clinically important. It can occur as the result of an increase in transmural pressure in the airways, which in itself can be due to raised pressure around the lung or to intrinsic narrowing of the airway wall. At relatively low inspiratory and expiratory positive pressures, there is good evidence to show that the small collapsible airways will tend to close, with a fall in lung volume. This is not a purely physical phenomenon because closure is more likely to occur in asthmatic subjects than in normal subjects at the same level of airways pressure [7]. Measurements obtained during continuous breathing of a gas mixture at a known inspired pressure show the change in lung volume and the associated partial expiratory flow—both on inspiration and on expiration. An increase in airway resistance increases the work of breathing, leading to mechanical fatigue and a decrease in alveolar ventilation. An increase in airway resistance may also cause or exacerbate respiratory failure. The effects of increased airway resistance on breathing and gas exchange make this the most important potential problem arising from high-pressure ventilation [8, 9].

21.3 Influence of High Pressures on the Nervous System

High-pressure nervous syndrome or high-pressure neurological syndrome (HPNS) [10] is characterized by neurological, psychological, and electroencephalographic (EEG) abnormalities during dives deeper than 150 meters with breathing helium-oxygen gas mixtures. Its signs and symptoms depend on both speed of compression and hydrostatic pressure, the faster the compression rate and the higher the pressure, the more severe the clinical presentation will be, the etiology of HPNS is still vague to some extent, but it could be explained by the compression effect of pressure, possibly in the lipid component of cell membranes of the central nervous system (CNS), which may also effect the molecular processes related to volume expansion. The main characteristics of HPNS are hyperexcitability of the CNS that involves neurological and psychological abnormalities, showing changes in EEG recordings. HPNS should be differentiated from other neurological symptoms which could be also related to deep diving as nitrogen narcosis, decompression sickness, and oxygen toxicity.

21.3.1 Tremors

Tremors are considered the most characteristic symptom of HPNS, which occurs at both rest and on movement. Tremors begin at the distal extremities and may spread to the whole body. The frequency of tremors is 8–12 Hz. The amplitude increases with faster compression speed and increasing hydrostatic pressure, and spontaneous constant eye oscillations in random directions(Opsoclonus) are one of the earliest signs of HPNS.

21.3.2 EEG Changes

ECG recordings of patients with HPNS were evaluated in several studies. This showed an increase in theta activity and a decrease in alpha waves in the EEG records of divers who suffered from HPNS. Authors like Rostain et al. reported a decrease in alpha frequencies from about 100 meters and an increase in theta frequencies in the frontal area at about 200 meters during a dive to 450 meters of seawater with the helium–nitrogen–oxygen gas mixture. Sleep EEG also displays specific alterations at high pressure, characterized by an increase in stages I and II, a decrease in the duration of stages III and IV, and a reduction of rapid eye movement (REM) periods.

21.3.3 Nitrogen Narcosis

Nitrogen narcosis [11] can be defined as changes in consciousness and neuromuscular functions which is caused by breathing compressed inert gas as breathing compressed air. While at atmospheric pressures greater than 1 ATM, the partial pressures of nitrogen increase, the severity of nitrogen narcosis varies according to individual sensitivity. At 100–150 fsw (30–45 msw), most divers will become lightheaded and euphoric with loss of fine discrimination, while deeper than 150 fsw (45 Msw), the symptoms progress to joviality and dizziness with uncontrolled laughter, loss of concentration, and mistakes in simple, practical, and mental tasks. Additional symptoms and signs include peripheral numbness and tingling and poor attention to personal safety. At 300 fsw (90 msw), mental depression and impaired neuromuscular coordination occur. At 350 fsw (105 msw), many divers lose consciousness. Severe narcosis may result in amnesia lasting for several hours.

21.4 High-Pressure Effects on the Cardiovascular System

One of the most serious effects of prolonged high pressures that divers are exposed to is the effect of the significant alterations of the autonomic nervous system (ANS). During descent, the hydrostatic pressure of the surrounding water balances the hydrostatic pressure within the systemic circulation and shifts the blood from the lower part of the body to the central circulation. This leads to an increase in the thoracic blood volume and alternation of ANS activity, further contributing to bradycardia, increased stroke volume and cardiac output, reduced muscle sympathetic nerve activity and systemic vascular resistance, and unaltered blood pressure [12].

21.4.1 *Impacts on Heart Function*

The physiological effects of pressure and the resulting changes in health status alter the body's circulatory system. The primary result of pressure on the circulatory system is a direct effect on the baroreceptors. A study by Marabotti et al. (2013) [13] using Doppler echocardiography showed left ventricular dilatation and diastolic impairment in SCUBA diving humans. Another study by Mariusz et al. 2018 [14] in a hyperbaric chamber to isolate the effect of high pressure from other effects as temperature found that there were significant reductions in heart rate and cardiac index with a parallel increase in total peripheral resistance after hyperbaric exposure. In addition, the left ventricle work index parameter significantly changed with reductions in left ventricular work index and ejection rate and increases in left ventricular ejection time.

21.5 High-Pressure Effects on the Musculoskeletal System

21.5.1 *Changes in Bone Density and Structure*

High pressures have an effect on human bone, but relevant information is limited to the response of bone to decreased density in space or immersion modeling in perfluorocarbons. No human high-pressure studies show alteration in bone density, nor are there any reported histological changes in bone for divers or caisson workers. Thus, it would seem that low pressure, rather than high, is the critical factor. Nevertheless, it has been suggested that aseptic bone necrosis reported in caisson workers at the turn of the century was due to nitrogen undersaturation and consequent microembolism formation when returning to ambient pressure [4, 5]. This is a speculative hypothesis, and there is no experimental evidence to support an increase in susceptibility of bone to "bend pressure" and microembolism formation at high partial pressures of gases, which cause alterations in bone tissue [15]. Considering the lack of hard information, it is important that further research is performed into the effects of high pressure on bone.

21.5.2 *Muscle Function and Strength*

Muscle function and strength can be affected by high pressure and also by pressure changes. This is a result of the incompressible nature of water, which makes the total pressure within living tissues at any depth the sum of the pressure due to the water and that due to the atmosphere.

21.5.3 *Joint Health and Mobility*

Cartilage, the material that provides a low-friction joint system, is damaged by degassing. This causes nitrogen bubbles to form in the joints in the same manner as decompression sickness. This causes great pain and inhibits movement. In rapid decompression incidents such as explosive decompression, decompression sickness and nitrogen embolism can be caused [5]. These can cause long-term damage and pain in joints.

21.6 Impact of High Pressures on the Digestive System

21.6.1 *Gastrointestinal Disturbances*

The most consistent effect of gases at pressure is distension of the bowel caused by the increased volume of gas. Gastrointestinal barotrauma is caused by the augmented volume of the gas stored in the gastrointestinal tract [3, 4]. During the ascent phase, gas expansion can result in symptoms such as cramping, pain, distention, and bloating. Modulation of food and liquid ingestion before diving is needed to avoid these effects.

21.6.2 *Nutrient Absorption and Metabolism*

At physiological pressures, around sea level, the nutrients ingested are absorbed and metabolized normally, but this is not the case when exposed to high pressures. The absorption and metabolism of nutrients take place in various parts of the gastrointestinal system. These nutrients are then transported to tissues and organs for metabolism and use for energy. High pressures have a profound effect on the solubility of gases in liquids, and nutrient transport is therefore greatly affected. It is known that the greater the pressure, the more soluble a gas is in a liquid. Energy transformations and use are affected by pressure in the overall metabolism of nutrients.

21.6.3 *Effects on the Liver and Pancreas*

Under physiological conditions, the liver receives approximately 25% of the cardiac output. Over 70% of this blood comes from the portal vein. In decompression sickness, the liver may be damaged as it is a common site for bubble formation. In an acute setting, severe damage may be sustained via obstruction of the proximal hepatic venules by gas emboli [15]. This causes ischemia in centrilobular areas, inflammatory cell infiltration, Kupffer cell activation, and damage to endothelial cells. Sublethal injury has been characterized by delayed erythrophagocytosis and prolonged catabolism of damaged erythrocytes, usually associated with hemolysis.

21.7 High-Pressure Effects on the Renal System

21.7.1 Kidney Function and Fluid Balance

The effect of pressure on the renal function and the resulting fluid retention is of major concern in underwater diving. Prolonged exposure of human divers to the hyperbaric environment leads to an increase in urine flow, which is greater during the compression phase as compared to the subsequent steady-state hyperbaric phase [16]. Early diuresis is often accompanied by a greater increase in excretion of osmotic substances and mild dehydration. Typically, this hyperbaric diuresis is isolated from any increase in glomerular filtration rate or daily fluid intake. The early hyperbaric diuresis could be triggered by the central pooling of blood, induced by breathing a denser gas, which increases the intrathoracic negative pressure during inspiration. During the early hyperbaric exposure leading to increased intrathoracic blood volume and inhibition of the antidiuretic hormone ADH system via the Gauer-Henry reflex, this initial hyperbaric diuresis results in activation of the plasma renin–angiotensin system during the steady-state hyperbaric phase. A study by Nakayama et al. [17] (1981) observed an increase in overnight urine flow in divers exposed to pressure exceeding 25 AT.

21.7.2 Electrolyte Imbalances

An increase in urine flow is often accompanied by increased excretion of osmotic substances such as Na, K, and inorganic phosphate. The rise in K excretion is due to facilitation of K secretion at the distal tubule as a result of increased aldosterone. The increase in Na excretion in the face of enhanced aldosterone secretion indicates that the Na transport in the proximal tubule is markedly inhibited (by an unknown mechanism). The phosphate excretion increases with no changes in plasma level of parathyroid hormone; thus, it may be due to an inhibition of Na phosphate cotransport in the proximal tubule. Ca increased excretion occurs secondary to the inhibition of Na transport at the proximal tubule [18].

21.8 The Influence of High Pressures on the Reproductive System

21.8.1 Fertility and Reproductive Hormones

Hyperbaric air pressure exposure has long been suggested to lower fertility rates or to cause decreased gonadal function [19]. High environmental pressures or clinical hyperbaric therapy have been associated with decreased fertility and an increased incidence of embryonic resorption in animal and human studies. Early reports by Buchanan and co-workers indicated that hyperbaric oxygen in increased environmental pressures acutely lowered plasma luteinizing hormone (LH) and follicle-stimulating hormone (FSH) levels in men while decreasing testosterone and ePiandrosterone excretion rates. LH and FSH levels remained low during the exposures, with transient testicular failure occurring in some of the subjects. Recovery to baseline hormone levels occurred after return to atmospheric pressure. These results were not confirmed by Pilmanis in a sea-level chamber study of men exposed to 3.7 ATA. A single 10-hour exposure was reported to have no effect on plasma testosterone levels, with significant increases noted for LH and FSH. Duration of exposure studies in man is also limited in scope, and none have assessed human fertility.

21.8.2 Pregnancy and High-Pressure Environments

The effects of raised atmospheric pressure on the health of pregnant women and their unborn children are matters of great concern [20], particularly since the use of SCUBA by women has become relatively common. While much of the available information pertains to diving at or near the sea surface, there are serious implications here for those living in high-pressure habitats, such as caisson workers or compression chamber attendants. Recommendations for pregnant women to avoid even moderate altitudes during the latter part of pregnancy add further impetus to a better definition of the maternal and fetal responses to hyperbaric conditions. Unfortunately, there is disagreement on some crucial issues, much of the available evidence is anecdotal, and experimentation in this group is clearly impractical. Several investigators have reported an increased risk of premature delivery or fetal distress in pregnancies occurring in or after high-altitude residence. However, many such reports come from geographical areas, such as the Andes or Himalayas, where malnutrition and infectious diseases are common, and such adverse influences could not be excluded. Experimental altitude studies on animals have shown conclusively that fetal growth is impaired by a reduction in maternal inspired oxygen tension.

The relations of hyperbaric exposure to this phenomenon are complex, but it has been suggested that in the early phase, the increased uterine blood flow caused by the vasodilator effect of inert gases might enhance the diffusion of oxygen from mother to fetus. Later, the direct splitting of inert gas molecules might decrease the oxygen tension in maternal blood and placental vessels, since this tension is a function of the partial pressure of other gases. Further research in this area is required.

21.9 Conclusion

High-pressure environments exert profound effects on human physiology, primarily through increased gas solubility and pressure-induced changes in bodily functions. Careful planning, proper training, and adherence to safety protocols are essential to prevent pressure-related injuries and ensure health and performance in high-pressure conditions.

References

1. Jones MW, Brett K, Han N, Cooper JS, Wyatt HA. Hyperbaric physics. In: StatPearls [Internet]. Treasure Island: StatPearls Publishing; 2024. PMID: 28846268.
2. Moon RE, Cherry AD, Stolp BW, Camporesi EM. Pulmonary gas exchange in diving. J Appl Physiol. 2008:91104.
3. Bosco G, Rizzato A, Moon RE, Camporesi EM. Environmental physiology and diving medicine. Front Psychol. 2018;9:319531.
4. Pendergast D, Moon R, Krasney J, Held H, Zamparo P. Human physiology in an aquatic environment. Compr Physiol. 2015;5:1705–50.
5. Vorosmarti J, Richard D, Vann PH. Chapter 30: Physics, physiology, and medicine of diving, medical aspects of harsh environments. In: Medical Aspects of Harsh Environments, vol. 2. Medical aspects of harsh environments textbooks of military medicine. United States Army; 2001.
6. Dugrenot E, Balestra C, Gouin E, et al. Physiological effects of mixed-gas deep sea dives using a closed-circuit rebreather: a field pilot study. Eur J Appl Physiol. 2021;121:3323–31.
7. Kennedy-Little D, Sharman T. Pulmonary Barotrauma. [Updated 2023 Jun 26]. In: StatPearls [Internet]. Treasure Island: StatPearls Publishing; 2024.
8. M Bennett AM, Cibis T. The underwater world and diving physiology. In: Engineering and medicine in extreme environments. Springer; 2022.
9. Bosco G, Rizzato A, Moon RE, Camporesi EM. Environmental physiology and diving medicine. Fron. Psychol. 2018;9:72.
10. Ozgok Kangal MK, Murphy-Lavoie HM. High pressure diving nervous syndrome. [Updated 2022 Oct 13]. In: StatPearls [Internet].
11. Kirkland PJ, Mathew D, Modi P, et al. Nitrogen narcosis in diving. [Updated 2023 Jul 31]. In: StatPearls [Internet]. Treasure Island: StatPearls Publishing; 2024.
12. Jain KK. Effects of diving and high pressure on the human body. In: Textbook of hyperbaric medicine. Cham: Springer; 2017.

13. Marabotti C, Scalzini A, Menicucci D, Passera M, Bedini R, L'Abbate A. Cardiovascular changes during SCUBA diving: an underwater Doppler echocardiographic study. Acta Physiol. 2013;209(1):62–8.
14. Kozakiewicz M, Slomko J, Buszko K, Sinkiewicz W, Klawe JJ, Tafil-Klawe M, Newton JL, Zalewski P. Acute biochemical, cardiovascular, and autonomic response to hyperbaric (4 atm) exposure in healthy subjects. Evid-Based Complement Alternat Med. 2018;2018:5913176, 8 pages.
15. Lee YI, Ye BJ. Underwater and hyperbaric medicine as a branch of occupational and environmental medicine. Ann Occup Environ Med. 2013;25:39.
16. Park YS, Claybaugh JR, Shiraki K, Mohri M. Renal function in hyperbaric environment. Appl Hum Sci. 1998;17(1):1–8.
17. Nakayama H, Hong SK, Claybaugh JR, Matsui N, Park YS, Ohta Y, Shiraki K, Matsuda M. Energy and body fluid balance during a 14-day dry Saturation dive at 31 ATA (Seadragon IV). In: Bachrach AJ, Matzen MM, editors. Underwater Physiology VII: Proceedings of the Seventh Symposium on Underwater Physiology. Bethesda: Undersea Medical Society; 1981. p. 541–54.
18. Hong SK, Claybaugh JR. Hormonal and renal responses to hyperbaria. In: Claybaugh JR, Wade CE, editors. Hormonal regulation of fluid and electrolytes. Boston: Springer; 1989.
19. Irgens A, Groning M, Irgens LM. Pregnancy outcomes in partners of male professional divers in Norway. Occup Med. 2016;66:600–6. https://doi.org/10.1093/occmed/kqw087.
20. Camporesi EM. Diving and pregnancy. Semin Perinatol. 1996;20(4):292–302. https://doi.org/10.1016/s0146-0005(96)80022-x. PMID: 8888455.

Chapter 22
Hyperbaric Oxygen Therapy: Role of Pressure

Ahsan Ahmed, Shreyans Agrawal, and Chayan Bhattacharya

22.1 Introduction

The pressure mechanism behind hyperbaric oxygen therapy (HBOT) lies well within the boundaries of the ideal gas laws. The Boyles law (p1v1 = p2v2) is seen to have direct correlation to HBOT, especially in relation to decompression sickness (DCS), where as the pressure elevates, the volume of the air bubble decreases substantially. The Charles law (p1v1/t1 = p2v2/t2) establishes a direct relation between the pressure, volume, and temperature of the system. This becomes extremely important to note that the temperature of the system is intended to increase when the vessel or the system is pressurized; this becomes a special concern when dealing with extremely sick patients and the pediatric population. Apart from the above two laws that compare the pressure, volume, and temperature relations, another law that affects the hyperbaric physiology is Henry's law which states that the amount of gas dissolved in a liquid is equal to the partial pressure of the gas exerted on the surface of the liquid; the clinical importance of the phenomenon lies in the fact that more oxygen can be dissolved within plasma when we increase the atmospheric pressure.

A. Ahmed (✉)
Department of Anesthesiology, KPC Medical College and Hospital, Kolkata, West Bengal, India

S. Agrawal
Intensive Care Unit, KPC Medical College and Hospital, Kolkata, West Bengal, India

C. Bhattacharya
Department of Anaesthesia & Critical Care, In-charge Critical Care Unit, B R Singh Hospital, Eastern Railway, Kolkata, India

A. G. D'Almeida, J. Hidalgo (eds.), *Evidence-Based Hyperbaric Medicine*, https://doi.org/10.1007/978-3-032-06346-5_22

22.2 Properties with Clinical Applications

Hyper-oxygenation of plasma	DCS , carbon monoxide poisoning, central retinal artery occlusion, compartment syndrome.
Boyle's law (p1v1 = p2v2)	Air embolism, gas embolism
Angiogenesis	Wound healing, poor graft/flap healing
Fibroblast synthesis	Delayed wound healing
Increase antibiotic synergy	Necrotizing soft tissue infection, refractory osteomyelitis

Breathing of 100% oxygen under elevated atmospheric pressure is the science behind HBOT. This form of treatment dates back to more than six centuries. When a patient is given 100% oxygen under increased atmospheric pressure, oxygen first dissolves in hemoglobin, saturating it completely, and then the blood becomes over-oxygenated when this oxygen starts to dissolve in plasma. HBOT has been known to treat various pathologies, including non-healing wounds, diving-associated injuries, and carbon-monoxide poisoning, as an adjuvant therapy for critical care patients under mechanical ventilation, to name a few. Recent studies have shown to expand the indication for HBOT, which include hypoxic brain injuries, inflammatory bowel diseases like ulcerative colitis, and Crohn's disease. It has also shown some promising trials toward moderate and severe COVID-19 pneumonitis. The effect of high pressure on 100% oxygen, as mentioned, touches various modalities; a few of them have been elaborated below.

DCS DCS occurs commonly after scuba diving, exposure to increased/decreased atmospheric pressures. When atmospheric pressure decreases rapidly, inert gases dissolved in blood form bubbles and cause mechanical blocks in blood vessels, which is followed by endovascular damage and activation of inflammatory responses, which further damage the vasculature. The bubbles formed in DCS are mainly formed of nitrogen. When a person is exposed to HBOT, the "oxygen-rich" blood is known to create a gradient between the bubble and the blood, causing the gas to come out and dissolve in the bloodstream, which ultimately causes a decrement in the bubble size, relieving the mechanical obstruction and re-establishing perfusion [1–3].

Carbon monoxide (CO) poisoning CO has 300 times greater affinity for Hb as compared to oxygen. When a person undergoes poisoning with the gas, he may experience headache, nausea, visual disturbances, seizures, loss of consciousness, and electrolyte abnormalities. CO takes close to 300 minutes to get replaced by oxygen at room air and around 90 minutes when treated with 100%oxygen. However, with HBOT, it takes just 32 minutes for the CO to be replaced with oxygen competitively. Apart from this, HBOT is also known to restore cytochrome oxidase aa3/c, which prevents lipid peroxidation [4, 5].

Non-healing wounds Non-healing wounds usually undergo ischemic damages due to the creation of a hypoxic environment within the tissue. HBOT has been known to have a multifactorial mechanism for wound healing, which includes angiogenesis and stimulation of fibroblasts and collagens, which are the mediators of healing. The patients are generally exposed to 2–2.4 atm of pressure with 100% oxygen for a repetitive period, depending on the response of the wound. HBOT also has a role in increasing penetration of several classes of antibiotics, creating a toxic environment for anaerobic bacteria, which are major colonizers of these wounds [6, 7].

Severe crush injuries Crush injuries are generally associated with very poor outcomes. HBOT has been known to cause hyper-oxygenation by increasing the solubility of oxygen in plasma. However, it also reduces the blood flow at the target, providing extra time for the capillaries to reabsorb excess fluid, thus decreasing edema. Another proposed mechanism for the same is that HBOT generates free radical scavengers. HBOT is also used as an adjuvant therapy in compartment syndrome. It is indicated in the symptomatic stage of compartment syndrome when features of pain and parasthesia start to set in. HBOT is also indicated post-fasciotomy to decrease morbidity [8, 9].

Refractory osteomyelitis Refractory osteomyelitis cases are known to cause complications such as non-healing wounds and formation of sinus tracts and may require aggressive modalities of treatment such as amputations and disarticulation. HBOT is shown to have a positive impact on osteoclasts' functioning, which is an oxygen-dependent process [10]. Neovascularization and increasing penetration of antibiotics are additional reasons for HBOT being evolved as a modern method of treatment for refractory cases of osteomyelitis [11].

Central retinal artery occlusion (CRAO) CRAO is a notorious cause of permanent vision loss, which presents as sudden painless loss of vision. CRAO is the most recently approved indication by the Undersea and Hyperbaric Medicine Society for HBOT [12, 13]. A recent study by Hertzog et al. [14] on a population with CRAO who were given HBOT at different time intervals has shown some success when it was given within the initial 8 hours of diminishment of vision. HBOT still sits in a gray zone as a treatment option for CRAO and requires further trials for establishment.

Acute anemia The indigenous transporter of oxygen for our human body is hemoglobin, which transports around 1.3 ml of oxygen per gram. When anemia occurs due to acute blood loss, hemoglobin falls sharply, leading to decreased oxygen transport to tissues. HBOT instantly increases dissolved oxygen in plasma and may improve tissue oxygen delivery temporarily [15]. An experiment performed in the 1960s by Borema concluded that pigs that had only plasma in their circulation were blue to sustain life under hyperbaric conditions [16]. This method can be indicative in patients who are waiting for blood product transfusion or are going into multiorgan failure acutely.

Sudden sensorineural hearing loss A review by Cochran et al. [17] concludes significant improvement in patients of sudden sensorineural hearing loss with HBOT. The proposed mechanism suggests an increased partial pressure of oxygen within the internal ear that causes betterment of the symptoms.

22.3 Newer indications for HBOT

Bisphosphonate-associated osteonecrosis Bisphosphonates are being used as first-line drugs for osteoporosis, Paget's disease, bone metastasis, and so on. The exact mechanism of osteonecrosis due to bisphosphonates is, however, unknown. Currently, there is no reliable treatment modality for this complication of bisphosphonates. Several trials involving HBOT are underway [18].

Ulcerative colitis and Crohn's disease Inflammatory bowel diseases have been a topic of concern for time immemorial, which are caused due to chronic inflammation and hypoxia. There are several treatment modalities involving corticosteroids, azathioprine, and other immunomodulatory agents. However, they do not work for everyone. HBOT has shown effects by its oxygenation improving potential and anti-inflammatory effects, which might be considered a treatment modality in the future [19, 20].

Traumatic brain injury Currently, there is no effective treatment modality for traumatic brain injury, leading patients with irreversible cognitive and behavioral impairment. For a long time, HBOT has been seen as a treatment option for traumatic brain injuries due to increased oxygenation, decrease in intra-cranial pressure, and promotion of neurogenesis and angiogenesis. There have been several cases reported concluding an improvement in cognition and sleep post HBOT [21].

SARS COVID-19 The COVID-19 pandemic caused by SARS COVID-19 virus engulfed the whole world and opened to windows to several new and old treatment modalities, and the symptoms ranged from asymptomatic to multiorgan failure and death. The exact mechanism of action is still not known. HBOT has been used off label as a treatment option for COVID-19-associated pneumonia associated with refractory hypoxia. The current treatment by HBOT is controversial but promising [22].

22.4 Complications of HBOT

Just like all other treatment modalities, HBOT has its own set of complications due to increased pressure effect. The most evident effect that needs to be illustrated is barotrauma (injury caused by unequalization of pressure within the system to the surrounding pressure). Middle ear dysfunction is the most common complication following HBOT, which may present acutely or after a few days [23]. Common symptoms include a decrease in hearing capacity, tinnitus, ear fullness, and ear pain. A blowout of the round or oval window may occur acutely, leading to immediate deafness, vertigo, and nystagmus. Sinus dysfunction may also be precipitated in the form of bleeding and pain. Chronic complications include dry cough, chest pain, and decreased vital capacity.

HBOT is also known to alter the morphology of our eye lens, leading to complications like progressive myopia, which generally resolves on its own. HBOT is also known to cause a decrease in seizure threshold, thus precipitating seizures in 0.7/10,000 population. The cause is thought to be due to oxygen toxicity. The patients should hence be removed from the oxygen source and be started on HBOT with less oxygen.

References

1. Brubakk A, Neuman T. Bennett and Elliott's physiology and medicine of diving. 5th ed. Great Britain: Elsevier Science Limited; 2003.
2. Navy Department. Diving Medicine and Recompression Chamber Operations. US Navy Diving Manual. Rev 4. Washington, DC: 1999. p. 5.
3. Spencer MP. Decompression limits for compressed air determined by ultrasonically detected blood bubbles. J Appl Physiol. 1976;40(2):229–35.
4. Brown SD, Piantadosi CA. Recovery of energy metabolism in rat brain after carbon monoxide hypoxia. J Clin Invest. 1992;89(2):666–72.
5. Feldmeier J. Hyperbaric Oxygen 2003: Indications and results- the Hyperbaric oxygen therapy committee report. Kensington: Undersea and Hyperbaric Medical Society.
6. Park MK, Myers RA, Marzella L. Oxygen tensions and infections: modulation of microbial growth, activity of antimicrobial agents, and immunologic responses. Clin Infect Dis. 1992;14(3):720–40.
7. Mader JT, Brown GL, Guckian JC, et al. A mechanism for the amelioration by hyperbaric oxygen of experimental staphylococcal osteomyelitis in rabbits. Infect Dis Clin N Am. 1990;4(3):433–40.
8. Skyhar MJ, Hargens AR, Strauss MB, et al. Hyperbaric oxygen reduces edema and necrosis of skeletal muscle in compartment syndromes associated with hemorrhagic hypotension. J Bone Joint Surg Am. 1986;68(8):1218–24.
9. Schraibman IG, Ledingham IM. Hyperbaric oxygen and local vasodilatation in peripheral vascular disease. Br J Surg. 1969;56(4):295–9.
10. Strauss MB, Malluche HH, Faugere MC. Effect of hyperbaric oxygen on bone resorption in rabbits. Seventh Annual Conference on Clinical Application of HBO. June 1982. Anaheim.
11. Mader JT, Brown GL, Guckian JC, et al. A mechanism for the amelioration by hyperbaric oxygen of experimental staphylococcal osteomyelitis in rabbits. J Infect Dis. 1980;142:915.

12. Rumelt S, Brown GC. Update on treatment of retinal arterial occlusions. Curr Opin Ophthalmol. 2003;14(3):139–41.
13. Canan H, Ulas B, Altan-Yaycioglu R. Hyperbaric oxygen therapy in combination with systemic treatment of sickle cell disease presenting as central retinal artery occlusion: a case report. J Med Case Rep. 2014;8(1):370.
14. Hertzog LM, Meyer GW, Carson S, et al. Central retinal artery occlusion treated with hyperbaric oxygen. J Hyperb Med. 1992;7:33–42.
15. Feldmeier J. Hyperbaric oxygen 2003: indications and results- the Hyperbaric oxygen therapy committee report. Kensington: Undersea and Hyperbaric Medical Society, Inc.; 2003.
16. Boerema I, et al. Life without blood. A study of the influence of high atmospheric pressure and hypothermia on dilution of the blood. J Cardiovasc Surg. 1960;19:133–46.
17. Bennett MH, Kertesz T, Perleth M, Yeung P, Lehm JP. Hyperbaric oxygen for idiopathic sudden sensorineural hearing loss and tinnitus. Cochrane Database Syst Rev. 2012;10:CD004739.
18. Al Hadi H, Smerdon GR, Fox SW. Hyperbaric oxygen therapy accelerates osteoblast differentiation and promotes bone formation. J Dent. 2014:382.
19. Dulai PS, Gleeson MW, Taylor D, Holubar SD, Buckey JC, Siegel CA. Systematic review: The safety and efficacy of hyperbaric oxygen therapy for inflammatory bowel disease. Aliment Pharmacol Ther. 2014;39(11):1266–75.
20. Bekheit M, Baddour N, Katri K, Taher Y, El Tobgy K, Mousa E. Hyperbaric oxygen therapy stimulates colonic stem cells and induces mucosal healing in patients with refractory ulcerative colitis: a prospective case series. BMJ Open Gastroenterol. 2016;3(1):e000082. https://doi.org/10.1136/bmjgast-2016-000082. PMID: 27195128; PMCID: PMC4860723.
21. https://www.uhms.org/resources/news-announcements/739-tbi-progress-report-a-new-paper-on-hyperbaric-oxygen-therapy-for-traumatic-brain-injury-has-beenpublished.
22. Paganini M, Bosco G, Perozzo FAG, Kohlscheen E, Sonda R, Bassetto F, et al. The role of hyperbaric oxygen treatment for COVID-19: a review. Adv Exp Med Biol. 2020.
23. McMonnies CW. Hyperbaric oxygen therapy and the possibility of ocular complications or contraindications. Clin Exp Optom. 2015;98(2):122–5.

Chapter 23
Complications of Hyperbaric Oxygen Therapy: Oxygen Toxicity

Ahsina Jahan Lopa and Payel Bose

23.1 Introduction

Oxygen is a vital but potent biochemical, and as such, it can be toxic depending on dose and exposure duration [1].

Hyperoxia describes any situation when cells, tissues, or organs are exposed to oxygen at a higher than normal partial pressure. There is no accepted clinical definition of hyperoxia or indeed normoxia. Hyperoxia can be defined as an arterial PO_2 value greater than the normal for that patient's age when breathing air. Hyperoxia may be "normobaric" when breathing a high inspired concentration at one atmosphere absolute pressure or "hyperbaric" when breathing at high atmospheric pressure. In the latter situation, inspired oxygen concentration may be normal (0.21) or lower but still result in hyperoxia.

In practice, hyperventilation of breathing air can raise arterial PO_2 to a maximum of around 16 kPa, but further increase can only be achieved by increasing the inspired oxygen concentration, increasing the ambient pressure, or both [2].

Hyperoxia could also describe a higher-than-normal blood oxygen content, for example, in a patient with polycythemia and a normal PaO_2, but most clinicians reserve the term for situations where PaO_2 is increased [3].

Hyperbaric oxygen therapy (HBOT), which utilizes both high pressure and high concentrations of oxygen, in multiple daily sessions per patient, has the potential to induce pulmonary oxygen toxicity (POT).

Physiological effects of hyperoxia include inhibition of hypoxic pulmonary vasoconstriction, promotion of atelectasis, and systemic vasoconstriction.

A. J. Lopa (✉)
Department of ICU and Emergency, Brahmanbaria ICU Specialized Hospital, Brahmanbaria, Bangladesh

P. Bose
Critical Care Medicine, Medica Superspecialty Hospital, Kolkata, West Bengal, India

A. G. D'Almeida, J. Hidalgo (eds.), *Evidence-Based Hyperbaric Medicine*,
https://doi.org/10.1007/978-3-032-06346-5_23

Adverse clinical effects of hyperoxia occur, including increased mortality, in intensive care, acute medicine, and perioperative medicine.

23.2 Pathophysiology of Oxygen Toxicity

Oxygen metabolism generates harmful reactive oxygen species (ROS), which are countered in all cells by ubiquitous antioxidant enzymes and molecules.

23.2.1 Reactive Oxygen Species

During cellular metabolism, elemental oxygen is reduced to water by the transport of electrons along a chain of enzymes in the mitochondria. As a result, hydrogen ions (protons) are also forced to move along the chain and across the mitochondrial membrane against their concentration gradient. This process, called chemiosmosis, involves electron donor molecules generated from the citric acid cycle, modifying the electrical charge of the mitochondrial enzymes until this forces the positively charged protons across the mitochondrial membrane. At the end of the mitochondrial chain, the protons reach a high enough energy level to combine with

molecular oxygen, and this results in the production of adenosine triphosphate. Not only high-energy electrons and hydrogen ions form water, but also a variety of other molecules are being generated with "leakage" from the enzyme chain, and these are collectively referred to as ROS. ROS were previously known as oxygen free radicals, being so named as they have one or more unpaired electrons, and are therefore "free" to interact with surrounding molecules, making them unstable and highly reactive.

The two most abundant ROS are the superoxide anion (O_2 produced by the reduction of molecular oxygen without the addition of any hydrogen ions) and hydrogen peroxide (H_2O_2), formed by the reduction of the superoxide anion.

Although the superoxide anion and hydrogen peroxide themselves have direct toxic effects, their interactions produce even more damaging ROS molecules. The Fenton or Habere–Weiss reaction results in the formation of two extremely reactive species, the hydroxyl radical (OH-) and singlet oxygen ($1O_2$, a high-energy, short-lived form of oxygen in which all electrons are paired), alongside the harmless hydroxyl ion.

The interaction between superoxide anion and hydrogen peroxide is the source of much of the oxygen-related damage to biological systems, because of continuously produced, toxic hydroxyl radicals. The hydroxyl radical is extremely unstable, immediately reacting with any molecule nearby, removing its electrons and thus generating a chain reaction for further ROS formation.

In all cells, a balance exists between oxidant and antioxidant molecular activity, which is highly regulated to ensure proper function. The development of defenses against hyperoxic damage is a central theme of animal evolution [4]. This balance between the detrimental effects of the ROS and the antioxidants that counter them is known as the redox state of the cell. Aside from their beneficial roles in the regulation of phagocytes and possibly in the killing of microorganisms, most effects of ROS are harmful.

ROS exert harmful effects on biological structures by multiple mechanisms. Examples are damaging DNA or RNA, impairing DNA repair systems, affecting transcription, or by lipid peroxidation, the last of which directly damages cell membrane structure. They may also interfere with protein function by direct oxidation of amino acids or oxidative deactivation of enzymes.

Hyperoxia will increase ROS formation, therefore overwhelming the antioxidant mechanisms' capacity, tipping the balance toward cellular oxidative stress, with the potential for tissue damage. Exposure time and PO_2 ultimately determine the cumulative oxygen "dose."

HBO is a relatively safe treatment but carries some risks. Possible complications include barotraumatic lesions, oxygen toxicity, confinement anxiety, and ocular effects. Oxygen toxicity can have effects on the central nervous system (CNS) (Paul Bert effect) and lungs (Lorraine Smith effect).

23.2.2 *HBOT and POT*

POT related to the high partial pressure of O_2 in the alveoli may impair respiratory function. Although the mechanisms of POT (also called the Lorrain Smith effect) [5] remain unclear, the increased production of reactive O_2 species during hyperoxic exposure presents a potential source of damage to lung parenchyma [6, 7]. Clinically, POT presents as tracheobronchiolitis, causing coughing, pleuritic chest pain, and dyspnea [8].

Clinical diagnosis is challenging due to a lack of unique objective findings: oftentimes, the only identifiable change in pulmonary function is a highly variable decrease in vital capacity (VC) [9, 10]. Other measures of pulmonary function, such as forced mid-expiratory flow and diffusion capacity, have been proposed as more sensitive markers of HBOT damage; however, none of these are highly specific [11].

An increase in local oxygen supply due to an increased gradient for diffusion is achieved by increasing the partial pressure of oxygen (PO_2) in inspired gas. This results in local stimulation of fibroblast proliferation and collagen synthesis, angiogenesis, and enhanced granulocyte function and peroxidase activity in ischemic tissue. There are two discrete phases of acute POT based on pathology of the lower respiratory tract: an acute, exudative phase characterized by reversible capillary endothelial cell damage, parenchymal edema, and the infiltration of inflammatory cells [12], and a subacute, proliferative phase in which type II pneumocytes and fibroblasts multiply and cause irreversible derangement of the lung architecture, including marked thickening of the blood–air barrier and pulmonary fibrosis with impaired gas exchange [13].

Toxic pulmonary effects of exposure to hyperoxia are well known. There is a dose-dependent reduction in VC with continuous exposure to a $PO_2 > 50$ kPa, as characterized by CLARK and LAMBERTSEN [14]. The concept of units pulmonary toxic dose (UPTD) as introduced by CLARK and LAMBERTSEN [14] is widely used for calculating acceptable oxygen exposure under different conditions, such as in diving procedures. It has also been shown that this effect is attenuated by intermittent exposure to up to the same cumulative dose of oxygen [15], and tolerance to the oxidative stress develops.

The safe threshold for hyperoxic exposure in humans before risking impairment in pulmonary function appears to be approximately double the ambient air pressure at sea level (0.21 ATA or 21 kPa) [16, 17]. However, this risk is proportional to both the inspired pressure and the duration of exposure [16, 17], so that with multiple longitudinal exposures, even small elevations of ATA above that threshold may pose considerable risks. Early, exploratory studies on human subjects reported that reversible symptoms of POT and associated changes in dynamic pulmonary function develop within approximately 3–16 hours of continuous exposure to 100% O_2 using ATAs in a range of 1.0–3.0 (101–304 kPa) [18, 19].

Two previous studies had conflicting results regarding the pulmonary toxicity effects of repetitive HBOT sessions.

In the Pott et al. study [20] in which 18 patients had 30 daily sessions in a monoplace chamber for 90 min at 2.4 ATA oxygen without air breaks, no significant changes in FVC or diffusing capacity were noticed. However, the Pott et al. study had a considerably smaller sample, where only 14 patients completed more than 20 sessions. The standard deviations of pulmonary functions were considerably large (over 20%); thus, small changes could have been missed.

The second study done by Thorsen et al. [21] included 20 patients treated in 21 HBOT daily sessions for 90 minutes of 2.4 ATA with 30: 5 air breaks; no significant changes in FVC, FEF25%, PEF, or diffusing capacity were noticed. However, there were significant reductions in FEV1 and FEF50–75%.

Harabin et al. [22] showed that intermittent delivery of HBOT (relatively long periods of hyperoxia interrupted by short periods of low oxygen pressure or normoxia) reduces pulmonary toxicity in animal models.

In order to quantify POT, UPTD has been introduced to predict impairment of pulmonary function [23]. As an example, hyperoxic exposures might be limited to 450 UPTD per day and 2250 UPTD per week, where each UPTD is the equivalent of 1 minute at 1 ATA (101 kPa) of 100% O_2. However, this model has several limitations, including a need for cumulative dose calculations to account for periods of recovery between exposures; hence, alternative metrics such as a POT index have been proposed [24].

With the HBO treatment protocols in common use, the daily exposure is equivalent to 275 UPTD, which is not expected to give changes in VC, and the exposure is interrupted by two periods of breathing air for 5 minutes. The cumulative exposure over approximately 5 days of treatment, 1425 UPTD, will give a mean reduction in VC of 10% if given continuously. Over a 3-week HBO treatment period, changes in VC are still not seen.

Oxygen toxicity is attenuated when the exposure is intermittent, implying that a cumulative dose, which would have resulted in a reduction in VC if given continuously, can be given intermittently without resulting in changes in VC. The mechanism of tolerance is mediated by inducing the lung enzyme superoxide dismutase (SOD), which functions as a free radical scavenger. Therefore, even though HBOT may increase free radical production, intermittent exposure actually induces SOD and other scavengers that reduce the net free radical concentrations and their potential toxic effects.

In conclusion, the reduction in pulmonary function after 3 weeks of hyperbaric oxygen treatment is not considered to be of any clinical significance unless repeated treatment series are considered or pulmonary function is reduced before treatment.

During the decompression phase of HBOT, acute pressure changes can cause pulmonary edema [25, 26]or pulmonary barotrauma, which may lead to arterial gas embolism [27], pneumomediastinum [28], or tension pneumothorax [29], although barotraumatic lung injury is very rare in the absence of high-risk features such as pre-existing respiratory disease [30].

23.2.3 HBOT and CNS Oxygen Toxicity

The CNS effects of oxygen toxicity are called the "Bert effect, " named after Paul Bert, who, in 1878, demonstrated convulsions in larks exposed to 15–20 ATA. The "Smith effect" is the pulmonary effects of oxygen toxicity, named after J Lorain Smith, who, in 1899, while trying to reproduce the "Bert effect, " noted fatal pneumonia in rats after 4 days of exposure to 73% oxygen at 1 ATA. The clinical settings of oxygen toxicity are broadly divided into two groups; in the first, the patient is exposed to very high concentrations of oxygen for a short duration, like in HBOT, and in the second, lower concentrations of the gas are used for a longer duration.

These two can result in the so-called "acute" and "chronic" oxygen toxicity, respectively. Acute toxicity has predominant CNS effects, while chronic toxicity has predominant pulmonary effects.

Although Bert originally reported that CNS toxicity occurred at oxygen pressures of >3 ATA, it may, however, occur at lower pressures if exposure is prolonged. An acute increase in oxygen saturation results in peripheral vasoconstriction, which leads to early manifestations of oxygen toxicity like twitching of the fingers and facial pallor. Continuation of exposure can lead to vertigo and nausea, followed by altered behavior, clumsiness, and finally convulsions. Some factors aggravating the CNS toxicity are raised pCO_2, stress, fatigue, cold, and dietary deficiency of trace elements such as selenium, zinc, and magnesium.

HBO seems to have some neurological risks due to oxygen neurotoxicity such as seizures. The exact incidence of oxygen toxicity seizures varies in the literature. While a study reported the rate as low as 0.002% [31], a 1990 study reported a surprising rate of 4.7% [32]. A recent study published in 2014 showed that the incidence of seizure is 1 in 2121 treatments (0.05%) [33]. In a 2016 study, retrospective analysis of 62, 614 HBO treatment sessions showed an overall seizure incidence of 0.011% [34]. Differences in patient selection, indications, and protocols make it difficult to compare the studies. For example, most of the studies in the literature included patients with carbon monoxide poisoning, which is itself a cause of seizures [35].

Suspected risk factors for oxygen toxicity include family history [36], conditions reducing the seizure threshold (like epilepsy, hypoglycemia, hyperthyroidism), and specific risk factors such as hypercarbia, acetazolamide, or disulfiram medication [37, 38].

Recent evidence suggests that O_2-induced seizures may result from an imbalance of excitatory and inhibitory synaptic neurotransmitters, glutamate, and GABA, respectively. The imbalance results in a greater relative decrease in presynaptic release of GABA than of glutamate [39], which suggests that the relative increase of excitatory neurotransmitters with respect to inhibitory neurotransmitters may be a basic mechanism of HBO_2 seizures.

Extracellular mediators of physiological functions such as NO also play a role in HBO_2 seizures. NO has been implicated in neurotoxicities resulting from excess glutamate stimulation in cultures of rat cortex, striatum, and hippocampus [40]. Neurons containing nitric oxide synthase (NOS), widespread throughout the cortex, react to HBO_2 by increasing NO production [41]. HBO_2-stimulated neuronal NO production promoted an imbalance between excitatory (glutamate) and inhibitory (GABA) synaptic activity. This, in turn, contributes to O_2-induced seizures in rats [39].

A long-standing question regarding hyperbaric oxygen seizures is whether certain regions of the CNS are more susceptible to HBO_2. Neuroanatomic studies have shown that centrally located regions of the brain are most affected by exposure to HBO_2, including the globus pallidus, substantia nigra, superior olivary nucleus, ventral cochlear nucleus, limbic structures, amygdala, and the spinal cord gray matter [42]. It is worth noting that the globus pallidus and substantia nigra are brain regions also susceptible to CO toxicity. Single-cell electrophysiology experiments have shown that hippocampus and brain stem neurons are disproportionately sensitive to increased PO_2 in surrounding tissues when exposed to HBO_2 [43].

CNS O_2 toxicity often presents acutely with little or no warning.

Common signs and symptoms of CNS O_2 toxicity are easily remembered using the mnemonic VENTID-C3 [44].

Visual symptoms: tunnel vision, blurred vision, or decreased peripheral vision
Ear symptoms: tinnitus, roaring, pulsing sounds, or perceived sounds not from an external stimulus
Nausea: often with vomiting and headache
Twitching/Tingling: of extremities, facial muscles
Irritability: or any change in mental status such as confusion, agitation, anxiety, or undue fatigue
Dizziness: or clumsiness, loss of coordination
Convulsions and death

Unfortunately, many of these symptoms are not exclusive to O_2 toxicity, and CNS O_2 toxicity does not usually proceed through any predictable sequence of the above signs. Convulsions, the most serious effect of O_2 toxicity due to its fatal potential if left untreated, may occur without warning or other accompanying signs. O_2-induced seizures are characterized as generalized tonic–clonic seizures, though focal seizures may be the only neurological manifestation at times [45]. After an O_2 toxicity convulsion, the individual usually remembers clearly the events up to the moment when consciousness was lost, but remembers nothing of the convulsion itself and little of the postictal phase [46]. Afterward, he or she often becomes suddenly alert and complains of no more than fatigue, muscular soreness, and possibly a headache.

Diagnosis of oxygen toxicity is based on the clinical symptoms. An electroencephalogram (EEG) is of no value in the monitoring of CNS toxicity.

The primary treatment for an O_2-induced seizure is to lower the inspired PO_2. This is accomplished by decreasing ambient pressure, switching to a breathing mixture with a lower percentage of O_2, or both. Decreasing inspired PO_2 may not immediately reverse the effects of CNS O_2 toxicity and is not without risk. It is believed that the biochemical processes responsible for the toxicity remain in place for a period after the PO_2 has been decreased in the ambient or inspired atmosphere. The individual experiencing the toxicity is not considered clear from danger until several minutes have passed after the PO_2 has been decreased [47].

In practice, the risk of acute O_2 toxicity is often mitigated by interspersing short periods of air amid the pure O_2 therapy at increased pressure, commonly referred to as "air breaks." [48]

Effects on the CNS attributed to increased hydrostatic pressure, such as high-pressure nervous syndrome [49], tend to occur at very high pressures, ranging from 15 to 70 ATA. This results from compression of cerebral spinal fluid, circulation, and extracellular and intracellular fluid compartments of the CNS. Cellular mechanisms most likely involve synaptic and membrane dynamic responses to severe and fast changes in pressure.

Treatment consists of monitoring the patient and supportive therapy until the symptoms resolve. Exogenous antioxidants, especially vitamin E and C, may be used prophylactically. The recommended dose of vitamin E is 100 mg/kg/day for 4–6 weeks. Adrenalectomy, hypophysectomy, and the hypothyroid state are associated with reduced severity of the toxicity, as is the use of alpha-adrenergic blockers. As dietary deficiency of trace elements is likely to worsen the toxicity, their supplementation may be helpful in deficient states.

Data support brain-derived neurotrophic factor, 7-nitroindozol, and NO as potential mechanisms for sensitization to repeated HBO_2 seizures [50]. MK-801, an NMDA receptor antagonist, has been shown to prevent EEG spikes associated with O_2 toxicity and O_2-induced seizures [51].

23.2.4 HBOT and Ophthalmic Oxygen Toxicity

Oxidative stress due to excess quantities of ROS can cause retinal ganglion cell (RGC) death [52]. With increased levels of oxygen, reversible constriction of the peripheral field of vision results in a progressive but reversible myopia, causing blurred vision. Several concomitant factors, such as increased ROS production and imbalance between pro-oxidative and antioxidant capacity, have been postulated as the crucial factors in early retinal injury, together with the reduced ocular perfusion pressure in the blood vessels [53]. Both vascular and mechanical theories help to explain the formation of ROS in glaucoma. The vascular theory is based on ischemia-induced production of ROS due to compromised blood flow in retinal vessels. The mechanical pressure theory for the formation of ROS involves elevated IOP inhibiting retrograde neurotrophin support for RGC axons. For both mechanisms, RGC death is due to oxidative stress.

A review of the literature found that in addition to cataract, age-related macular degeneration, and kerato-conus, there may be other ocular diseases for which the pathology involves ROS and so for which exposure to HBOT-related oxidative stress could be significantly adverse [54]. For example, a patient with a ruptured retinal arterial macroaneurysm experienced acute development of severe macular edema 2 days after the seventh HBOT treatment [55].

Yonekawa and coauthors recommended that HBOT could be contraindicated for retinovascular diseases. The involvement of oxidative stress in glaucomatous pathology [56] suggests that patients with glaucoma could be contraindicated for HBOT.

There has been increasing evidence that glaucomatous neurodegeneration is analogous to other neurodegenerative diseases in the CNS, such as Alzheimer's disease [57]. To the extent that oxidative stress may reach pathological levels which are above the cell's antioxidant capacity, dietary antioxidant supplements such as Vitamin E and compound extract Ginkgo biloba may be of benefit in protecting RGCs.

23.2.5 Hyperoxia: Miscellaneous Effects

Oxygen also has toxic effects on the ears and red blood cells. Serous otitis media and dysbaric osteonecrosis were seen in astronauts during space flight. Prolonged oxygen exposure can change RBC morphology, and hemolysis occurs.

During neonatal resuscitation, unintentional hyperoxia leads to retinopathy and broncho-pulmonary dysplasia.

The routine use of oxygen in patients with suspected myocardial infarction (MI) and SpO_2 more than 90% does not reduce mortality at 1 year. Rather, hyperoxia increases infarct size, leading to recurrent MI and arrhythmia [58].

Recent trial suggests no benefit from oxygen in patients with stroke if SpO_2 is more than 93% and hyperoxia increases disability and mortality [59].

23.3 Conclusion

Oxygen remains the best treatment for any patient with hypoxemia, but evidence continues to accumulate of a lack of benefit of oxygen in many conditions not associated with hypoxemia, and of harm from hyperoxia.

References

1. Thomson L, Paton J. Oxygen Toxicity; 2014, 15
2. Lumb A. Nunn's applied respiratory physiology. 8th ed. Edinburgh: Elsevier; 2017.
3. British Thoracic Society Emergency Oxygen Guideline Development Group. BTS guidelines for oxygen use for adults in healthcare and emergency settings. Thorax. 2017;72:ii1.
4. Jackson RM. Pulmonary oxygen toxicity. Chest. 1985;88(6):900–5. https://doi.org/10.1378/chest.88.6.900. PMID: 3905287.
5. Smith JL. The pathological effects due to increase of oxygen tension in the air breathed. J Physiol. 1899;24(1):19. https://doi.org/10.1113/jphysiol.1899.sp000746. PMID: 16992479.
6. Klein J. Normobaric pulmonary oxygen toxicity. Anesth Analg. 1990;70(2):195–207. https://doi.org/10.1213/00000539-199002000-00012. PMID: 2105672.
7. Fisher AB, Forman HJ, Glass M. Mechanisms of pulmonary oxygen toxicity. Lung. 1984;162(1):255–9. https://doi.org/10.1007/BF02715655. PMID: 6392761.
8. van Ooij PJAM, Sterk PJ, van Hulst RA. Oxygen, the lung and the diver: friends and foes? Eur Respir Rev. 2016;25(142):496–505. https://doi.org/10.1183/16000617.0049-2016. PMID: 27903670.
9. Wingelaar TT, Brinkman P, van Ooij PJAM, et al. Markers of pulmonary oxygen toxicity in hyperbaric oxygen therapy using exhaled breath analysis. Front Physiol. 2019;10(APR):475. https://doi.org/10.3389/fphys.2019.00475. PMID: 31068838.
10. Wingelaar TT, van Ooij PJAM, van Hulst RA. Oxygen toxicity and special operations forces diving: hidden and dangerous. Front Physiol. 2017;8(JUL):1263. https://doi.org/10.3389/fpsyg.2017.01263. PMID: 28790955.
11. Edmonds C, Bennett M, Lippmann J, Mitchell S. Oxygen toxicity. In: Diving and subaquatic medicine. 5th ed. CRC Press; 2015. p. 242.
12. Davis WB, Rennard SI, Bitterman PB, Crystal RG. Pulmonary oxygen toxicity. Early reversible changes in human alveolar structures induced by hyperoxia. N Engl J Med. 1983;309(15) https://doi.org/10.1056/NEJM198310133091502. PMID: 6888481.
13. Robinson FR, Casey HW, Weibel ER. Animal model: oxygen toxicity in nonhuman primates. Am J Pathol. 1974;76(1):175. PMID: 4210278.
14. Clark JM, Lambertsen CJ. Pulmonary oxygen toxicity: a review. Pharmacol Rev. 1971;23:37–133.
15. Hendricks PL, Hall DA, Hunter WL Jr, Haley PJ. Extension of pulmonary oxygen tolerance in man at 2 ATA by intermittent oxygen exposure. J Appl Physiol. 1977;42:593–9.
16. Miller JN, Winter PM. Clinical manifestations of pulmonary oxygen toxicity. Int Anesthesiol Clin. 1981;19(3):179–99. https://doi.org/10.1097/00004311-198119030-00011. PMID: 6169647.

17. Schaefer KE. Oxygen in closed environmental systems. In: Gilbert DL, editor. Oxygen and living processes. Springer; 1981. p. 343–57. https://doi.org/10.1007/978-1-4612-5890-2_15.
18. Clark JM, Lambertsen CJ, Gelfand R, et al. Effects of prolonged oxygen exposure at 1.5, 2.0, or 2.5 ATA on pulmonary function in men (predictive studies V). J Appl Physiol (1985). 1999;86(1):243–59. https://doi.org/10.1152/jappl.1999.86.1.243. PMID: 9887137.
19. Fisher AB, Hyde RW, Puy RJ, Clark JM, Lambertsen CJ. Effect of oxygen at 2 atmospheres on the pulmonary mechanics of normal man. J Appl Physiol. 1968;24(4):529–36. https://doi.org/10.1152/jappl.1968.24.4.529. PMID: 5643400.
20. Pott F, Westergaard P, Mortensen J, Jansen EC. Hyperbaric oxygen treatment and pulmonary function. Undersea Hyperb Med. 1999;26(4):225–8.
21. Thorsen E, Aanderud L, Aasen TB. Effects of a standard hyperbaric oxygen treatment protocol on pulmonary function. Eur Respir J. 1998;12(6):1442–5.
22. Harabin AL, Survanshi SS, Weathersby PK, Hays JR, Homer LD. The modulation of oxygen toxicity by intermittent exposure. Toxicol Appl Pharmacol. 1988;93(2):298–311.
23. Harabin AL, Homer LD, Weathersby PK, Flynn ET. An analysis of decrements in vital capacity as an index of pulmonary oxygen toxicity. J Appl Physiol (1985). 1987;63(3):1130–5. https://doi.org/10.1152/jappl.1987.63.3.1130. PMID: 3654459.
24. Arieli R. Calculated risk of pulmonary and central nervous system oxygen toxicity: a toxicity indexderived from the power equation. Diving Hyperb Med. 2019;49(3):154. https://doi.org/10.28920/dhm49.3.154-160. PMID: 31523789.
25. Weaver LK, Churchill S. Pulmonary edema associated with hyperbaric oxygen therapy. Chest. 2001;120(4):1407–9. https://doi.org/10.1378/chest.120.4.1407. PMID: 11591590.
26. Obiagwu C, Paul V, Chadha S, Hollander G, Shani J. Acute pulmonary edema secondary to hyperbaric oxygen therapy. Oxf Med Case Rep. 2015;2015(2):183–4. https://doi.org/10.1093/omcr/omv002. PMID: 25988073.
27. Rivalland G, Mitchell SJ, van Schalkwyk JM. Pulmonary barotrauma and cerebral arterial gas embolism during hyperbaric oxygen therapy. Aviat Space Environ Med. 2010;81(9) https://doi.org/10.3357/ASEM.2783.2010. PMID: 20824998.
28. Jaeger N, Brosious J, Gustavson R, et al. Pneumomediastinum following hyperbaric oxygen therapy for carbon monoxide poisoning: case report. Undersea Hyperb Med. 2013;40(6):521–3. PMID: 24377195.
29. Unsworth I. Pulmonary barotrauma in a hyperbaric chamber. Anaesthesia. 1973;28(6):675–8. https://doi.org/10.1111/J.1365-2044.1973.TB00555.X. PMID: 4759876.
30. Brenna CTA, Khan S, Djaiani G, Buckey JC, Katznelson R. The role of routine pulmonary imaging before hyperbaric oxygen treatment. Diving Hyperb Med. 2022;52(3):197–207. https://doi.org/10.28920/dhm52.3.197-207. PMID: 36100931.
31. Yildiz S, Aktas S, Cimsit M, Ay H, Toğrol E. Seizure incidence in 80, 000 patient treatments with hyperbaric oxygen. Aviat Space Environ Med. 2004;75(11):992–4.
32. Sloan EP, Murphy DG, Hart R, Cooper MA, Turnbull T, Barreca RS, et al. Complications and protocol considerations in carbon monoxide-poisoned patients who require hyperbaric oxygen therapy: report from a ten-year experience. Ann Emerg Med. 1989;18(6):629–34.
33. Heyboer M, Sharma D, Santiago W, McCulloch N. Hyperbaric oxygen therapy: side effects defined and quantified. Adv Wound Care (New Rochelle). 2017;6(6):210–24. https://doi.org/10.1089/wound.2016.0718.
34. Hadanny A, Meir O, Bechor Y, Fishlev G, Bergan J, Efrati S. Seizures during hyperbaric oxygen therapy: retrospective analysis of 62, 614 treatment sessions. Undersea Hyperb Med. 2016;43(1):21–8.
35. Seidel R, Carroll C, Thompson D, Diem RG, Yeboah K, Hayes AJ, et al. Risk factors for oxygen toxicity seizures in hyperbaric oxygen therapy: case reports from multiple institutions. Undersea Hyperb Med. 2013;40(6):515–9.
36. Binnetoğlu A, Yumuşakhuylu AC, Demir B, Bağlam T, Derinsu U, Sarı M. Association between family history and idiopathic sudden sensorineural hearing loss. J Int Adv Otol. 2015;11(1):30–2. https://doi.org/10.5152/iao.2015.607.

37. Plafki C, Peters P, Almeling M, Welslau W, Busch R. Complications and side effects of hyperbaric oxygen therapy. Aviat Space Environ Med. 2000;71(2):119–24.
38. Manning EP. Central nervous system oxygen toxicity and hyperbaric oxygen seizures. Aerosp Med Hum Perform. 2016;87(5):477–86. https://doi.org/10.3357/AMHP.4463.2016.
39. Demchenko IT, Piantadosi CA. Nitric oxide amplifies the excitatory to inhibitory neurotransmitter imbalance accelerating oxygen seizures. Undersea Hyperb Med. 2006;33(3):169–74.
40. Dawson VL, Dawson TM, Bartley DA, Uhl GR, Snyder SH. Mechanisms of nitric oxide-mediated neurotoxicity in primary brain cultures. J Neurosci. 1993;13(6):2651–61.
41. Moskvin AN, Zhilyaev SY, Sharapov OI, Platonova TF, Gutsaeva DR, et al. Brain blood flow modulates the neurotoxic action of hyperbaric oxygen via neuronal and endothelial nitric oxide. Neurosci Behav Physiol. 2003;33(9):883–8.
42. Vion-Dury J, LeGal La Salle G, Rougier I, Papy JJ. Effects of hyperbaric and hyperoxic conditions on amygdala-kindled seizures in rat. Exp Neurol. 1986;92(3):513–21.
43. Garcia AJ 3rd, Putnam RW, Dean JB. Hyperbaric hyperoxia and normobaric reoxygenation increase excitability and activate oxygeninduced potentiation in CA1 hippocampal neurons. J Appl Physiol (1985). 2010;109(3):804–19.
44. Naval Sea Systems Command, United States Department of the Navy. Navy diving manual, 5th ed. Washington, DC: U.S. Government Printing Office; 2005.
45. Seckin M, Gurgor N, Beckmann YY, Ulukok MD, Suzen A, Basoglu M. Focal status epilepticus induced by hyperbaric oxygen therapy. Neurologist. 2011;17(1):31–3.
46. Kindwall EP, Whalen HT. Hyperbaric medicine practice. 2nd ed. Flagstaff: Best Publishing Company; 2004.
47. Davis JC, Hunt TK, editors. Hyperbaric oxygen therapy. Bethesda: Undersea Medical Society, Inc.; 1977.
48. Bitterman N. CNS oxygen toxicity. Undersea Hyperb Med. 2004;31(1):63–72.
49. Dean JB, Mulkey DK, Garcia AJ, Putnam RW, Henderson RA. Neuronal sensitivity to hyperoxia, hypercapnia, and inert gases at hyperbaric pressures. J Appl Physiol (1985). 2003;95:883–909.
50. Jellestad FK, Gundersen H. Behavioral effects of 7-nitroindazole on hyperbaric oxygen toxicity. Physiol Behav. 2002;76(4–5):611–6.
51. Demchenko IT, Boso AE, O'Neill TJ, Bennett PB, Piantadosi CA. Nitric oxide and cerebral blood flow responses to hyperbaric oxygen. J Appl Physiol (1985). 2000;88(4):1381–9.
52. Kumar DM, Agarwal N. Oxidative stress in glaucoma: a burdenof evidence. J Glaucoma. 2007;16:334–43.
53. Nita M, Grzybowski A. The role of the reactive oxygen species and oxidative stress in the pathomechanism of the age-related ocular diseases and other pathologies of the anterior and-posterior eye segments in adults. Oxidative Med Cell Longev. 2016:3164734. https://doi.org/10.1155/2016/3164734.
54. McMonnies CW. Hyperbaric oxygen therapy and the possibilityof ocular complications or contraindications. Clin Exp Optom. 2015;98:122–5.
55. Yonekawa Y, Hypes SM, Abbey AM, Williams GA, Wolfe JD. Exac-erbation of macular oedema associated with hyperbaric oxygentherapy. Clin Experiment Ophthalmol. 2016;44:625–6.
56. Chrysostomou V, Rezania F, Trounce IA, Crowston JG. Oxidativestress and mitochondrial dysfunction in glaucoma. Curr Opin Pharmacol. 2013;13:12d–5d.
57. Cheung W, Guo L, Cordeiro MF. Neuroprotection in glaucoma:drug-based approaches. Optom Vis Sci. 2008;85:406–16.
58. Hofmann R, James SK, Jernberg T, et al. For the DETO2XSWEDEHEART investigators. Oxygen therapy in suspected acute myocardial infarction. N Engl J Med. 2017;377:1240e9.
59. Roffe C, Nevalle T, Sim J, et al. Effect of routine low-dose oxygen supplementation on death and disability in adults with acute stroke: the Stroke Oxygen Study randomized clinical trial. JAMA. 2017;318:1125e35.

Index

A. G. D'Almeida, J. Hidalgo (eds.), *Evidence-Based Hyperbaric Medicine*,
https://doi.org/10.1007/978-3-032-06346-5

H

I

L

M

N

O

P

R

S

MIX
Papier aus verantwortungsvollen Quellen
Paper from responsible sources
FSC® C105338

If you have any concerns about our products,
you can contact us on
ProductSafety@springernature.com

In case Publisher is established outside the EU,
the EU authorized representative is:
Springer Nature Customer Service Center GmbH
Europaplatz 3, 69115 Heidelberg, Germany

Printed by Libri Plureos GmbH
in Hamburg, Germany